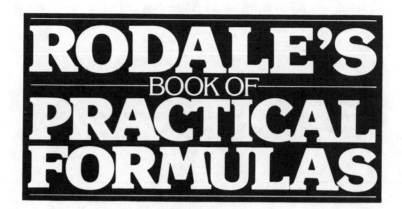

RODALE'S BOOK OF PRACTICAL FORMULAS

Paula Dreifus Bakule, Editor

Contributing Writers

Michael Castleman
Kate Delhagen
Patricia Fisher
Linda A. Gilkeson, Ph.D.

Diane K. Gilroy
Judith Benn Hurley
Walter Jowers
Leslie Spraker May

Susan H. Pitcairn, M.S.
Cindy Ross
Mort Schultz
Trisha Thompson

MJF BOOKS

NEW YORK

The information in this book has been carefully researched, and all efforts have been made to ensure accuracy. Rodale Press, Inc., assumes no responsibility for any injuries suffered or damages or losses incurred during use of or as a result of following this information. All directions should be carefully studied and clearly understood before taking any action based on the information and advice presented in this book.

Senior Managing Editor: Margaret Lydic Balitas
Editor: Paula Dreifus Bakule
Copy Editor: Lisa D. Andruscavage
Administrative Assistant: Stacy A. Brobst
Special Assistance by Cheryl Winters Tetreau and Nancy J. Ondra
Book Design by Rhoda M. Krammer, Plus Graphics
Interior Illustrations by Robin Brickman and Jean Gardner

Published by MJF Books
Fine Communications
POB 0930
Planetarium Station
New York, NY 10024-0540

Library of Congress Catalog Card Number 93-80926
ISBN 1-56731-046-X

Published by Arrangement with Rodale Press, Inc.
Manufactured in the United States of America

MJF Books and the MJF colophon are trademarks of Fine Creative Media, Inc.

10   9   8   7   6   5   4   3   2

Contents

About the Writers

Michael Castleman, author of the health chapter, is the former editor of *Medical Self-Care* magazine as well as numerous books on health-related topics. A Phi Beta Kappa graduate from the University of Michigan, Castleman holds a master's degree in journalism from the University of California at Berkeley. His most recent books include *Before You Call the Doctor: The Family Physician's Guide to Home Treatment of Everyday Health Problems,* with Anne Simmons, M.D., and Bobbie Hasslebring, and *The Healing Herbs.*

Kate Delhagen, coauthor of the outdoor life chapter and former professional triathlete, completed the 1988 Hawaii Ironman Triathlon. Now a top-ranked triathlon competitor, she is currently the senior health and fitness editor for *Runner's World* magazine.

Patricia Fisher, author of the housekeeping chapter, has for the past ten years written the nationally syndicated household hints column "Polly's Pointers." As author of *1081 Helpful Household Hints for Making Everything Last Longer,* Fisher developed many of her household hints from firsthand experience. She works from home in New Paltz, New York, managing not only a full-time writing career but also a busy household that includes her happy carpenter husband, three children, and two cats.

Linda A. Gilkeson, Ph.D., coauthor of the gardening chapter, holds a doctorate in entomology from McGill University, Montreal, Canada. She has written frequently about natural insect controls for gardeners both for Canadian regional garden publications and for *Harrowsmith* magazine. Her extensive gardening experience includes ten years as owner of Rosmarinus Herbs, a Prince Edward Island herb farm. She is research director for Applied Bionomics, a Canadian research and development firm that specializes in rearing beneficial insects for commercial growers. She currently lives and gardens with her dog, Xi'n, on Vancouver Island, British Columbia.

Diane K. Gilroy, author of the crafts chapter, is a crafts writer and editor at Rodale Press. For the past five years, she has served as associate editor of Rodale's holiday craft publication *Have a Natural Christmas.* Gilroy holds a master's degree in secondary education, and her special interest is in adapting complex crafts to suit the skills of school-age children.

Judith Benn Hurley, author of the cooking chapter, is a nationally syndicated columnist for the *Washington Post* and award-winning author of

Rodale's Garden-Fresh Cooking and *Healthy Microwave Cooking* and co-author of *The Healing Foods*. In addition to her journalism background, Hurley has studied cooking in dozens of countries, including Zimbabwe, Egypt, Malaysia, Hong Kong, Italy, and France.

Walter Jowers, author of the home repair and remodeling chapter, is a writer and renovation consultant based in Nashville, Tennessee. His previous work includes contributions to *Rodale's Projects for Outdoor Living* as well as articles on old home restoration for *Fine Homebuilding* and *Practical Home-owner* magazines. He also wrote the "Restoration Primer" column for the *Journal of Light Construction* and worked as a contributing editor for *Old House Journal*. He currently owns a renovation and restoration consulting company called Straight Talk.

Leslie Spraker May, coauthor of the gardening chapter, holds a master's degree in ornamental horticulture and is former publications editor for Longwood Gardens in Kennett Square, Pennsylvania. May has written about and given numerous workshops on creating Christmas ornaments from natural materials. She has also written on such diverse topics as vegetable gardening, gardening in the city, and home landscaping.

Susan H. Pitcairn, M.S., author of the pet-care chapter, is also coauthor of *Dr. Pitcairn's Complete Guide to Natural Health for Dogs and Cats*. She is founder and former editor of the *California Holistic Veterinary Medical Association Newsletter*. As an assistant to her husband, holistic veterinarian Richard Pitcairn, D.V.M., she has developed numerous handbooks and teaching aids for seminars in veterinary homeopathy and holistic medicine. She lives in Oregon with her husband and a white, blue-eyed cat named Ming.

Cindy Ross, coauthor of the outdoor life chapter, is author of the "Everyday Wisdom" column of *Backpacker* magazine. A veteran of over 6,000 trail miles, including both the Appalachian and Pacific Crest trails, Ross wrote and illustrated *A Woman's Journey on the Appalachian Trail* and *Journey on the Crest: A 2,600 Mile Walk from Mexico to Canada*.

Mort Schultz, author of the car-care chapter, is also author of more than a dozen how-to books on subjects ranging from car repair to appliance repair and home wiring. As creator of the "Car Clinic" column in *Popular Mechanics* magazine, Schultz has written on car-care issues for more than 25 years. His most recent book is *Keep Your Car Running Practically Forever*.

Trisha Thompson, author of the beauty chapter, is the former beauty columnist of *Medical Self-Care* magazine. Currently, Thompson is the health and psychology editor at *Self* magazine. She's also author of a guide to good health for teenagers entitled *Maintaining Good Health*.

Introduction

On these pages, you'll find a rich collection of recipes—a sort of alchemist's journal for making everything from potpourri to potting soil. The alchemists of twelfth-century Europe pursued the tantalizing goal of transforming a base metal, usually copper or lead, into gold. Theirs was an art practiced in secrecy, with formulas and procedures written in code, a sort of early precursor to our modern-day patent system. After all, rendering your competitors unable to read about your discoveries prevented them from profiting from them.

Even though we may smile at the muddled thinking that surrounds the mystical conversion of lead to gold, we are all alchemists at heart. Each time we transform a piece of fabric into a suit, a packet of seeds into a row of lettuce, or paper and sticks into a kite, we are indulging in the universal human pleasure of creating something fine or useful from something ordinary. And each time we save money by using a homemade product instead of a store-bought one, we are making our own gold out of everyday lead.

This collection of recipes and formulas offers a simple step-by-step route to making your own mixtures, potions, preparations, and compounds—for performing your own homemade alchemy. Using the collection here, you'll find out how to make brass polish from ketchup, furniture scratch remover from pecans and a dab of mineral oil, and paper preservative from milk of magnesia and club soda. You'll also discover some weird and wonderful formulas that really do work—like Christmas tree ornaments from applesauce, facial cleanser from cucumbers and milk, paint stripper from wood ashes, and dog shampoo from oatmeal.

So before you patch a hole in your wall, go on a diet, deflea your dog, plant a rosebush, or polish your silver, check through these pages. There's a formula here to help you. You'll not only save money or a trip to the store but also perform your own conversion of common lead into fine gold.

Paula Dreifus Bakule
Editor

Chapter One

Car Care

by Mort Schultz

You don't need this book to find out how to wash or polish your car. Your owner's manual or any general car-care book will give you all the advice you need. And, there are dozens of special cleaning agents especially formulated for every conceivable part of your car.

The purpose of this chapter is to help you solve a few tough problems often not covered in car-care books. For example, suppose tree sap has dripped and hardened on the hood of your car. How can you get rid of windshield scratches? Or restore worn-looking velour upholstery? Try the formulas on pages 3, 6, and 11. You'll be pleased with the results.

If you go to an amusement park and someone puts an unsightly bumper sticker on your brand-new, super-duper sports car, what then? You're stuck. Or are you? Read "Good Idea!" on page 8 to find out.

Each of the many formulas in this chapter will help you to perform a useful task that commercial products probably won't accomplish.

- Your manually operated radio antenna has corroded and become difficult to raise and lower. The formula on page 12 will free up the mast.
- The simulated-wood panels of your station wagon are covered with a milky haze, making your car look like it's headed for the junkyard. You think your options are to keep feeling embarrassed, sell the car, or have a high-priced body shcp restore the panels. But there's a fourth choice. You'll find it in "Good Idea!" on page 4.
- Your brand-new windshield wiper blades are chattering as they sweep across the windshield. You're discouraged because you bought them to replace the old blades that were chattering. Obviously, the blades aren't to blame. See "Windshield Wiper Chatter" on page 11 for the easy-as-pie solution to this common problem.
- You may have noticed a haze all over the windows of your brand-new car. A commercial window cleaner may have little effect, but that haze can't withstand the formula on page 10.

There's one more thing you should know about each of the formulas in this chapter. They've all been tested to see if they work. They do!

CAR-CARE BASICS

The formulas here will keep your car looking great and your garage in tip-top shape. You'll find a useful collection of simple tricks for solving annoying problems like chattering windshield wiper blades or frozen door locks.

Tree Sap Remover

As you notice it on your car, remove sap with a soft cloth dampened with rubbing alcohol. Then rinse with water. If sap has hardened and rubbing alcohol doesn't work, try this formula. This formula works for sugar-based saps, like maple, but not for resinous saps, like pine.

INGREDIENTS

laundry detergent (*not* laundry soap)
very hot tap water
auto body polish

SUPPLIES

rubber spatula
bucket
rubber work gloves
clean, soft cloths (terry cloth is ideal)
garden hose

Press the spatula against the edge of a blob of sap to break the bond. Mix a sudsy solution of detergent and water in the bucket. Dip a cloth into the water, scooping up suds. Lay the hot, sudsy cloth on the residue and rub, pressing as hard as you can. Repeat until the residue disappears. If the soapy water cools, mix more. After removing the residue, spray the area with cold water. Let dry, then polish it with auto body polish as directed on the label.

GOOD IDEA!

To remove dried **wax spots from your car's black plastic bumper strips,** mix a slurry of 1/2 cup baking soda in 1 cup turpentine or mineral spirits. Apply the slurry to the entire bumper strip and scrub vigorously with a brush. Rinse with water. Spots usually disappear with one or two applications.

GOOD IDEA!

To restore hazy simulated-wood panels on your car, all you need is scouring powder and shoe polish. To remove the milky haze, first scrub the panels with bleach-free scouring powder. Rinse and dry the panels. Then apply brown shoe wax (not liquid polish) and buff the panels to a shine.

Simulated Convertible Top Cleaner

A simulated convertible cloth top, sometimes called a cambria cloth top, needs special cleaning. Don't use regular vinyl-top cleaner or abrasives, such as scouring powder. You may damage it.

SUPPLIES

small bar of mild, nondetergent soap or 1 cup nondetergent laundry soap flakes

pocketknife (optional)

bucket

garden hose

clean, soft-bristle brush, such as a horsehair shoe brush

If you're using bar soap, cut the bar into shavings with the pocketknife. Place shavings or flakes in the bucket. Using strong water pressure from the hose, make a thick, sudsy, soap solution. Dip the brush into the suds and lightly scrub the top. Don't press hard. Rinse the top with plain water and allow it to air-dry. Don't use a hair dryer. It can damage the top.

Good Battery Maintenance

Your battery may be "maintenance-free," but it still requires your care and attention to operate efficiently. Twice a year, inspect the terminals and connectors, and check the electrolyte level. Also check the case, terminals, and connectors for acid deposits.

Acid gas escapes from the interior of the battery through small vent openings in the battery case. Moisture on the battery surface absorbs the acid gas and forms a white crust around the terminals and connectors. Sometimes the acid and moisture form a thin, sticky residue but not a full-blown crust. If you touch this residue, be sure to wash your hands immediately.

When you check your battery, look for an accumulation of white acid crust. If you see it on the surface, neutralize it using the formula on page 5. And clean your battery terminals and connectors at least once a year, even if no crust is evident.

Battery Life Extender

To prolong the life of a "maintenance-free" battery, clean it two times a year with this formula.

INGREDIENTS

½ box baking soda
2 quarts cold water

SUPPLIES

rubber work gloves

rubber apron

goggles, safety glasses, or face shield

bucket

scrub brush

water

clean, absorbent rag

petroleum jelly

☛ **BE SAFE.** The deposits and film on the outside of the battery are corrosive. Also, gases given off by a battery are explosive. Wear rubber gloves, a rubber apron, and goggles. Do not smoke. Remove jewelry before doing this job. Any metal object hitting both battery terminals may cause a spark that can explode the battery. To safely disconnect the cables from the terminals, always disconnect the negative cable first. When reconnecting the cables to the battery, always connect the negative cable last.

Wearing the proper saftey gear, disconnect the connectors from the terminals following the safety note above. Mix baking soda with water in the bucket and scrub the top of the battery, the terminals, the connectors, and the sides that you can reach. If acid residue is present, the solution will make a sizzling sound as you apply it. Rinse the battery with plain water and repeat the scrub and rinse cycle until the sizzling sound stops. Dry the battery with a clean rag. To prevent corrosion of the terminals, spread a thin coating of petroleum jelly on these parts.

GOOD IDEA!

For extra-thorough **battery maintenance,** remove the battery from the car and clean the underside as well as the battery tray. To accomplish this task, purchase a battery carrier and appropriate wrenches for safely removing the battery from the car. You may also want to install corrosion-resistant rings at each terminal. You'll find these supplies at auto supply stores.

Windshield Scratch Remover

Grit on windshield wiper blades can cause scratches, which may be hazardous when you drive at night. Light from oncoming cars or from overhead reflectors can be dispersed by the scratches and shine into your eyes. Before replacing a badly scratched windshield, try this.

INGREDIENTS

jewelers' rouge

4 ounces ammonia

1 gallon water

SUPPLIES

portable electric drill mounted with a lamb's-wool buffing pad

heavy-duty extension cord

rubber work gloves

bucket

sponge

paper towels

☛ **BE SAFE.** Wear rubber gloves to protect your hands. If working outdoors, the extension cord should be rated for outdoor use by the Underwriters Laboratories. Make sure no puddles of water are on the ground where you're working.

Rub jewelers' rouge onto the buffing pad until it appears to be coated with powder. Place the pad against the windshield where scratches are present. Turn on the drill. If the scratches are not too deep, the jewelers' rouge will restore the windshield. After polishing, Put on rubber gloves and mix ammonia and water in the bucket. Wash the windshield with a sponge. Dry with paper towels.

➻ **Note:** Jewelers' rouge is a generic name for a number of polishing compounds used on gemstones and precious metals. You can usually purchase the rouge from a jeweler who makes settings and mounts stones. Rouge comes in varying degrees of polishing power or abrasiveness. Be sure to ask for a grade of rouge suitable for polishing glass.

Aluminum Alloy Wheel Cleaner

If a commercially available wheel cleaner doesn't eliminate corrosive deposits from the aluminum alloy wheels on your car, try this method.

SUPPLIES

rubber work gloves

aluminum pot and pan cleaner

pads of #000 steel wool (*not* steel wool soap pads)

garden hose

clean rags

☞ **BE SAFE.** *Wear rubber gloves to protect your hands.*

Wearing rubber gloves, scoop aluminum cleaner onto a pad of steel wool. Gently polish off corrosion using a circular motion. Don't press. Aluminum wheels may be made of solid aluminum or they may be steel wheels with an anodized aluminum coating. If your wheels are anodized aluminum over steel, heavy pressure may rub off much of the anodizing from the wheel.

When corrosion has been eliminated, spray the wheel with water. Then, dry the wheel with clean rags or let it air-dry.

GOOD IDEA!

To keep your aluminum alloy wheels looking great for months, spray on a coat of clear lacquer after cleaning. The clear lacquer coat will help keep the shine for a few months, but it's not permanent. Eventually, it will lose its shine and protective qualities. You can then remove it with lacquer thinner, clean your wheels again, and reapply.

GOOD IDEA!

To remove stubborn stickers from your car's bumper or trunk, all you need is some shortening and a little dishwashing detergent.

First rub shortening into the edge of the unwanted sticker. When the sticker edge looks greasy and transparent, lift it with your fingernail and draw it away from the bumper or panel. As you meet resistance, apply more shortening. Continue in this manner until you can remove the entire sticker. Wash away the remaining adhesive residue with a solution of very hot water and dishwashing detergent.

Adhesive-Backed Sticker Removal for Rear Window Defroster Grids

If a decal has been placed over the grid of a rear window defroster, scraping or pulling it off can cause the defroster to malfunction. That's because each grid is instrumental in circulating electric current to the other grids. Pulling on one grid may tear or loosen it, causing an interruption in the current and failure of the entire rear window defroster. Follow this formula to remove the decal without destroying the grid.

INGREDIENTS

spray can of 3M Wood Grain and Stripe Remover

fingernail polish remover

warm water

laundry detergent (*not* laundry soap)

SUPPLIES

plastic tablecloth or rubber sheet

single-edged razor blade

rubber work gloves

clean, absorbent rags

bucket

☛ **BE SAFE.** Wear rubber gloves to protect your hands. Read and follow the safety directions on the can of 3M Wood Grain and Stripe Remover. Be sure the car is well-ventilated.

Cover the rear deck and rear upholstery of the car with the tablecloth or sheet to protect them from the 3M Wood Grain and Stripe Remover, which may drip as it's being applied. Using the razor blade, make two or three horizontal slices in the decal. *Be careful not to nick a grid with the razor.* Wearing rubber gloves, saturate a rag with the 3M Wood Grain and Stripe Remover. Lay the damp rag on the decal. *Do not rub.* Instead, hold the rag steady and allow the solvent to saturate the decal. It will begin to disintegrate. Repeat the process as often as necessary until all the decal material is gone. The 3M Wood Grain and Stripe

Remover will dissolve the decal material but not the adhesive, which will remain on the glass. To remove that, saturate a clean rag with fingernail polish remover and lay it on the adhesive. Eventually, the adhesive will dissolve onto the rag. To protect the grids, do not rub or scrape the adhesive. Finally, mix a sudsy solution of water and detergent in the bucket and carefully wash the spot.

➤ **Note:** *3M Wood Grain and Stripe Remover is a product that is used to remove vinyl stripes from car bodies. It is available at auto supply stores.*

Driveway Cleaner

This formula works for oil, grease, or transmission fluid that drips from your car onto a concrete surface. Note that your car shouldn't leak any of these fluids. Be sure to have the leak fixed so you don't have to do this job again.

SUPPLIES

paint thinner
new cat litter
stiff-bristle push broom

☛ **BE SAFE.** *If you're treating a garage floor, open the garage door to ventilate the area. Paint thinner is highly flammable. Avoid open flames. Do not smoke. Wrap grease-soaked cat litter in newspaper and dispose of according to your municipality's regulations.*

Pour paint thinner directly from the can onto the spots. Saturate the spots as well as an area 6 to 12 inches beyond them. Then, spread a thick layer of cat litter over the entire treated area so that none of the concrete surface is visible.

Let the cat litter stand for about an hour to absorb the greasy stains. Then use the broom to sweep up the soiled cat litter. Some stains may require two applications.

Glass Haze Remover

Car windows may develop a haze on the inside surface from gases given off by interior vinyl. Vinyl usually contains a softener (called a plasticizer), which keeps the vinyl pliable as it ages. When vinyl gets hot, it gives off plasticizer as a gas that settles on the glass as a hazy film. This formula will clear that haze from windows.

INGREDIENTS

1 ounce liquid dishwashing detergent
2 quarts warm water
4 ounces ammonia
1 gallon cold water

SUPPLIES

bucket
soft, clean, absorbent rags (terry cloth is ideal)
sponge
paper towels

☛ **BE SAFE.** *Wear rubber gloves to protect your hands.*

Mix detergent and warm water in the bucket to form a sudsy solution. Using a soft rag, wash all vinyl surfaces inside the car—seats, door panels, sun visors, and headlining, as well as the padded dash. The detergent solution washes off excess plasticizer from the surface of the vinyl. Wipe the vinyl dry with clean rags. Keep the doors of the car open an hour or two to get rid of dampness.

To remove haze from the inside of windows, mix ammonia and cold water together in the bucket. Wash the windows using the sponge. Dry with paper towels. Commercial window washing solution also works. Be aware that windows may cloud up again as more plasticizer is released from the vinyl. Depending upon the average ambient temperature in your area, this treatment will last for three months to a year. Repeat the treatment as often as necessary.

Velour Upholstery Refresher

Velour upholstery that looks worn out is usually just crushed. This procedure restores velour to like-new condition.

SUPPLIES

steam iron filled with water

heavy-duty extension cord

clean, soft-bristle brush, such as a horsehair shoe brush

☞ **BE SAFE.** If working outdoors, the extension cord should be rated for outdoor use by the Underwriters Laboratories. Make sure no puddles of water are on the ground where you're working.

Let the iron heat until it's steaming heavily. Using care not to press the iron directly to the cloth, moisten an area 1½- to 2-feet square. The fabric should be moist, but not soaking wet. Now use the brush to stroke the upholstery *against* the direction in which the pile has been crushed. Next, move the brush in a circular motion to work the pile back and forth. As the first section dries, repeat the procedure in an adjoining section. After all the upholstery has been treated, check it. If there are any spots that are still crushed, give it another treatment.

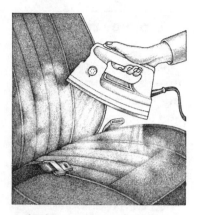

Refreshing velour upholstery with a steam iron

Windshield Wiper Chatter

Windshield-wiper-blade chatter often results when wax applied at an automatic car wash gets on the blades and windshield. Before deciding to purchase new blades, remove the old wax from both the blades and the windshield.

To get the wiper blades into a working position where you can reach them, turn on the ignition and the windshield wiper switch. When the wipers sweep to mid-windshield position (or within easy reach), turn off the ignition switch.

Mix 4 ounces ammonia and 1 gallon cold water in a bucket. Lift each blade off the windshield and wash the rubber with a paper towel that has been saturated with ammonia-water solution. Dry each blade with a fresh paper towel. To clean the windshield, wash the glass using a sponge soaked in the ammonia-water solution. Dry the windshield with paper towels.

GOOD IDEA!

To keep your car's power antenna assembly in top shape, clean and lubricate the antenna every three months. First, clean the fully extended antenna with a soft rag dampened with rubbing alcohol (70 percent isopropyl). Raise and lower the antenna several times, and repeat the alcohol cleansing. Next, wipe the antenna with a rag dampened with lightweight machine oil, such as 3-in-1 oil or sewing machine oil. Finally, retract and fully extend the antenna and wipe it with a clean rag to remove excess oil. This simple routine will prevent burnout of the antenna motor or breakage of the antenna cable.

Corrosion Prevention for Manual Radio Antennas

A manually operated (nonpower) antenna can corrode badly enough to make it difficult to raise and lower the mast. To prevent this from happening, apply the following formula once a year.

SUPPLIES

rubber work gloves

pad of #000 steel wool (*not* steel wool soap pad)

turpentine, mineral spirits, or rubbing alcohol (70 percent isopropyl)

clean, absorbent rag

waxed paper

☛ **BE SAFE.**   Wear rubber gloves to protect your hands.

Raise the antenna to its highest point. Wearing rubber gloves, moisten the steel wool pad with turpentine, mineral spirits, or rubbing alcohol and use it to clean all parts of the antenna. When the antenna is clean, dry it with a rag. Lubricate the antenna by rubbing waxed paper over all the metal parts. The paraffin from the waxed paper will be transferred to the antenna. Then, raise and lower the antenna three times. In addition to lubricating the antenna, paraffin prevents corrosion.

➻ **Note:**   Buy mineral spirits at paint supply stores and hardware stores.

Rust Inhibitor

This technique prevents the spread of rust that's already established. Treat rust spots as soon as you notice them. The longer rust remains, the farther it spreads.

SUPPLIES

small, hand-held electric grinder mounted with a
    conical grinding stone

heavy-duty extension cord

garden hose

2 artist's brushes (optional)

1 small bottle of auto body primer

1 small bottle of touch-up paint

paint thinner (optional)

☛ **BE SAFE.** If working outdoors, the extension cord should be rated for outdoor use by the Underwriters Laboratories. Make sure no puddles of water are on the ground where you're working.

Using care not to disturb the surrounding paint, carefully remove rust using the grinder and grinding stone. Grind until the rust disappears, even if you have to go down to the bare metal. Wash the area well with plain water and allow it to air-dry completely. Use an artist's brush to apply a thin coat of primer to the exposed area. Some brands of primer and touch-up paint include a small brush as part of the cap.

Allow primer to dry according to the directions on the bottle, or at least 24 hours. Next, apply touch-up paint over the primer. To save the brushes for later touch-ups, clean them with paint thinner.

➡ **Notes:** Hand-held electric grinders and grinding stones are available in hobby stores. Auto body primer and touch-up paint color-matched to your car are available at auto supply stores.

GOOD IDEA!

To prevent your car door lock from freezing, simply inject two drops of synthetic motor oil, such as Mobil 1, into the keyhole. Push the car door key into the lock and move it in and out several times to distribute the oil. Remove the key and wipe it clean. Be sure to use synthetic motor oil because conventional engine oil or regular household oil will thicken in cold weather and make it difficult to operate the lock.

Chapter Two

Cooking

by Judith Benn Hurley

Does this ever happen to you? You're whipping up dinner, the chicken's almost done, and you want to microwave the broccoli. Except you're in a rush and can't remember the correct microwave time to cook broccoli. Or you're planning a party and need to know how much ground beef to buy for a crowd. How about coming face-to-face with a bushel of garden-fresh to-matoes? Where can you find the easiest way to preserve them while keeping their flavor intact?

If you cook, you probably have dozens of cookbooks. While books with spectacular food photos are nice to look at, and recipes that contain ingredi-ents from Pago Pago are exotic, the cookbook that most of us turn to again and again is the one with easy, basic information.

That's the point of this chapter. It provides a wealth of easy recipes for everyday meals as well as more elaborate recipes for holidays and celebra-tions. In the healthy eating department, you'll discover ways to add zip with-out adding salt to meats, poultry, and fish. Low-fat marinades are also in-cluded as well as a baked potato topping and low-fat frozen dessert. For holidays, choose from a wealth of recipes—everything from a red-white-and-blue cheesecake tart for the Fourth of July to a warm Christmas cider.

What about everyday home cooking—the no-fuss, no-time meals most of us want to prepare daily? To make dinner from just about anything you have on hand in the refrigerator, try the quick stir-fry recipe. Or use the fast but delicious recipes for fish, poultry, and vegetables. For more easy home-cooking ideas, check out the healthful sandwich chart, on page 21, and the pastas and toppings chart, on page 23. And for the weekday morning rush hour, see the opposite page for a nourishing breakfast you can make in 1 minute flat.

HOME-COOKING BASICS

Home cooking for your grandmother probably meant an entire day devoted to preparing a tummy-warming supper. Home cooking today can still conjure up those old images of love, security, and ease, but the all-day preparation time and the heavy emphasis on fat, salt, and sugar are no longer necessary.

The health-wise, easy recipes here offer all of the old-fashioned goodness associated with a thick, hearty stew or a chewy oatmeal cookie. But now the stew is thickened with a medley of vegetables instead of fat and flour, and the oatmeal cookies are for breakfast instead of dessert.

The 1-Minute Breakfast

Despite its colorful name, buttermilk contains very little butterfat. In fact, buttermilk has almost the same calorie count and fat content as skim milk. This instant shake combines tangy buttermilk and sweet fruit for a low-fat, tasty breakfast.

Yield: 1 serving

INGREDIENTS

½ cup cold orange juice
1 banana, quartered
½ cup cold buttermilk
¼ cup vanilla low-fat or nonfat yogurt

SUPPLIES

blender or food processor
8-ounce chilled mug

Combine all ingredients in the blender or food processor and whiz until thick and smooth. Pour into the mug and enjoy.

❧ **Variation:** Instead of banana, use ½ cup berries or 2 peaches, peeled, pitted, and pureed.

GOOD IDEA!

To brown cookies lightly and easily without using fat on the cookie sheet, line the pan with baking parchment, available at kitchen and cooking supply stores. If you don't use baking parchment, try a nonstick cooking spray, but watch the cookies closely so the bottoms don't overbrown.

For the best texture when making whole-grain cookies, have all ingredients at room temperature before mixing.

Make-Ahead Breakfast Cookies

These treats have no refined sugar or salt.

Yield: about 16 cookies

INGREDIENTS

  1   tablespoon canola oil or rice bran oil
  ½   cup all-fruit apple butter
  3   tablespoons plain nonfat yogurt
  1   teaspoon vanilla extract
  2   egg whites
1¼   cups whole wheat pastry flour (about 5 ounces)
  ½   teaspoon baking soda
  ¼   teaspoon baking powder
  1   teaspoon ground cinnamon
  1   cup rolled oats or oat and dried fruit muesli

SUPPLIES

electric mixer
baking parchment
wire cooling rack
sealable container

Preheat the oven to 375°F. In a medium bowl, combine oil, apple butter, yogurt, vanilla, and egg whites. Beat with the mixer until well-combined. In a large bowl, combine remaining ingredients. Mix well with a wooden spoon. Add wet ingredients and combine. Don't overmix.

Line a large cookie sheet with baking parchment. Drop well-rounded spoonfuls of dough onto the sheet, leaving a bit of space between. Bake until cooked through, about 14 minutes. Let cool on the wire rack. Store tightly sealed. They'll last about three days.

➬ **Note:** Both canola oil and rice bran oil are mono-unsaturated, a characteristic that promotes heart health. Both are available at most supermarkets and specialty food stores. Check labels; you may already have canola oil in your pantry.

Easy Berry Omelette

This omelette has a fresh, fruity flavor.

Yield: 2 servings

INGREDIENTS

¼ cup sliced fresh strawberries, blueberries,
    or raspberries
½ teaspoon finely grated orange peel (no white pith)
1 teaspoon canola oil or rice bran oil
2 eggs
   splash of water

SUPPLIES

10-inch nonstick sauté pan
pastry brush

In a small bowl, combine berries with orange peel and set aside. Heat the pan on medium-high and brush the bottom with oil. Whisk together eggs and water. Pour into the pan and swirl it around a bit for even cooking. Add berry mixture. Continue to cook and swirl until eggs are set, about 2 minutes.

Use a spatula to coax the edges of the omelette from the pan. Tip the omelette onto a plate, folding it over as you serve.

✿ **Variation:** If you're cutting back on saturated fat and cholesterol, substitute two egg whites for one of the whole eggs.

➻ **Notes:** Using a real sauté pan, which has sloped sides, makes it easier to remove the finished omelette from the pan. Both canola oil and rice bran oil are mono-unsaturated, a characteristic that promotes heart health. Both are available at most supermarkets and specialty food stores. Check labels; you may already have canola oil in your pantry.

> **GOOD IDEA!**
>
> **F**or a special breakfast treat, garnish a berry omelette with fresh orange sections and mint sprigs. For an easy suppertime omelette, add leftover stir-fried vegetables instead of berries and orange peel.

Supper's On

The recipes here provide health-wise, tasty dinnertime fare with little fuss. For a quick supper using whatever vegetables and meats you have on hand, see the stir-fry on page 20. For a hearty, all-in-one-dish supper, try the casserole below.

Basic Beef Casserole

In the old-fashioned sense, a casserole is simply a slow way of cooking fresh food in a covered dish in the oven. Casseroles have little to do with processed foods thrown together and topped with crumbs.

Yield: 4 servings

INGREDIENTS

1 pound cubed lean beef
1 medium yellow onion, chopped
1 stalk celery, chopped (leaves, too)
1 carrot, chopped
1 bay leaf
1 teaspoon dried thyme
1 teaspoon dried rosemary
1½ cups defatted beef stock
crusty bread

SUPPLIES

3-quart covered casserole dish or clay cooker

Preheat the oven to 325°F. Combine all ingredients in the casserole dish or clay cooker. Cover and bake until the beef is tender, about 3 hours. Remove bay leaf. Serve warm accompanied with crusty bread.

✿ **Variations:** To make a chicken casserole, use chunks of skinless chicken meat and chicken stock instead of beef stock. For extra zest, substitute some dry white wine for the stock.

GOOD IDEA!

To serve beef casserole for company, prepare it a day ahead of your party and refrigerate in a microwave-safe covered container. Reheat just before serving. Overnight cooling actually improves flavor. Your guests will notice the great taste, and you'll appreciate the peace of mind brought by having your main dish prepared early.

White Bean and Eggplant Stew

Beans are a great source of low-fat fiber. Eggplant is noted for its hospitable way of accepting and blending all the flavors in a recipe.

Yield: 4 servings

INGREDIENTS

1 tablespoon olive oil

1 medium yellow onion, minced

2 cloves garlic, mashed through a press

¼ cup minced fresh celery leaves

2 cups cubed unpeeled eggplant

6 Italian plum tomatoes, peeled and seeded

2 cups defatted chicken stock

½ teaspoon dried thyme

½ teaspoon dried rosemary

1 cup cooked tiny white beans, such as cannellini, marrow, or navy

2 tablespoons freshly grated Parmesan cheese

SUPPLIES

4-quart or larger soup pot

Warm the pot over medium heat, then add oil. When it's warm, add onions, garlic, and celery leaves and sauté until fragrant and just wilted, about 3 minutes. Add eggplant and tomatoes, cover, and let simmer for about 7 minutes. Stir in stock, thyme, and rosemary and continue to simmer until eggplant is tender, about 20 minutes. Add the beans, heat through, and serve hot, sprinkled with the Parmesan.

GOOD IDEA!

To improve the **flavor of vegetable-based stews,** add plenty of celery leaves. Their robust flavor is a wonderful salt substitute, and they add vitamins as well as roughage to any dish.

GOOD IDEA!

To ensure even cooking in a stir-fry dish, cut all ingredients the same size. To keep the ingredients from sticking, heat the wok well before you add the oil.

Basic Stir-Fry

With this basic formula, you can create a stir-fry at a moment's notice, using ingredients you have on hand.

Yield: 4 servings

INGREDIENTS

1 tablespoon soy sauce

2 tablespoons defatted chicken stock or water

1 tablespoon dry sherry

1 teaspoon honey

1 clove garlic, mashed through a press

½ teaspoon grated gingerroot

1 teaspoon cornstarch dissolved in 1 tablespoon water

2 teaspoons cornstarch

12 ounces sliced chicken, beef, pork, or lamb

2 tablespoons canola oil or rice bran oil

2 cups sliced vegetables, such as bell peppers, onions, green beans, bok choy, or carrots

SUPPLIES

wok

Combine soy sauce, stock or water, sherry, honey, garlic, ginger, and dissolved cornstarch in a small bowl, whisk well, and set aside.

Heat a wok on high for about a minute. Meanwhile, toss cornstarch with chicken, beef, pork, or lamb until all the slices are lightly coated. When the wok is hot, pour in 1 tablespoon oil and heat for another 30 seconds. Tip in coated meat and stir constantly until cooked through, about 2 minutes for thin slices. Remove meat and keep it handy.

Heat remaining tablespoon of oil for about 30 seconds and toss in vegetables. Stir constantly until almost cooked through, about 1 minute for thin slices. Return meat to the wok and add soy sauce mixture, stirring constantly until all ingredients are well-coated and shiny. Serve warm.

➥ **Note:** Both canola oil and rice bran oil have a high smoke point, which means these oils can get very hot without burning. This characteristic allows quick cooking on high heat without breakdown of the oil. Also, both oils are mono-unsaturated, a characteristic that promotes heart health. Both are available at most supermarkets and specialty food stores. Check labels; you may already have canola oil in your pantry.

Here's to Healthy Lunches

Brown bags carry everyday lunches, but they don't have to carry everyday fare. It's just as easy to fill a brown bag with a healthful and delicious sandwich as it is to toss in a boring, unhealthful one. Here are a few ideas.

SANDWICH BAR Bread and Filling Combos That Taste Great	
Bread	**Filling**
Crisp taco shell	Marinated bean salad
	Tuna in a lemon vinaigrette
Crusty French bread	Sliced tomato and part-skim mozzarella
5-grain bread, toasted	Peanut butter and all-fruit apple butter
Flour tortilla	Cooked beans and rice
Rye bread	Lean roast beef and mustard
Whole wheat bread	Sprouts and sliced avocado
Whole wheat English muffin	Sliced tomato and a poached egg
Whole wheat pita	Chopped marinated vegetables
	Pasta salad or brown rice salad

Supper Italian Style

No matter which country our ancestors came from, most of us think of Italian fare as fun, filling, and delicious. The recipes that follow provide authentic, home-cooked taste without special ingredients or an entire day spent in the kitchen.

Easy Homemade Pizza

How long does it take to mix the whole-grain dough and bake? Only 20 minutes.

Yield: one 11-inch pizza or 4 servings

INGREDIENTS

  1 teaspoon quick-rise dry yeast (about ½ package)
 ½ cup warm water (115°F)
  1 tablespoon olive oil
1¼ cups whole wheat pastry flour (about 5 ounces)
 ½ teaspoon salt
 ½ cup tomato sauce
  1 cup shredded part-skim mozzarella cheese

SUPPLIES

pizza pan or cookie sheet with a perforated bottom
nonstick cooking spray

Preheat the oven to 500°F. In a medium bowl, combine yeast, water, and oil and mix well. Stir in flour and salt and mix well. Let the dough rest for about 5 minutes.

Spray the pizza pan or cookie sheet with nonstick spray. Set the dough on it and shape into an 11-inch round. Spread on sauce, sprinkle with cheese, and bake until the crust is cooked through, about 12 minutes.

✿ **Variation:** *Instead of tomato sauce and mozzarella cheese, simply sprinkle the crust with dried rosemary and freshly grated Parmesan cheese.*

GOOD IDEA!

To make a pizza with a crispy crust, use a perforated pizza pan. The holes allow air to circulate, making a crisp crust without the need for extra oil. If you bake pizza on black cookie sheets, reduce the temperature to 450°F. For easy pizza slicing, use kitchen shears.

Low-Fat Meatballs

These can be an appetizer or entrée.

Yield: 4 to 6 servings

INGREDIENTS

1 pound lean ground beef or turkey

2 egg whites

2 cloves garlic, mashed through a press

1 leek, topped, tailed, and minced

1 carrot, grated

1 cup brown rice or unhulled barley, cooked

1 tablespoon minced fresh thyme or 1 teaspoon dried

1 tablespoon minced fresh basil or 1 teaspoon dried

SUPPLIES

cookie sheet with sides

Preheat the oven to 350°F. Combine all ingredients in a large bowl. Lightly wet your hands and form walnut-size balls. Set them on the cookie sheet and bake until cooked through, about 30 minutes. Serve hot or cold.

> **GOOD IDEA!**
>
> **To make Italian suppers a breeze,** keep a bag of meatballs in your freezer. Place freshly mixed meatballs on a waxed-paper-covered cookie sheet and store in your freezer until just frozen—about an hour. Then store them in plastic bags in your freezer. At serving time, you can easily remove just the number you need. These keep in your freezer for up to six months.

THAT'S ITALIAN **Pastas and Toppings That Taste Great**	
Pasta	**Toppings**
Angel's hair	Chopped ripe, flavorful tomatoes and fresh crushed herbs; oriental-style peanut sauce
Bow-ties and medium shells	Medium-bodied tomato-mushroom sauces; vinaigrettes and fresh vegetables
Dumplings and gnocchi	Medium-bodied tomato sauces; bell pepper purees; herbed white sauces
Fettuccine and linguine	Clam sauces; herb-scented white sauces; olive oil and fresh crushed garlic
Rigatoni and mostaccioli	Medium- to heavy-bodied tomato sauces; meat sauces; cheesy sauces

GOOD IDEA!

Use homemade to-mato sauce as a tasty ketchup substitute on sandwiches or as a condi-ment to meats. You can also enjoy homemade sauce without meatballs in a variety of ways, such as over baked eggplant or over pasta sprinkled with cheese.

Homemade Tomato Sauce

Why bother to make it yourself? To enjoy fresh to-mato flavor without unnecessary salt, fat, and preservatives.

Yield: 2 pints

INGREDIENTS

5 pounds fresh Italian plum tomatoes (about 25)
1 tablespoon olive oil
1 medium onion, minced
2 cloves garlic, mashed through a press
2 stalks celery, minced (leaves, too)
2 tablespoons finely chopped fresh parsley
2 tablespoons minced fresh basil or 2 teaspoons dried

SUPPLIES

food processor
5-quart or larger soup pot

Core tomatoes with a sharp paring knife. Place batches in a food processor and whiz until pureed. Heat the pot on medium-high and add oil. Add onions, garlic, and celery and sauté until fragrant and just wilted, about 3 min-utes. Add tomatoes, parsley, and basil and simmer, loosely covered, until thick, about an hour. Freeze in portion-size containers for up to a year.

Freezing Tomatoes

Freeze extra summer tomatoes for use in wintertime sauces and soups. To freeze, first fill a large soup pot with water and bring to a boil. Meanwhile, core fresh tomatoes with a sharp paring knife. Place a few tomatoes in a wire mesh strainer and set the whole thing in the boiling water. Let blanch for about 2½ minutes for medium-size tomatoes. Small ones, like Italian plums, require 2 minutes, and large, beefsteak types need 3 minutes.

Remove the strainer full of tomatoes and immediately set into ice water for about 25 seconds to stop the cooking. When the toma-toes are cool enough to handle, peel them and pack into freezer containers or freezer bags. They'll keep in the freezer for up to a year.

Smart Substitutions

What do you do when your favorite cookie recipe calls for white sugar, but you prefer the subtle taste of honey? How about when you forgot to buy buttermilk for your favorite cornbread recipe? It's simple. Use the chart here to fill in the gaps and make that special recipe come out right anyway.

IN A PINCH	
Food Substitutions That Work	
Food	**Substitution**
1 cup buttermilk	½ cup plain nonfat yogurt mixed with ½ cup skim milk
1 cup skim milk	1 cup water mixed with 2 Tbs. instant nonfat dry milk
1 cup fruit juice for cooking	1 cup brewed spicy herb tea
1 cup beef stock	1 cup water plus 2 tsp. tamari or soy sauce
1 Tbs. fresh herbs	1 tsp. dried herbs
1 cup cooked dried beans	1 cup canned beans, rinsed well
1 Tbs. butter for sautéing	1 Tbs. olive oil
1 whole egg for baking	2 egg whites
1 cup sour cream for a dip	1 cup plain nonfat yogurt
1 Tbs. lemon juice	1 Tbs. vinegar
¼ cup dry white wine	¼ cup dry white vermouth
1 cup refined sugar for baking	½ to ⅔ cup honey or pure maple syrup (plus 3 Tbs. extra flour)
1 Tbs. cornstarch	1 Tbs. arrowroot
1 Tbs. baking powder	1½ tsp. baking soda plus 1½ tsp. cream of tartar
1 cake of baking yeast	1 package (2½ tsp. granulated baking yeast)
1 tsp. prepared mustard	¼ tsp. dried mustard plus ¾ tsp. vinegar

FESTIVE COOKING

Make merry on your next anniversary or holiday with one of the special recipes here. Many of them celebrate the taste of seasonal fruits while others offer health-wise versions of traditional recipes.

New Year's Good-Luck Salad

Tradition holds that eating black-eyed peas on New Year's Day brings good luck.

Yield: 4 servings

INGREDIENTS

2 cups cooked black-eyed peas (from dried peas)
1 sweet red pepper, cored, seeded, and chopped
1 sweet yellow pepper, cored, seeded, and chopped
1 tablespoon reduced-calorie mayonnaise
1 tablespoon plain nonfat yogurt
2 tablespoons freshly squeezed lemon juice
1 teaspoon hot-pepper sauce, or to taste
1 tablespoon minced fresh thyme or 1 teaspoon dried
1 tablespoon minced fresh basil or 1 teaspoon dried
1 clove garlic, mashed through a press
curly leaf lettuce

Combine peas and peppers in a medium serving bowl and keep them handy. In a small bowl, whisk together mayonnaise, yogurt, lemon juice, hot-pepper sauce, thyme, basil, and garlic to make dressing.

Pour dressing over peas and peppers and toss well to combine. Serve at room temperature or very slightly chilled on curly lettuce leaves. This keeps for several days in the refrigerator.

GOOD IDEA!

To make a salad with canned black-eyed peas instead of dried, be sure to drain the peas and rinse them well to rid them of salt and gooey liquid. To prepare cooked black-eyed peas from dried, rinse and drain the peas. Then cover with 4 cups water per cup of peas. Let soak overnight. The following day, bring the peas to a slow boil in the water in which they were soaked. Reduce heat, cover, and simmer until tender, about 1 hour.

Valentine's Day Apricot Confections

Here's a heart-healthy sweet for your sweetheart.

Yield: 6 confections

INGREDIENTS

1½ cups rolled oats

12 dried apricots

3 dried dates, pitted

2 egg whites

3 tablespoons all-fruit apricot preserves

1 cup grated carrot

SUPPLIES

food processor

paper baking cups

microwave-safe muffin pan or six 4-ounce glass
     custard cups

large frying pan (optional)

Toss oats, apricots, and dates into the food processor and whiz until apricots and dates are finely chopped and all ingredients are about the same size. With the motor running, pour in egg whites and preserves and combine well. Add carrots and whiz until well-combined.

To microwave, insert baking cups into custard cups or into each well of the muffin pan. Add dough and smooth out the tops to make them even. Microwave, uncovered, on full power until cooked through and dry to the touch, about 4 minutes for a 700-watt microwave. Confections do *not* rise or brown like muffins. Let stand at least 3 minutes.

To cook without a microwave, add the dough directly into custard cups. Fill a large frying pan with ½ inch water. Bring water to a boil and place filled custard cups in the boiling water. Steam them, uncovered, in the water for about 12 minutes.

> ### GOOD IDEA!
>
> **T**o top treats without adding a lot of sugar or extra fat, try drizzling them with vanilla yogurt. Yogurt is tasty and healthy, too!

Easter Fruit Salad

Enjoy this salad as part of an Easter brunch or even as a light dessert after an Easter feast.

Yield: 4 to 6 servings

INGREDIENTS

3 ripe Anjou or Bartlett pears, cored and chopped into 1-inch pieces

2 cups red or green seedless grapes

¼ cup toasted, shredded coconut

juice of 1 lime

Combine all ingredients in a medium bowl and toss well to combine. Serve at room temperature or very slightly chilled.

✿ **Variation:** Substitute chopped apples for pears. Golden Delicious or Cortland apples are good choices because they retain a fresh color longer than other varieties.

Mother's Day Strawberry Tart

An easy, make-ahead dish for Mother's Day brunch or dessert.

Yield: 6 servings

INGREDIENTS

½ cup whole wheat pastry flour (about 2 ounces)

½ cup unbleached flour (about 2 ounces)

2 tablespoons canola oil or rice bran oil

½ cup low-fat cottage cheese

splash of water (optional)

1 cup vanilla low-fat yogurt

2 cups fresh strawberries, halved

½ cup all-fruit apricot preserves

GOOD IDEA!

To preserve the flavor of fresh berries, don't wash them. Simply brush them off with a pastry brush. Freezing berries keeps them available in off seasons. Use defrosted berries in blender fruit shakes, in fruit salads, or mixed half-and-half with vanilla nonfat yogurt.

SUPPLIES

food processor
10-inch tart pan with removable bottom
nonstick cooking spray
wire cooling rack
small saucepan or small microwavable dish

Preheat the oven to 375°F. To make the crust, combine both flours and oil in the food processor and whiz until the mixture looks like cornmeal. With the motor running, add cottage cheese and continue to process until the mixture forms a ball. If no ball is formed after 6 seconds, add a splash of water and process to the ball stage.

Spray the tart pan with nonstick spray. Press the dough into the bottom and sides until you have a smooth, even crust. Bake until golden and cooked through, about 25 minutes. Place the pan on the wire rack, and let the shell cool completely before proceeding to the next step.

To fill the shell, spread yogurt over the bottom. Then arrange berries over the yogurt. Meanwhile, melt preserves in the saucepan over low heat or in the dish in the microwave, uncovered, on full power for about 30 seconds. Spoon melted preserves over the berries and refrigerate until well-chilled, at least an hour. Store leftover tart in the refrigerator.

➺ **Note:** Both canola oil and rice bran oil are mono-unsaturated, a characteristic that promotes heart health. Both are available at most supermarkets and specialty food stores. Check labels; you may already have canola oil in your pantry.

GOOD IDEA!

To enjoy cheesecake at your Fourth of July picnic without a lot of work, prepare the cheesecake ahead of time and freeze it without the fruit topping. Defrost the cheesecake overnight in the refrigerator. Take the berries along and add before serving.

Fourth of July Cheesecake Tart

The perfect patriotic dessert—it's red, white, and blue.

Yield: 8 servings

INGREDIENTS

4 ounces graham crackers
2 tablespoons canola oil or rice bran oil
1 cup low-fat cottage cheese
1 cup plain nonfat yogurt
1 teaspoon vanilla extract
3 tablespoons maple syrup
1 egg or 2 egg whites
   fresh blueberries and strawberries

SUPPLIES

food processor
9-inch tart pan with removable bottom
nonstick cooking spray

Preheat the oven to 325°F. To make the crust, combine crackers and oil in the food processor and whiz until crumbly. Spray the bottom and sides of the tart pan with nonstick spray. Press crumbs into the bottom and sides.

To make the filling, combine cottage cheese, yogurt, vanilla, syrup, and egg in the food processor and whiz until smooth. Scoop into the crust and bake until set, about 30 minutes. Let cool thoroughly in the pan before removing. Serve at room temperature or very slightly chilled, garnished with fresh berries.

➡ **Note:** Both canola oil and rice bran oil are mono-unsaturated, a characteristic that promotes heart health. Both are available at most supermarkets and specialty food stores. Check labels; you may already have canola oil in your pantry.

Moist Halloween Pumpkin Cake

A Halloween treat that also offers up a healthy dose of vitamin A.

Yield: 8 servings

INGREDIENTS

⅓ cup cake flour (about 1 ounce)

⅓ cup finely ground date sugar or brown sugar

1 teaspoon baking powder

½ teaspoon pumpkin pie spice

pinch salt

2 cups grated fresh pumpkin

¼ cup canola oil or rice bran oil

all-fruit apple butter (optional)

SUPPLIES

4½ × 8½-inch loaf pan

nonstick cooking spray

wire cooling rack

Preheat the oven to 350°F. In a medium bowl, combine flour, sugar, baking powder, pumpkin pie spice, and salt. Stir until well-combined. Add pumpkin and oil and stir to combine. Spray the loaf pan with nonstick spray and pour in the batter. Bake on a mid-oven rack until cooked through, 20 to 25 minutes. Let cool for 5 minutes, then carefully turn the cake out onto the wire rack to cool completely. Slice and serve plain or, if desired, top with a bit of apple butter.

➻ **Note:** *Both canola oil and rice bran oil are mono-unsaturated, a characteristic that promotes heart health. Both are available at most supermarkets and specialty food stores. Check labels; you may already have canola oil in your pantry.*

GOOD IDEA!

For the best flavor in pumpkin cake, buy neck pumpkin. Traditional jack-o'-lantern pumpkins lack the robust flavor needed to make a good-tasting cake. If you can't find neck pumpkin, substitute butternut squash.

GOOD IDEA!

To lightly brown challah without adding grease to the baking pan, line the pan with baking parchment, available at kitchen supply stores and specialty food stores.

Hanukkah Challah

A quick way to make a traditional holiday bread.

Yield: 2 loaves

INGREDIENTS

1 package quick-rise dry yeast

6 to 7½ cups unbleached flour (24 to 30 ounces)

½ teaspoon salt

1½ cups hot water (125°F)

⅓ cup canola oil or rice bran oil

1 tablespoon honey

3 eggs, beaten, or 6 egg whites

1 egg beaten with a splash of water

SUPPLIES

plastic wrap

baking parchment

pastry brush

wire cooling rack

waxed paper

In a large bowl, combine yeast, 6 cups flour, and salt. Pour in water, oil, honey, and egg and combine well using your hands or a large spatula.

Turn the dough out onto a lightly floured surface and knead for about 6 minutes, gradually kneading in extra flour if the dough is sticky. The final dough should be smooth and a bit stiff for easy braiding.

Set the dough in a large, lightly oiled bowl and roll it over to coat all sides with oil. Cover the bowl with plastic wrap and let rise until double in size, about 30 minutes.

Punch the dough down and slice into halves, then thirds. Flour your hands. On a lightly floured surface, roll each third into a 14-inch log. Braid together three logs and pinch the ends closed. Repeat for the second loaf. Set both loaves on a large cookie sheet lined with baking parchment. Let rise until double in size, 30 to 40 minutes.

Preheat the oven to 350°F. Before baking, brush loaves with the egg/water glaze. Bake until golden, 45 to 50 minutes. Let cool on the wire rack. Store at room temperature, wrapped in waxed paper.

↦ **Note:** *Both canola oil and rice bran oil are mono-unsaturated, a characteristic that promotes heart health. Both are available at most supermarkets and specialty food stores. Check labels; you may already have canola oil in your pantry.*

Christmas Cider

Keep this cider warm in a fondue pot, deep chafing dish, or crock pot. Be sure to make the spice mixture ahead of time so that it has time to dry.

Yield: 1 quart

INGREDIENTS

2 Tbs. plus 2 tsp. maple sugar, date sugar, or brown sugar

1 teaspoon ground cinnamon

¼ teaspoon freshly ground nutmeg

6 whole cloves

1 lemon, halved

2 cups cranberry juice

2 cups apple cider

SUPPLIES

wire cooling rack

In a small bowl, mix together sugar, cinnamon, nutmeg, and cloves. Remove all of the interior part of the lemon. Use a spoon to pack half the spice mixture into each empty lemon shell. Tamp it down tightly. Set shells on the wire rack and leave in a cool, dry place for about a week.

To make the cider, combine the dried shells, cranberry juice, and cider in a medium saucepan and simmer for at least an hour. Serve warm.

GOOD IDEA!

To make a thoughtful but inexpensive holiday gift, stuff lemon shells with brown sugar, cinnamon, nutmeg, and cloves and dry for a week. Place stuffed shells in a small basket along with a decorative card with instructions for making a holiday cider. Decorate with a festive bow.

GOOD IDEA!

To get the greatest volume out of beaten eggs, the eggs should be at room temperature. To get cold eggs quickly to room temperature, place the eggs in a saucepan filled with warm tap water. Eggs will be ready to beat within 10 minutes.

Anniversary Cake

This cake is great for birthdays and other celebrations as well.

Yield: 10 to 12 servings

INGREDIENTS

½ cup whole wheat pastry flour (about 2 ounces)
½ cup unbleached white flour (about 2 ounces)
6 eggs, separated
½ cup warm maple syrup
1 teaspoon vanilla extract
⅛ teaspoon cream of tartar
1 cup all-fruit apricot preserves or lemon curd
2 cups raspberries

SUPPLIES

9-inch springform pan
waxed paper
electric mixer
wire cooling rack

Preheat the oven to 350°F. Butter the bottom of the springform pan and line it with waxed paper. Then butter and flour the waxed paper. Lightly butter and flour the sides of the pan.

Sift both flours together and set aside. In a large mixing bowl, beat egg yolks with the mixer at high speed until light and lemon colored. Gradually beat in 6 tablespoons of syrup and continue beating until the mixture is very thick and smooth, 12 to 15 minutes. Beat in vanilla.

In another large bowl, beat egg whites with clean beaters until foamy. Add cream of tartar and beat until soft peaks form. Gradually beat in remaining syrup and continue to beat until stiff peaks form. Gently fold one-quarter of egg whites into yolk mixture. Fold in remaining whites.

Fold in flour mixture gently but thoroughly, one-third at a time. Pour batter into the prepared pan and bake until the top springs back when lightly touched and a cake tester comes out clean, 35 to 40 minutes. Let cake cool in the pan for 10 minutes. Remove the sides of the pan and invert cake onto the wire rack. Remove the bottom of the pan and the waxed paper and allow the cake to cool completely.

Slice the cake into two layers. Set one layer on a plate. Spread the top of it with about ⅔ cup preserves or lemon curd. Add the second layer and spread remaining preserves on top of the cake. Arrange raspberries on top.

➥ **Note:** *Lemon curd is available at most supermarkets.*

BETTER THAN STORE-BOUGHT

Make your own convenience foods and save your money as well as your health. Some recipes here are just as easy to prepare as store-bought mixes, plus they're less expensive and don't contain the salt and preservatives of boxed mixes. Other recipes provide healthful alternatives to some empty-calorie convenience foods.

Irish Soda Bread

Keep dry mix handy to make bread anytime.

Yield: enough dry mix for 4 loaves

INGREDIENTS
FOR DRY MIX

16 cups whole wheat bread flour (about 4 pounds)
 1 teaspoon salt
 ¼ cup baking powder
 2 teaspoons baking soda

To make the bread mix, combine all ingredients well in a large bowl. Store tightly covered in the refrigerator.

> **GOOD IDEA!**
>
> **For a festive topping for an unfrosted cake,** whip 1 cup heavy cream with 1 tablespoon preserves or maple syrup. Spread on top layer of cake and sprinkle with fresh berries.

> **GOOD IDEA!**
>
> **To make Irish soda bread with a distinct flavor,** add 2 teaspoons crushed caraway seed, ⅓ cup raisins, or ¼ cup finely minced fresh herbs to the mixed dough. Fresh herbs that taste especially good include basil, rosemary, and sage.

(continued)

INGREDIENTS

4 cups dry mix

   about 2 cups low-fat buttermilk

1 tablespoon honey

SUPPLIES

4½ × 8½-inch loaf pan

nonstick cooking spray

wire cooling rack

To make one loaf of bread, preheat the oven to 425°F. Spray the pan with nonstick spray. Combine all ingredients in a large bowl and mix well. When the dough becomes sticky, mix with your hands. If dough is too wet, knead in a bit of dry mix. Knead just until the dough is smooth and the ingredients are well-combined. Place the dough in the pan and use a sharp knife to cut a ½-inch slash down the middle of the dough. This keeps the bread from cracking as it bakes. Bake until cooked through, 30 to 40 minutes. Let cool on the wire rack.

GOOD IDEA!

For a festive dessert or party snack, stuff large dried figs or pitted prunes with yogurt cheese. Roll the stuffed fruits in toasted coconut before serving on a party platter.

Yogurt Cheese

Use this nonfat cheese as you would cream cheese.

Yield: about 1½ cups

SUPPLIES

4 cups plain nonfat yogurt

large fine-meshed strainer lined with a paper towel or
   large colander lined with two layers of cheesecloth

sealable container

Set the lined strainer or colander in the sink. Scoop in yogurt and let drain overnight. Refrigerate yogurt cheese in a tightly covered container for up to a week.

✿ **Variation:** For a vegetable dip or sandwich spread, add dill and garlic to yogurt cheese.

Oatmeal Refrigerator Muffins

Store the mixed batter, tightly covered, in the refrigerator for up to two weeks. Make as needed.

Yield: 12 muffins

INGREDIENTS

1 cup whole wheat pastry flour (about 4 ounces)
1½ cup rolled oats
2 teaspoons baking powder
½ teaspoon baking soda
1 teaspoon ground cinnamon
1 egg or 2 egg whites
1 cup low-fat buttermilk
1 tablespoon canola oil or rice bran oil
3 tablespoons maple syrup

SUPPLIES

electric mixer
muffin tins
nonstick cooking spray

Preheat the oven to 375°F. In a medium bowl, combine flour, oats, baking powder, baking soda, and cinnamon and stir well. In another medium bowl, combine remaining ingredients and use the mixer to combine well. Pour into the dry ingredients and mix by hand, about 15 strokes. Don't overmix.

Spray muffin tins with nonstick spray and fill each well three-quarters full. Bake until cooked through, about 18 minutes.

✿ **Variation:** Add ¼ cup raisins, chopped dates, or chopped pecans to the batter.

➾ **Note:** Both canola oil and rice bran oil are monounsaturated, a characteristic that promotes heart health. Both are available at most supermarkets and specialty food stores. Check labels; you may already have canola oil in your pantry.

GOOD IDEA!

For a quick and nutritious breakfast, bake muffins ahead and freeze them tightly sealed in a plastic bag. To serve for breakfast, cover frozen muffins with a dry, cotton napkin and leave out overnight. To thaw and warm two frozen muffins in the microwave, cover the muffins with a damp paper towel and microwave on high for 40 seconds.

Freezer Apple-Bran Muffins

Enjoy these hearty breakfast muffins right away, or make ahead and freeze.

Yield: 18 muffins

INGREDIENTS

      1 cup unbleached flour (about 4 ounces)
      1 cup whole wheat pastry flour (about 4 ounces)
      2 cups wheat bran
      2 teaspoons baking powder
      1 teaspoon baking soda
      1 teaspoon ground cinnamon
      1 egg or 2 egg whites
      1 tablespoon canola oil or rice bran oil
   1½ cups low-fat buttermilk
     ½ cup all-fruit apple butter

SUPPLIES

electric mixer
muffin tins
nonstick cooking spray

Preheat the oven to 375°F. In a large bowl, combine the flours, wheat bran, baking powder, baking soda, and cinnamon. In a medium bowl, combine remaining ingredients with the mixer. Add to the dry mixture and combine well by hand, about 15 strokes. Don't overmix.

Bake in muffin tins coated with nonstick spray. Bake until cooked through, about 18 minutes. Cool on a wire rack. Store in a tightly sealed plastic bag to freeze.

➡ **Note:** Both canola oil and rice bran oil are mono-unsaturated, a characteristic that promotes heart health. Both are available at most supermarkets and specialty food stores. Check labels; you may already have canola oil in your pantry.

Hot Cereal

A high-fiber breakfast with no added fat or refined sugar.

Yield: enough mix for 14 servings

INGREDIENTS
FOR DRY MIX

3 cups medium bulgur

3 cups oat bran

1 cup chopped raisins or dried apricots

Combine all ingredients in a large jar. Cover and refrigerate for up to six months.

INGREDIENTS

½ cup dry mix

½ cup apple juice or skim milk

SUPPLIES

small saucepan

For one serving, combine dry mix and juice or milk in the saucepan. Bring to a boil over high heat, stirring occasionally. Reduce the heat and simmer until cereal is soft and all the liquid has been absorbed, about 4 minutes. Serve warm.

✿ **Variation:** You may substitute regular cracked wheat for the bulgur, but cooking time will be slightly longer.

➴ **Note:** Bulgur is preboiled cracked wheat available at many supermarkets, specialty food stores, and bulk food stores.

GOOD IDEA!

For a quick supper dish with bulgur, simply sauté a cup of mixed, finely chopped fresh vegetables in a tablespoon of oil. Good vegetables to try include minced celery (leaves, too), green peppers, scallions, and carrots. Stir in 1 cup bulgur, 1 ⅓ cups boiling water, and one bay leaf. Reduce heat, cover, and cook over very low heat for about 15 minutes. Remove bay leaf before serving.

GOOD IDEA!

For a great-tasting pancake topping, combine 1/3 cup vanilla low-fat yogurt sweetened to taste with maple syrup. For an interesting texture, place toasted sesame seeds or slivered almonds in the pan and pour the batter over them.

Freezer Peach Pancakes

Peaches add sweetness without adding refined sugar. Keep a stack in your freezer for quick breakfasts.

Yield: 4 servings

INGREDIENTS

1 cup whole wheat pastry flour (about 4 ounces)
1½ teaspoon baking powder
2 tablespoons wheat germ
2 tablespoons all-fruit peach preserves
½ teaspoon vanilla extract
1 egg or 2 egg whites
1 cup skim milk
1 peach or 2 plums, pitted and finely chopped

SUPPLIES

nonstick skillet or griddle
nonstick cooking spray
plastic wrap or aluminum foil (optional)

In a medium bowl, combine flour, baking powder, and wheat germ. In another medium bowl, combine remaining ingredients. Add to the dry ingredients and use a large spatula to combine well, about 12 strokes. Don't overmix.

Spray a nonstick pan with nonstick spray and heat on medium. For each pancake, drop in about 2 tablespoons of batter and cook until bubbles appear on top, about 3 minutes. Flip and cook about 3 minutes more.

To freeze, wrap the pancakes in foil or plastic wrap. To reheat, preheat the oven to 500°F. Set pancakes directly on the oven racks and bake until heated through, about 2 minutes. Or, for each pancake, microwave on high for 30 seconds.

✿ **Variation:** To make waffle batter, use 1⅔ cups skim milk.

Basic Vanilla Ice Cream

No commercial ice cream even comes close to the taste of homemade.

Yield: about 2 quarts

INGREDIENTS

5 cups light cream, whole milk, or skim milk
1 vanilla bean
¾ cup mild-flavored, light-colored honey

SUPPLIES

small saucepan
ice cream maker

Pour 2 cups of cream or milk into the saucepan. Add vanilla bean. Heat on medium, stirring constantly, until the cream is scalded, about 10 minutes. Properly scalded cream smells cooked but not burned. Remove from the heat. Scrape the seeds and pulp from the vanilla bean and discard the pod. Add seeds and pulp to the scalded cream. Then, in a large bowl, combine scalded cream, remaining cream or milk, and honey. Chill in the refrigerator for at least 1 hour. Process in an ice cream maker according to manufacturer's directions.

✿ **Variations:** Stir in fruit chunks, fruit puree, or small whole berries when you stir in the honey. To make maple-flavored ice cream, substitute maple syrup for the honey.

GOOD IDEA!

To enjoy the best flavor in homemade ice cream, eat it within a day or so of making it. Because it lacks food additives, it doesn't keep well in the freezer. Store tightly covered in the coldest part of the freezer for no longer than one month.

GOOD IDEA!

To perk up a cake without icing, top with strawberry syrup. A low-sugar strawberry syrup also tastes great on ice cream, frozen yogurt, or fruit salad, not to mention pancakes, waffles, and biscuits.

Strawberry Syrup

Keep sealed in the refrigerator for up to three weeks.

Yield: 1 cup

INGREDIENTS

1 cup ripe, flavorful strawberries
¼ cup white grape juice
1 teaspoon finely grated orange peel

SUPPLIES

blender or food processor
small saucepan

Combine all ingredients in the blender or food processor and whiz until smooth. Cook in the saucepan on medium-high until slightly thickened, about 3 minutes.

GOOD IDEA!

When picking raspberries, bring along small, shallow containers, no more than 2 inches deep. Raspberries are extremely fragile. Those at the bottom of a deep container will turn to mush.

Don't wash fresh berries because they fall apart and lose flavor quickly. Before eating, simply brush them off with a pastry brush.

Raspberry Fruit Spread

Refrigerate, tightly covered, and use for up to a month.

Yield: 2 cups

INGREDIENTS

4 cups fresh raspberries
½ cup apple juice
½ cup freshly squeezed orange juice
  juice and pulp of 1 lemon
¼ cup light honey

SUPPLIES

12-inch, deep frying pan

Tip berries into the pan and mash them coarsely with a spatula. Add remaining ingredients and bring to a boil. Continue to boil, stirring frequently, until thick and syrupy, about 15 minutes.

Apricot-Pecan Cookies

Make the batter ahead and keep it tightly covered and refrigerated for up to two weeks. Bake as many cookies as you like at one time.

Yield: about 18 cookies

GOOD IDEA!

If you're sensitive to sulfites, be sure to ask for unsulfured apricots. Try substituting dried peaches for apricots in cookie recipes.

INGREDIENTS

- 1/4 cup unsalted butter
- 3/4 cup all-fruit apricot preserves
- 1 egg or 2 egg whites, lightly beaten
- 1/2 cup unbleached flour (about 2 ounces)
- 1/2 cup whole wheat pastry flour (about 2 ounces)
- 1 teaspoon baking powder
- 3/4 teaspoon freshly grated orange peel (no white pith)
- 1/2 teaspoon ground cinnamon
- 1/2 cup chopped pecans
- 1 cup chopped dried apricots

SUPPLIES

- electric mixer
- baking parchment
- wire cooling rack

In a medium bowl, combine butter, preserves, and egg. Beat with an electric mixer until smooth. Combine both flours and baking powder in a medium bowl and stir well. Add orange peel, cinnamon, pecans, and apricots. Pour the wet ingredients into the dry and combine well by hand, about 15 strokes. Don't overmix.

To bake cookies, preheat the oven to 350°F. Drop tablespoons of dough onto parchment-lined cookie sheets and bake until cooked through, 12 to 15 minutes. Let the cookies cool on the wire rack.

Note: *You can use nonstick cooking spray instead of baking parchment, but watch that the bottoms don't overbrown.*

HERE'S TO YOUR HEALTH

Put away your salt shaker and your butter dish. Flavoring foods with salt and butter is not only a poor choice for healthful eating, it's also old hat. Each of the no-fat marinades and no-salt spice mixes here provides a bouquet of flavors to make plain broiled or roasted meats truly special.

GOOD IDEA!

To flavor meat without salt, try sprinkling on one of these combinations.
- Lemon juice, minced fresh rosemary, and freshly ground black pepper
- Minced fresh thyme, ground cloves, grated orange peel, and freshly ground black pepper
- Minced garlic, herbed vinegar, and freshly ground black pepper

No-Salt Spice Mix for Meat

To cut back on salt, keep this convenient mix on your kitchen counter instead of your salt shaker. It compliments the flavor of any red meat.

Yield: about ¼ cup

INGREDIENTS
2 tablespoons black peppercorns, such as tellicherry
1 tablespoon white peppercorns
1½ teaspoons whole coriander seed
1½ teaspoons whole allspice

Combine all ingredients in a pepper mill. Use to flavor marinades and sauces for meats or as a condiment to sprinkle on before eating.

➦ **Note:** Since this spice mix is intended to eliminate the need for salt, it's important to buy the best-quality spices available. Tellicherry peppercorns are imported from Malabar in India and have a distinctive fruity aroma. Check labels to make sure this is what you are buying.

No-Salt Spice Mix for Poultry

This mix is especially good for chicken cutlets.

Yield: about ¼ cup

INGREDIENTS

1 tablespoon dried rosemary leaves
1 tablespoon dried sage leaves
1 tablespoon dried thyme leaves
1 tablespoon dried lemon peel

SUPPLIES

jar with lid
mortar and pestle or electric spice grinder

Combine all ingredients in a jar, seal, and keep in a cool, dry place for up to six months. To use, grind a teaspoon of the mixture in the mortar and pestle or spice grinder and sprinkle on cooked poultry. One teaspoon is enough for two servings.

✿ **Variation:** *Dried orange peel, instead of lemon peel, is especially tasty with turkey.*

No-Fat Marinade for Poultry Cutlets

Keeps poultry moist and tender without oil or butter.

Yield: enough for 1 pound or 4 servings

INGREDIENTS

½ cup plain nonfat yogurt
2 teaspoons chili powder or curry powder
2 cloves garlic, mashed through a press

Combine all ingredients in a small bowl and stir well. Spread on poultry cutlets and let marinate, covered and refrigerated, for at least an hour. Overnight is fine. Then grill, broil, bake, or microwave.

GOOD IDEA!

To keep grilled chicken moist, *grill it with the skin on. The skin helps protect the tender meat against the harsh heat of the fire. To avoid unwanted fat, you can remove the skin at serving time.*

For flavoring grilled chicken, place a spice mixture between the skin and the flesh. Grill with the skin in place. Remove skin just before serving.

GOOD IDEA!

To enhance the flavor of fish without adding fat, combine equal parts dried basil, thyme, Greek oregano (rigani), and dillweed. Store in a sealed jar. To use, grind about a teaspoon in a mortar and pestle or electric spice grinder and sprinkle on cooked fish or fish salad. One teaspoon flavors two servings.

No-Fat Marinade for Fish

Great for flounder, haddock, shrimp, or scallops.

Yield: enough for 1 pound or 4 servings

INGREDIENTS

2 teaspoons soy sauce
1 teaspoon finely grated gingerroot
1 tablespoon dry sherry
2 teaspoons orange juice concentrate
   juice of 1 lemon or lime

Combine all ingredients in a small bowl and whisk well to combine. Rub into fish fillets, peeled shrimp, or scallops. Let marinate, covered and refrigerated, for about 30 minutes. Then grill, broil, bake, or microwave.

➡ **Note:** Never add salt to fish before cooking. It makes fish dry and flavorless.

GOOD IDEA!

To add texture to a baked potato, garnish with a low-fat topping and sprinkle on shredded raw carrots or beets. Top it all off with lightly toasted sunflower seeds.

Low-Fat Baked Potato Topping

A delicious substitute for fatty sour cream.

Yield: 4 servings

INGREDIENTS

¼ cup nonfat cottage cheese or farmer's cheese
¼ cup plain nonfat yogurt
2 tablespoons skim milk
1 tablespoon minced fresh chives

Combine all ingredients in a medium bowl and beat well by hand. Scoop onto baked potatoes.

✿ **Variation:** Add snipped dill and use as a vegetable dip.

Low-Fat Easy Mayonnaise

Slash calories and fat from sandwich spreads and dressings with this quick-to-make alternative.

Yield: about ¾ cup

INGREDIENTS

10½ ounces silky-type or soft-texture tofu (about ¾ cup)
 1 tablespoon white vinegar
 1 tablespoon freshly squeezed lemon juice
 ½ teaspoon Dijon-style mustard
 1 tablespoon canola oil or olive oil
  pinch of salt

SUPPLIES

blender or food processor
jar with lid

Combine all ingredients in the blender or food processor and whiz until smooth. Refrigerate overnight to allow the flavors to mingle. Keep refrigerated in the covered jar for up to two weeks.

✿ **Variation:** Flavor the mayonnaise with herbs and spices to add interest to sandwiches and salads. Curry powder, dill, tarragon, or toasted ground cumin are tasty additions.

➩ **Note:** Canola oil is mono-unsaturated, a characteristic that promotes heart health. It is available at most supermarkets and specialty food stores. Check labels; you may already have canola oil in your pantry.

GOOD IDEA!

To add flavor to fish, baste the skin side with low-fat mayonnaise before grilling. The mayonnaise not only adds flavor, it helps keep the fish moist during cooking.

To reduce the fat content of a traditional sour cream dip, substitute low-fat mayonnaise for a quarter of the sour cream.

GOOD IDEA!

To prevent oil and vinegar dressing from separating, add a few drops of egg white to the dressing, shake, and serve.

Lemon Vinaigrette

Great on mixed greens or as a marinade for blanched broccoli and carrots.

Yield: 4 servings

INGREDIENTS

1 tablespoon apple-cider vinegar
1 tablespoon balsamic vinegar
1 tablespoon olive oil
¼ teaspoon Dijon-style mustard
¼ teaspoon finely grated lemon peel (yellow part only)
   freshly ground black pepper (optional)

SUPPLIES

blender or food processor

Combine all ingredients in the blender or food processor and whiz until well-combined. Toss with salad.

GOOD IDEA!

For a yogurt treat appealing to children, spoon newly frozen yogurt into Popsicle molds, freeze, and serve. For variety, place chopped nuts or whole berries in the bottom of each mold before adding the yogurt. If you don't have Popsicle molds, pour the yogurt into small paper cups and insert wooden Popsicle sticks.

Low-Fat Frozen Berry Yogurt

A delicious frozen dessert without the fat and refined sugar of typical commercial ice cream.

Yield: 4 servings

INGREDIENTS

1 cup fresh blueberries
1 cup fresh strawberries
¼ to ⅓ cup orange juice concentrate
2 cups plain nonfat yogurt
1 teaspoon vanilla extract

SUPPLIES

blender or food processor
ice cream maker

Toss berries and concentrate (amount depends on sweetness of berries) into a blender or processor and whiz until smooth. Place berry puree in a medium bowl and fold in yogurt and vanilla. Process in an ice cream maker according to manufacturer's instructions. Serve in chilled dishes or crepes, or sandwiched between big oatmeal cookies.

COOKING FOR A CROWD

Family reunions and Memorial Day picnics should be fun for the cook as well as the guests. The buying tips and the recipes that follow are designed to take all the guesswork out of cooking for a party.

Under the theory that the cook would rather keep company with the guests than with the stove, all the dishes here are simple to prepare. Before you make up your shopping list for your next backyard bash, check out these food-buying guidelines and recipes.

Party Beverage Buying Tips

Perfect planning helps the host enjoy the party as much as the guests. These tips on buying beverages for a crowd take the guesswork out of party planning.

- When planning a party, pick up a pound of ice per person. Yes, this does mean buy 16 pounds of ice for 16 guests. And if you'll be chilling beverages in an ice bucket, you'll need more.
- To make coffee for 25 people, use about ½ pound coffee to 3½ quarts water. The same goes for tea.
- If you're serving carbonated beverages, be sure to stock up on club soda, sparkling mineral water, tonic water, and ginger ale.
- Popular juices to serve include apple, tomato, orange, and cranberry. In fact, many people are choosing apple juice and club soda mixed together rather than an alcoholic cocktail.
- Don't forget beverage garnishes—lime and lemon wedges, orange sections and peel, olives, and bitters. Also important are party napkins, stirrers, and shakers.

How Much Should You Buy?

The U.S. Department of Agriculture says that one serving of meat should weigh about 4 ounces, uncooked. But buying bony cuts makes buying the right amount complicated. One pound of vegetables will serve four as a side dish, right? Well, not always. The portion planners below take all the guesswork out of shopping for your next party.

THE MAIN EVENT
Meat Portions for Serving a Crowd

Meat	To Serve		
	8	12	16
Boneless cuts, like brisket, chuck, flank steak, ground meats, ham, rib roast, tenderloin, top sirloin, veal breast, veal cutlets	2 lb.	3 lb.	4 lb.
Boneless poultry cutlets and fish fillets	2 lb.	3 lb.	4 lb.
Bony cuts like pork ribs	6 lb.	9 lb.	12 lb.
Cuts with bones, like ham, lamb chops, pork chops, porterhouse steaks, T-bone steaks, and pork and beef roasts	2⅔ lb.	4 lb.	5½ lb.
Whole poultry with bones	8 lb.	12 lb.	16 lb.

GREENS, ROOTS, AND PODS
Vegetable Portions for Serving a Crowd

Vegetable	To Serve		
	8	12	16
Broccoli, cabbage, carrots, cauliflower, eggplant, mushrooms, okra, shelled peas, squash	2 lb.	3 lb.	4 lb.
Greens that shrink during cooking, like cress, collards, kale, sorrel, spinach	4 lb.	6 lb.	8 lb.
Large vegetables, like baking potatoes, corn on the cob, globe artichokes	8 pieces	12 pieces	16 pieces
Vegetables to be shelled, like peas in the pod and shell beans	4 lb.	6 lb.	8 lb.

Vegetarian Chili

A low-fat but tasty alternative to traditional chili.

Yield: 18 servings

INGREDIENTS

¼   cup olive oil
3   large yellow onions, chopped
3   cups dried lentils
4   cups bulgur
3   quarts plus 1½ cups defatted stock or water
⅓   cup chili powder, or to taste
5   cloves garlic, mashed through a press

SUPPLIES

4-quart or larger soup pot

Heat oil in the pot over medium heat. Add onions and cook until lightly browned, about 7 minutes. Add remaining ingredients. Bring to a boil. Simmer, loosely covered, until lentils are tender and most of the liquid has been absorbed, about 40 minutes. Serve piping hot.

➻ **Note:** *Bulgur is preboiled cracked wheat available at many supermarkets, specialty food stores, and bulk food stores.*

Party Punch

Refreshing for brunch, lunch, or a light dinner.

Yield: 12 servings

INGREDIENTS

6   cups purple grape juice
6   cups freshly squeezed orange juice
6   cups seltzer water or sparkling mineral water

Combine all ingredients in a large punch bowl and serve over crushed ice.

GOOD IDEA!

For a great finishing touch, garnish chili with freshly grated cheese, such as Monterey Jack, and minced scallions. It's a tasty topping for any chili.

GOOD IDEA!

To spruce up your party punch, add thin slices of lemon. For a more exotic look, try garnishing with pink nasturtiums.

GOOD IDEA!

To serve any casserole or stew to a crowd where seating is limited, prepare the dish with all meats and vegetables cut into bite-size pieces that can be eaten with a fork alone. Guests who are standing won't have to contend with cutting utensils to enjoy the meal.

Easy Beef Stew

Great for winter weekends.

Yield: 12 servings

INGREDIENTS

 2 tablespoons olive oil
1½ pounds lean stew meat, cut into 1-inch pieces
 2 tablespoons flour
 2 cups water
 2 cups tomato juice
 3 cloves garlic, mashed through a press
 1 tablespoon Worcestershire sauce, or to taste
12 pearl onions
 5 medium carrots, cut into 1-inch chunks
 4 medium waxy-type potatoes, cut into 1-inch chunks

SUPPLIES

4-quart soup pot

Heat oil in the pot over medium-low heat. Toss meat with flour and add to the pot. Let brown slowly for about 15 minutes. Then add remaining ingredients and simmer until vegetables are tender, about 1½ hours. Serve warm.

Party-Time Hints

To serve a crowd easily, plan serving details as well as you plan the menu. Here are some party-tested strategies for entertaining.

Before you write out the guest list, calculate how many people your ground floor can accommodate comfortably. You can accommodate roughly twice as many people for an open house as you can for a single party.

The week before your party, remove nonessential furniture to allow guests more room to circulate. Set up a beverage or snack center in a little-used downstairs room. Both of these strategies will encourage guests to mingle.

Plan on five to seven hors d'oeuvres per guest. For the earliest guests, have cold canapes ready. As the crowd increases, warm hors d'oeuvres in a microwave.

Early on the day of the party, fill your coffeemaker with water and coffee, and set a timer to turn it on automatically about mid-way through the party. When dessert time rolls around, fresh coffee will be waiting.

Apple Crisp

For best results, choose Granny Smith or McIntosh.

Yield: 18 servings

INGREDIENTS

5 pounds cooking apples, peeled, cored, and chopped into 1-inch pieces

juice of 3 lemons

1 cup all-fruit apple butter

about ½ cup flour

¼ cup canola oil or rice bran oil

3½ cups rolled oats

SUPPLIES

12 × 24-inch deep baking pan

nonstick cooking spray

aluminum foil

Preheat the oven to 350°F. Combine apples, lemon juice, and ½ cup apple butter in a large bowl. If apples are juicy, add all the flour. If dry, add only a small amount. Mix well. Apples are properly coated when they are dry and smooth to the touch. Coat the inside of the pan with nonstick spray, add the apple mixture, and level it.

In a medium bowl, combine remaining apple butter, oil, and oats and mix well. Spread over apples and cover with foil. Bake on a mid-oven rack until just bubbly, about 40 minutes. Remove the foil and continue to bake until the oats have gently browned, 15 to 20 minutes more. Serve warm or very slightly chilled.

✿ **Variations:** For a richer topping, use half oats and half chopped nuts. Substitute Anjou pears for half the apples.

➦ **Note:** Both canola oil and rice bran oil are mono-unsaturated, a characteristic that promotes heart health. Both are available at most supermarkets and specialty food stores. Check labels; you may already have canola oil in your pantry.

GOOD IDEA!

To keep stored apples at peak flavor and condition, place them in plastic bags in the refrigerator and spray with water from a plant mister once a week. Apples stored this way will keep four to six weeks. However, one bad apple will spoil the whole bunch, so be sure to check your apple stores frequently.

GOOD IDEA!

To make the preparations for your party less hectic, plan ahead. One thing you can do is prepare some foods ahead of time. Casseroles can be prepared and assembled early in the day. As party time nears, preheat the oven and bake just before serving time.

Mixed-Vegetable Casserole

A good side dish for roast turkey, flank steak, or hamburger.

Yield: 12 servings

INGREDIENTS

3 cups chopped tomatoes
3 cups chopped zucchini
3 medium onions, chopped
3 cloves garlic, mashed through a press
¼ cup minced fresh parsley
¼ cup minced fresh basil or 1 tablespoon dried
1 cup grated part-skim mozzarella cheese
2½ cups bread crumbs

SUPPLIES

12 × 24-inch deep baking pan
spoon or paddle
nonstick cooking spray

Coat the pan with nonstick spray and add tomatoes, zucchini, onions, garlic, parsley, and basil. In a small bowl, combine cheese and bread crumbs. Combine 1½ cups of this mixture with the vegetables. Level vegetables in the pan and cover the top with remaining cheese/bread crumb mixture. Refrigerate until just before serving time, up to 24 hours, or preheat oven to 350°F and bake immediately. Bake until cooked through and vegetables are tender, about 55 minutes. Serve warm.

Whole Wheat Stuffing with Toasted Walnuts

Serve with roast turkey, roast chicken, or roast beef.

Yield: 12 servings

INGREDIENTS

⅔ cup chopped walnuts

1 tablespoon olive oil

2 stalks celery, chopped (leaves, too)

1 large onion, chopped

3 cloves garlic, mashed through a press

2 loaves whole wheat bread,
    torn into bite-size pieces

¼ cup minced fresh basil or 2 teaspoons dried

4 to 5 cups defatted chicken stock or beef stock

SUPPLIES

large, nonstick sauté pan

12 × 24-inch deep baking pan

aluminum foil

Preheat the oven to 350°F. Add walnuts to the sauté pan and stir constantly over medium-high heat until toasted, about 3½ minutes. Set nuts aside, put the pan back on the heat, and add oil. When oil is hot, add celery, onions, and garlic and sauté until partially browned and fragrant, about 8 minutes.

Place bread pieces in the baking pan. Add the celery mixture, nuts, and basil and toss well to combine. Slowly pour on the stock, taking care that the bread absorbs all the liquid. If the bread is very dry, you'll need the full 5 cups.

Cover with foil and bake until cooked through, about 35 minutes. For a drier texture, remove the foil midway through baking.

> ## GOOD IDEA!
>
> **To toast nuts perfectly,** place a dry non-stick pan on medium-high heat and add the nuts. Stir constantly until just browned, 2½ to 3½ minutes. Watch them carefully to prevent burning.

Chapter Three

Gardening

by Linda A. Gilkeson, Ph.D., and Leslie Spraker May

Most gardeners use at least one home remedy for controlling pests, and even a casual researcher could probably come up with a dozen home remedies just for aphids. Every keen gardener has at least heard of garlic or soap spray, of rhubarb leaf or horsetail tea, even if he hasn't actually used them. Once included as standard recipes in early-1900s gardening books, many of these formulas are now passed from person to person as part of gardening folklore. As usually happens with such information, specific methods and quantities gradually change or are forgotten as the information is passed along. This chapter provides an updated handbook of all that over-the-back-fence information that gardeners have been collecting and exchanging forever. It includes a wide collection of pest and disease control recipes, helpful tips, and general gardening formulas for such tasks as planting roses and storing dahlia tubers.

Not only are homemade formulas usually cheaper than their commercial equivalents, they come in just the quantity you need to get the job done, without leaving leftovers sitting from year to year in the garden shed. Making your own sprays and traps is also a way to conserve resources, cut down on wasteful packaging, and ensure that biodegradable and least-toxic ingredients are used.

This chapter has something for everyone—from the rose devotee to the fruit enthusiast. You'll find a broad range of insecticides and fungicides as well as a selection of special needs formulas, such as a special formula for preparing rose beds or for preserving Christmas trees. You'll find a nice selection of traditional recipes for such indispensable items as horsetail tea, pyrethrum sprays, sticky trap lures, tree band glue, and slug bait. For those gardeners who love to experiment, there are plenty of variations on basic formulas to leave room for fun. What's more, this chapter offers the best ideas from a rich variety of sources—from antique gardening books to the most recently published scientific papers. A few recipes, such as neem spray and the potato starch spray, are homemade versions of modern commercial products that are only just now coming on the market.

Some of these recipes, such as the one for grafting wax, may be fun to make just to see if you can do it, but they aren't likely to be cheaper than old-fashioned commercial grafting wax from a garden center. Others, like tree band glue to capture gypsy moths, are easy to make, work just as effectively, and cost less than the commercial product. With the exceptions of the bordeaux and nicotine preparations, sprays in this section are much less poisonous than commercial chemical pesticides. They are also not as long-lasting, which means that you may need to use them more frequently to control a severe infestation.

As with any insecticide, no matter how nontoxic the ingredients, use these homemade insect formulas only as a last resort, when other control measures, such as sticky traps, handpicking, tree bands or barriers, don't give satisfactory control. No-spray gardening preserves native beneficial predators (like insects, birds, mites, and toads). Few people realize just how common and widespread beneficial insects are and that they do the best pest control job of all if they are allowed to live in your garden.

How to Use These Formulas

For all the sprays or dusts in this chapter (whether for insects or diseases), always try a small amount of the formula on a few leaves first. No recipe has been tried on all the possible kinds of plants and under the range of conditions found in yards and gardens. Checking for leaf damage before treating the whole plant will prevent heartbreaking and needless loss of a sensitive plant. Follow the directions and the list of ingredients exactly. Plants are extremely sensitive. For example, the inclusion of extra soap in a formula (a seemingly harmless practice), may severely burn or even defoliate some plants. Do not substitute ingredients unless they're specifically mentioned as an acceptable variation on the original formula. And be sure to label and safely store all your bottles, boxes, and cans of ingredients as well as the final formulas. None of these recipes would make great food for your cat, and some of them offer enough potential harm to be kept locked away from children. In almost every formula, you'll find plenty of advice on handling and storing all ingredients safely. Take the advice seriously, follow the directions precisely, and enjoy the good results and great gardening experiences that follow.

ORGANIC FERTILIZERS

The rich soil of a well-maintained organic garden meets the needs of most plants admirably. Because organic fertilizers tend to release nutrients throughout the growing season, fertilizing plants in midseason is not as important as it is in a conventional garden. Occasionally, however, you will need to provide a dose of readily available plant nutrients, either to stimulate increased growth or to help crops overcome stress factors like disease or insect pests.

Homemade Organic Fertilizer

If you send a soil sample to a soil testing lab, your soil report may recommend applying 25 pounds of 5-10-10 fertilizer per 1,000 square feet of garden. A commercial 5-10-10 fertilizer is 5 percent nitrogen, 10 percent phosphorus, and 10 percent potassium. Instead of buying a bag of chemical fertilizer, mix an organic fertilizer that accomplishes the same results.

Yield: the equivalent of 25 pounds of 5-10-10 commercial fertilizer

INGREDIENTS

17 pounds cottonseed meal
 8 pounds colloidal phosphate
45 pounds granite dust

SUPPLIES

large wheelbarrow or plastic drop cloth
shovel

Simply place all ingredients in the wheelbarrow or on the drop cloth and mix.

➡ **Note:** Cottonseed meal, colloidal phosphate, and granite dust are sold at farm supply stores and some garden centers. See page 444 for other sources.

GOOD IDEA!

To get a reliable soil analysis, collect soil samples properly. Late autumn is a good time to collect samples from at least three different areas in your garden. For each area, scrape away the surface litter and use a trowel to dig a 6-inch hole. Take a slice of soil from one side of the hole. Place all samples in the same clean plastic container. Mix the samples and let them dry. Remove any stones or plant pieces. Place required amount of soil into the sample bag provided by the lab and close. Results take four to six weeks, or longer in spring.

Sam Dunbarr's Fertilizer Tea Barrel

Sam Dunbarr of Lemon Grove, California, has used this special flower and vegetable fertilizer for 25 years.

Yield: 50 gallons

INGREDIENTS

   green plant residue from yard and garden
4 gallons manure
2 cups fish emulsion
2 cups seaweed extract
1/2 gallon blackstrap molasses
   water

SUPPLIES

heavy screen, cut to fit inside barrel
several bricks
50-gallon barrel with a spigot near its base
burlap sack

Place the screen on the bricks in the bottom of the barrel, so that it rests about 1 inch above the spigot. The screen acts as a filter to prevent solids from clogging the spigot. Fill the barrel to within a foot of the rim with plant residue. Dump manure into the burlap sack and place on top of plant material. Add fish emulsion, seaweed extract, and molasses. Finally, fill the barrel with water. Allow to steep for several days before drawing liquid off via the spigot. Use undiluted as a soil drench.

➥ **Notes:** Fish emulsion is a concentrated brown liquid made from fish oils and water. Seaweed extract is liquefied kelp. Buy both at well-stocked garden supply stores and through mail-order suppliers. See page 444 for other sources. Blackstrap molasses is the liquid left after extraction of sugar from sorghum. Buy it at farm supply stores or livestock feed dealers.

GOOD IDEA!

To help control disease and insect pests, add an onion/garlic infusion to fertilizer tea. Pour boiling water over two handfuls chopped green onions or 4 bruised garlic cloves. Cover and allow to steep for up to a day. Add 1/2 cup of the strained solution to each 50 gallons of fertilizer tea.

Comfrey and Nettle Fertilizer

Both comfrey and stinging nettle contain significant
amounts of nitrogen. Comfrey is also high in potassium,
and nettle contains iron. Together, they make an excellent
stimulant for developing plants.

Yield: varies by amount of ingredients chosen

INGREDIENTS

comfrey leaves
leaves from *young* shoots of stinging nettle
water (preferably rainwater)

SUPPLIES

thick leather gloves
open-weave bag, such as an old stocking or mesh bag
bucket

☛ **BE SAFE.** Stinging nettles applied to bare skin cause an unpleasant sting. To avoid stings and even possible allergic reactions, wear gloves and protective clothing when gathering nettles. When touched, nettle hairs give off formic acid, the same
substance that makes an ant bite memorable.

Wearing gloves, fill the bag with a mixture of comfrey
and nettle leaves and place it in the bucket. Cover with
water. Set the bucket outside (it will stink). Allow the mixture to soak for three to four weeks, until the leaves have
rotted. Strain the liquid off and use it as a fertilizing drench.

➥ **Note:** Stinging nettle (Urtica dioica) is a perennial weed
common throughout the northern half of the United States. It is
recognizable by its squarish stem, covered with many fine, bris-
tling hairs that give a smart sting to bare skin. For this formula,
gather only the young, immature growth.

Making Compost

Making compost is essentially a method of speeding up the natural decay processes that usually occur without our help. In nature, decay occurs wherever there is a supply of organic material, an active community of decay-causing microorganisms, and optimum amounts of both carbon and nitrogen for the microorganisms to feed upon. All organic material contains carbon and nitrogen in varying amounts, although in both plants and animals, carbon is far more abundant than nitrogen.

Decay-causing microbes work by using the carbon for food and the nitrogen to reproduce themselves. Organic material with a relatively high nitrogen content breaks down very quickly because the abundant nitrogen supply encourages a miniature population explosion of decay-causing microbes, each of which feeds on the organic material. Conversely, material relatively low in nitrogen breaks down very slowly because while the microorganisms have carbon for food, they don't have enough nitrogen to multiply quickly. Generally, hard organic materials like wood, dried leaves, and straw are relatively low in nitrogen, and soft materials like grass clippings and manure are relatively high in nitrogen.

Microorganisms do the work of composting best when the overall ratio of carbon to nitrogen (called the C-to-N ratio and written C:N) in the compost pile is about 25 or 30 to 1. When the ratio is much higher than that, the microorganisms do not multiply, and the composting process is slow. When the ratio is significantly lower than that, abundant nitrogen is available, the bacteria multiply quickly, and the compost pile gets very hot. Excess nitrogen is often released as ammonia, an offensive-smelling gas.

To build an effective compost pile, simply layer materials high in nitrogen alternately with soil and with materials high in carbon. The soil supplies the microorganisms that do the composting. See "How Fast Will It Rot?" on page 62 for ideas on selecting compost materials.

HOW FAST WILL IT ROT? Relative Carbon and Nitrogen Content for Compost Materials			
Composts Slowly		**Composts Quickly**	
High Carbon	**C:N**	**High Nitrogen**	**C:N**
Cornstalks	60:1	Alfalfa hay	12:1
Leaves	40:1 to 80:1	Kitchen scraps	15:1
Oat straw	80:1	Fruit wastes	35:1
Paper	170:1	Grass clippings	19:1
Sawdust	500:1	Humus	10:1
Straw	80:1	Legume-grass hay	25:1
Sugar cane residues	50:1	Mature sweet clover	23:1
Wood	700:1	Rotted manure	20:1

GOOD IDEA!

To produce a free, high-quality organic fertilizer and mulch, recycle garden wastes. Compost provides major nutrients for plant growth and improves soil structure. It also encourages a balanced population of soil-dwelling creatures, such as fungi and earthworms, which contribute to plant health. Compost is a far better fertilizer and soil conditioner than any commercial product.

Basic Compost

A classic compost pile combines leaves, grass clippings, and soil in a standard ratio.

Yield: varies by amount of ingredients chosen

INGREDIENTS

leaves
grass clippings
soil
water

SUPPLIES

lawn mower with collection bag or shredder
shovel
garden fork

Make compost by starting with about 6 inches of leaves. Onto this, place 2 inches of grass clippings, then about 1/8 inch of soil. Repeat the layering until you have a substantial pile. Dampen the pile evenly as you build it.

Compost microorganisms need moist but not wet conditions to thrive. A handful of fresh composting material should feel like a squeezed out sponge, damp but not wet.

For faster composting, shred leaves either by collecting them in the bag of a lawn mower or running them through a shredder. Do include, however, some coarse, unshredded material to help the pile to aerate. The bacteria that compost most efficiently need oxygen to thrive. A pile that is too finely shredded packs down tightly, excludes air, and slows down the work of the oxygen-loving microbes. Some gardeners ensure aeration by building the compost pile over a layer of brush or old cornstalks.

Every few days, turn the pile. Composting is complete in about two weeks, when all the materials are uniformly dark and crumbly and have a fresh, earthy odor.

Choose an out-of-the-way spot in your yard for your compost pile. To keep the compost from blowing around, enclose the area with chicken wire or other fencing. The area should be about 9 square feet in area by 3 feet high. If you build the pile too high, the weight of the additional materials will exclude air and slow the process.

Cold Compost

The basic compost formula on the opposite page makes compost quickly by encouraging heat buildup within the pile. Some researchers think that high-temperature compost lacks some beneficial microorganisms that help control soil-borne diseases. Evidently, heat kills the desirable microorganisms. Low-temperature compost, made slowly over a period of months, seems to be more effective in suppressing soil-borne diseases. To keep your soil healthy, try mixing a little low-temperature compost into every batch of high-temperature compost. To make low-temperature compost, simply rake damp, unshredded leaves together, piling them no higher than about 3 feet. During hot weather, turn the pile once a month. In cold weather, leave the pile unturned. Low-temperature compost takes six to nine months to be ready to use.

Seaweed Compost Accelerator

Many so-called compost activators simply introduce specific microorganisms to the compost pile, but it's really not necessary to buy a commercial compost starter at all. The addition of high-nitrogen organic materials, such as cottonseed meal, dried blood, or manure, will trigger a sluggish pile.

One compost activator that does seem to work well is seaweed. Used as the core of a compost heap, seaweed promotes decay in the entire pile. If you do not have enough seaweed to use as a main ingredient in your compost, you can make your own seaweed-based compost accelerator.

Yield: 1 gallon

INGREDIENTS

2 pounds dried seaweed
1 gallon water

SUPPLIES

mortar and pestle or food processor
2-gallon bucket
8-quart pot
candy thermometer

Crush or grind seaweed with a mortar and pestle or food processor. Place it in the bucket. Place water in the pot. Insert the thermometer and heat water to 140°F. Pour the hot water over the seaweed and allow to steep overnight. To activate a large compost pile, pour the entire batch over the pile. If you're only making a small amount of compost (less than 50 cubic feet), you may want to experiment, using only half of the activator.

✿ **Variation:** You can use fresh seaweed instead of dried. Chop it first, then soak it overnight in water that has been heated to 160° to 180°F.

PROPAGATION BASICS

This section covers propagation from seeds, cuttings, and grafting. Successful seed starting requires paying close attention to only three conditions: temperature, light, and soil mix. The seeds of each species have unique requirements for light and temperature conditions in order to break dormancy. But after the first bursting of the seed coat, the soil mix becomes just as important as light and temperature. The soil mixes and soil treatments here should help you enjoy great success with many different seed types. The additional information on rooting cuttings and grafting will help you expand your propagation techniques to new areas.

Anti-Fungal Compost Tea

Researchers at the University of Bonn in West Germany report that soaking seeds in tea made from well-rotted compost containing both animal and plant material results in a much lower incidence of damping-off.

Yield: varies by amount of ingredients chosen

INGREDIENTS

1 part well-rotted compost (made from a mixture of plant material and manure)
6 parts water

SUPPLIES

stiff stirring stick
1-gallon bucket or other container, such as a milk jug
strainer lined with cheesecloth

Stir compost and water together in the bucket or other container. Allow the mixture to steep for a week, then strain. Soak seeds overnight in the tea before sowing.

GOOD IDEA!

To use compost tea as a liquid fertilizer, dilute it to a light brown color before watering houseplants and garden plants with it. Spread the compost strained from the tea around your plants as a mulch, or return it to the compost pile.

G O O D   I D E A !

To prevent damping-off, drench the soil of a seedling flat with a garlic infusion before sowing seeds. Peel a single garlic clove and puree it with a quart of water in a blender. Allow the mixture to steep for 24 hours, then strain. Apply the liquid as a soil drench before sowing seeds or as a spray on germinating seedlings.

Soil Sterilizer with Chamomile Flowers

Some gardeners swear by this chamomile infusion as a protection against damping-off.

Yield: 1 quart

INGREDIENTS

2   handfuls fresh chamomile flowers or 2 tablespoons dried
1   quart boiling water

SUPPLIES

2-quart covered saucepan or casserole
strainer lined with cheesecloth or large coffee filter

Place flowers in the saucepan or casserole and pour boiling water over them. Cover and allow flowers to soak for a minimum of 15 minutes, preferably 24 hours. Strain and use as a drench on newly germinated seedlings.

➩ **Note:** If you don't grow chamomile in your garden, buy it in health food stores and herb shops.

Homemade Propagation Containers

Recycle clear, plastic food containers and milk cartons for use as propagation containers. Carry-out salad containers are ideal for starting seeds. Simply punch a few drainage holes in the bottom half and fill it to ½ inch from the rim with seed-starting mix. Plant your seeds and close the lid to provide a humid, greenhouse-like atmosphere. Cuttings need deeper containers for proper growth. Cut the upper half off of a quart or half-gallon milk carton and poke several holes in the remaining base for drainage. Fill the carton to ½ inch from the rim with a soilless mix and insert your cuttings. Clear plastic bags are ideal covers for maintaining humidity around cuttings. Ventilate closed containers (of either seeds or cuttings) several times a week, by opening the lid or bag for an hour or two. You can reuse plastic containers a few times by disinfecting them after each use. Milk cartons are only good for one use.

Seed-Starting Mix

Seeds generally require only warmth and moisture to germinate. After the first small root and tiny leaves have appeared, they also need light and a growing mix that provides sufficient nutrients for continued growth. This formula makes a good all-purpose seed-starting mix suitable for almost any type of seed.

Yield: varies by amount of ingredients chosen

INGREDIENTS

1 part sterilized topsoil
1 part vermiculite
1 part sterilized sand

SUPPLIES

clean container, such as a bucket or washtub
stiff stirring stick
clean plastic garbage bag (optional)

Children's play sand is usually sterilized. If you need to sterilize the sand yourself or are using your own topsoil, see "Easy Soil Sterilization" on page 68. Simply combine equal parts of all ingredients in a suitably sized container. To avoid introducing unwanted soil-borne fungi into the mix, do not stir with a garden tool, such as a shovel or hoe. For best results, use this seed-starting mix in flats or pots that have been sterilized. Use immediately or store in a sealed plastic garbage bag.

✿ **Variation:** Substitute sterilized finished compost for the topsoil and peat moss for the vermiculite.

➦ **Notes:** Buy vermiculite, which is simply air-filled mica granules, and sand at garden centers. Sterilized sand is often available at toy stores.

GOOD IDEA!

An **easy way to sterilize a flat of soil** for seedlings or cuttings is to drench it with boiling water. Use 1 gallon boiling water to sterilize a standard 21 × 11-inch flat. Or try putting 2 to 10 pounds of moist garden soil in a microwavable plastic bag with the top twisted partly closed (bag needs to be vented). Do not use a twist-tie. Process on full power—2 1/2 minutes for a 2-pound batch and 7 minutes for a 10-pound batch. Remove the bag from the oven and open very carefully. Cool before using. Microwave sterilization also works for sand.

GOOD IDEA!

To help prevent damping-off, cover the soil surface of seedling flats with a thin layer of milled sphagnum moss. Bacteria that live in the sphagnum moss produce chemicals that prevent damping-off. Be sure to apply the moss only after sterilizing the soil. Another way to prevent damping-off is to plant seedlings in sterilized containers—soaked in 1 part chlorine bleach to 10 parts water—and use only sterile ingredients for soil mixes.

Seedling Transplant Soil Mix

As soon as true leaves appear, move seedlings to a soil slightly richer than seed-starting mix.

Yield: varies by amount of ingredients chosen

INGREDIENTS

3 parts sterilized topsoil

2 parts peat moss

2 parts sand

2 parts finished compost

SUPPLIES

bucket, washtub, or plastic drop cloth

garden spade or hand shovel

clean plastic garbage bag (optional)

If you are using your own topsoil, see "Easy Soil Sterilization" below. Combine all ingredients in the bucket or washtub or on the drop cloth. Mix thoroughly. Use immediately or store in a sealed plastic garbage bag.

❀ **Variation:** Add a little alfalfa meal or cottonseed meal to each bushel of this mixture to give plants a nutritional boost.

➥ **Note:** Alfalfa meal and cottonseed meal are available at farm supply stores and some garden centers. See page 444 for other sources.

Easy Soil Sterilization

To avoid damping-off, use sterile soil mixes for seeds and seedlings. Sterilize small amounts of soil in your oven. This process can create quite a smell, so ventilate the area. Place 4 to 6 cups of loose, fertile topsoil in a large oven bag; make it no more than three-quarters full. Add ½ to 1 cup water (enough to moisten the soil thoroughly) and mix well until uniformly wet. Close the bag very loosely; insert a meat thermometer through the bag and into the soil. Bake at low heat until the thermometer registers about 170°F. Turn heat down or even off, if necessary, to maintain the soil temperature at 170°F for 30 minutes. Don't allow the soil temperature to go above 180°F, as substances toxic to plants may be formed. Remove and open the bag very carefully. Cool before using. This procedure works for sterilizing sand, too.

Pot Sterilizer

Damping-off begins when soil-borne fungi attack newly germinated seedlings at the soil surface. Typical symptoms include sudden wilting and a ring of dead tissue around the base of the seedling stem. An entire flat of seedlings may die within a matter of hours. To prevent damping-off and other soil-borne diseases, sterilize pots and seedling flats.

Yield: 11 gallons, enough for about forty-five 3½-inch plastic pots plus 10 large plastic seedling flats

INGREDIENTS

10 gallons water
 1 gallon chlorine bleach

SUPPLIES

galvanized metal washtub, large laundry sink, or small
   child's swimming pool
warm water
dish detergent
scrub brush
stiff stirring stick

First fill the washtub, sink, or pool with plenty of warm water and dish detergent. Scrub the pots and flats clean. Be sure to remove old fertilizer salts that may have accumulated around the pot rims. Drain the soapy water and rinse everything thoroughly in clean water. Then fill the washtub, sink, or pool with 10 gallons of water. Stir in bleach. Place plastic pots or flats in the bleach solution and allow to soak for 10 minutes. Remove and rinse. Reuse the bleach solution for succeeding batches of pots or flats.

✿ **Variation:** *If you'd like to disinfect only a few pots or flats, simply use the ratio of 1 part bleach to 10 parts water. One cup of bleach plus 10 cups of water makes about 3 quarts of sterilizing solution.*

GOOD IDEA!

To disinfect clay or metal plant containers, just immerse them in boiling water or heat them briefly in a 180°F oven. Allow them to cool; store in a clean, dry place. Before planting in clay pots, soak them in clean water for a few hours; otherwise they will draw water out of the potting mix and possibly harm your plants.

GOOD IDEA!

To sow very tiny seeds evenly, try using sand. Sowing tiny seeds can often be tricky, even for the most careful gardener. Add a few teaspoons of clean white sand to the seed packet; hold the packet closed and shake it to mix the sand and seeds. Spread this mixture evenly over the prepared container. Besides helping to distribute the seeds evenly, the sand also provides good germination conditions.

Cornell University Soilless Mix

Many professional plant propagators prefer a seed-starting mix containing no soil at all. Composed primarily of peat moss and vermiculite or perlite, these so-called soilless or peat-lite mixes are lightweight, compaction resistant, freely draining, and virtually disease-free. The first soilless mixes were developed at Cornell University in the 1960s.

Yield: 4 gallons

INGREDIENTS

2 gallons vermiculite or perlite
2 gallons shredded peat moss
2 tablespoons superphosphate
2 tablespoons ground limestone
8 tablespoons dried cow manure or steamed bonemeal
   water

SUPPLIES

clean 5-gallon plastic bucket or washtub
clean plastic garbage bag (optional)

Combine all ingredients in the bucket or washtub. You must completely moisten the mix before sowing seeds. An easy way to do this is to place the mix in a plastic garbage bag and add water a little at a time, squeezing and kneading the plastic bag with each addition of water. When the mix is thoroughly dampened, it's ready for seed sowing.

•• **Notes:** Vermiculite is simply air-filled mica granules. Perlite is simply air-filled granules of volcanic sand. Both are sterile and both have great water-holding capacity. You'll find them at garden centers. Buy bonemeal at garden centers and through mail-order suppliers. See page 444 for other sources.

Brooklyn Botanic Garden Soilless Mix for Transplants

Propagator Robert Hays of the Brooklyn Botanic Garden recommends a soilless, compost-based mix for transplants.

Yield: varies by amount of ingredients chosen

INGREDIENTS

10	parts compost
3	parts sand
1½	parts peat moss
1½	parts perlite

SUPPLIES

bucket, washtub, or plastic drop cloth

shovel

clean plastic garbage bag (optional)

Combine all ingredients in the bucket or washtub or on the drop cloth. Use immediately or store in a sealed plastic garbage bag. Fertilize transplants growing in this mix with a fish emulsion starter solution (see page 73) every 1½ to 3 weeks.

➤ Notes: *Perlite is simply air-filled granules of volcanic sand. It is sterile and has great water-holding capacity. You'll find it at garden centers.*

GOOD IDEA!

To boost the light intensity reaching your windowsill seedlings, surround them with foil-covered cardboard sheets or other shiny materials. Providing adequate light for seedlings is often the most difficult part of raising seedlings indoors. Bright natural light is the ideal for strong seedlings. Foil or other shiny materials will reflect more light onto the seedlings, helping them grow straight and strong.

Seed Starting Indoors

Raising seedlings indoors is an easy way to get the plants you want at a low price. Buy good-quality, current seed; last year's seed is no bargain! Follow package directions for germination. Seedlings need warm soil—set seed trays on top of your refrigerator or on a board over a radiator. Check every day; keep the flats moist but not wet. Clear plastic over the trays can help maintain a humid atmosphere for the germinating seeds; be sure to ventilate the trays for an hour or two several times a week. Once the seeds sprout, remove the plastic and move them to a slightly cooler area with plenty of light. Gradually expose the seedlings to outdoor conditions before planting them in the garden after the last frost.

Soil Cylinders for Starting Seedlings

These cylinders make inexpensive substitutes for commercial peat pellets sold for seed starting. In this formula, gelatin binds the soil, stabilizes the cylinders even after repeated waterings, and supplies nitrogen for the young seedlings.

Yield: 80 to 100 two-inch-high soil cylinders

INGREDIENTS

20 pounds soil mix of your choice
2 envelopes unflavored gelatin
1 quart water

SUPPLIES

5-gallon bucket or other suitable mixing container
2-quart saucepan
spoon or paddle
clean 6-ounce tomato paste can with both ends removed (save one end)
empty seed flat

Place soil mix in the bucket. Place water in the saucepan, bring to a boil, remove from heat, and add gelatin, stirring until thoroughly dissolved. Cool. Add enough of the gelatin mixture to the soil mix so that a handful forms a small clod when squeezed.

Place the tomato paste can upright at one end of a seed flat and fill it about two-thirds full of the soil mix. Cover the mix with one of the can's cut-off ends and push down to compact the soil slightly. Push again, gently, to eject the newly formed soil cylinder from the can. Continue making soil cylinders in this manner until the seed flat is full. Allow an hour or two for the soil cylinders to set before planting seeds.

✿ **Variation:** Depending on the type of soil mix you choose, you may need more or less gelatin. One quart of gelatin mixture will set 20 pounds of fairly dry loam and perlite.

Fish Emulsion and Seaweed Extract Starter Solution

Most seedlings respond well to a weak "starter solution," which provides a quick dose of readily available nutrients. Starter solutions help young plants recover quickly from the shock of transplanting. You can use a compost tea as a starter solution or try the following.

Yield: 1 cup

INGREDIENTS

½ cup fish emulsion
½ cup seaweed extract

SUPPLIES

stirrer
small disposable container, such as a coffee can
8-ounce jar or bottle with lid

Mix fish emulsion and seaweed extract together in the container. Pour into a jar or bottle, seal tightly, and store in a cool, dark place. To use, add 3 tablespoons of starter solution to 1 gallon of water. Use as a soil drench at transplanting time or as a spray for foliar feeding.

Notes: Fish emulsion is a concentrated brown liquid made from fish oils and water. Seaweed extract is liquefied kelp. Buy both at well-stocked garden supply stores and through mail-order suppliers. See page 444 for other sources.

GOOD IDEA!

To provide the necessary moisture without hurting seedlings, mist gently with a spray bottle. Pouring or sprinkling water over the seedlings can knock them down and flood some areas of the tray while missing others. Besides misting, another "low-impact" method of watering is watering from below. Place the pot or flat in a shallow pan containing water or a nutrient solution. Let the seedling pot soak up water until the top of the soil is moist. Remove and let drain.

Manure-Tea Starter Solution

If you have a readily available source of poultry, horse, or cow manure, try this starter solution for your young transplants. Fill a large barrel, garbage can, or other waterproof container one-eighth full of manure. Then fill the container to the top with water. Allow to steep for a day or two; stir the mixture several times during this period. Dip off the liquid with a clean can and dilute it with water to a light amber color. Water each transplant with clear water, then pour about a cup of this solution around the base of each. Repeat at 10- to 14-day intervals to encourage vigorous growth.

Rooting Garden Cuttings

For good results with cuttings, use a rooting stimulant, a substance applied to the cutting to induce root formation, and a proper rooting medium, a mix that both supports the cutting and keeps it moist during the root formation. Rooting mediums for cutting propagation must provide support, good air circulation, and adequate moisture. No nutrients are necessary until the new plant is established and has begun growth.

Willow Water for Rooting Cuttings

For over 50 years, professional plant propagators have induced root formation on cuttings by applying various chemicals. There is a good deal of evidence that cuttings of certain easily rooted plants release a strong rooting stimulant when they stand in water. Willow yields the most thoroughly studied rooting stimulant, but cotoneaster, holly, and honeysuckle cuttings also yield similar results.

Yield: 1 quart

SUPPLIES

1-quart jar
water
handful of foot-long, soft-wood willow shoots
flat of sterile rooting mix
clear plastic

Fill the jar with water. Stand willow shoots in water for 24 hours. Remove them and place softwood cuttings to be rooted in the jar of willow water. Remove after 24 hours. Insert them into the flat of rooting mix. Cover with clear plastic to prevent the cuttings from drying out. Check the flat often, adding water, as necessary, to keep the medium evenly moist but not wet. During the rooting period, be sure to remove dead leaves or other debris that may carry disease organisms.

Rooting Stimulant
from Germinating Wheat or Barley

Germinating grain produces an effective rooting stimulant. A jar of sprouted wheat or barley is an old-fashioned propagating tool that still works.

Yield: 1 cup

SUPPLIES

1 cup wheat or barley seeds

1-quart, wide-mouthed jar or similar container

water

8-inch square of cheesecloth

1 rubber band

Place seeds in the jar and cover with water. Soak seeds overnight. The next day, cover the mouth of the jar with cheesecloth, secure with a rubber band, and turn it upside down to drain. Rinse and drain the seeds with warm water several times in this manner, removing broken seeds that float. Place the jar in a warm place and rinse the seeds several times a day until the majority have begun to sprout.

When most of the seeds have sprouted, you may use them as a rooting stimulant for cuttings. Take cuttings to be rooted and swirl the cut ends through the sprouted grain just before planting. To avoid rubbing the rooting stimulant off as you push the cuttings into the rooting medium, make a narrow trench first with a pencil or thick knife.

➡ **Note:** *Use only untreated seed for this formula. You can usually find untreated barley or wheat at health food stores.*

GOOD IDEA!

Try this old-fashioned rooting trick: Place a grain seed into the split end of a cutting before placing it in the rooting medium. Grain can also be used to encourage rooting of plants propagated by air layering.

GOOD IDEA!

To prevent cuttings from drying out as you collect them, place them in a plastic bag as soon as you cut them. Keep the bagged cuttings at a moderate temperature by placing each bagful in a covered foam ice chest. (Don't put ice in the chest.) To gently cushion each bag of cuttings, blow air into the bag and seal it like a balloon. The air cushion will keep the cuttings from being crushed as the chest is filled.

Soilless Mix for Rooting Cuttings

This soilless mix is fine for rooting cuttings, but you will need to move the newly rooted plants to a richer mix as soon as they show any sign of growth.

Yield: varies by amount of ingredients chosen

INGREDIENTS

1 part peat moss or vermiculite
1 part perlite or sterilized sand
water

SUPPLIES

clean plastic garbage bag

Combine all ingredients in the plastic garbage bag and mix thoroughly. Work a small amount of water into the mix by kneading the closed plastic bag. Repeat until mix is evenly moist. Place mix in a flat for receiving cuttings or seal and store in a cool, dark place.

✿ **Variation:** If you are propagating acid-loving plants like rhododendron, be sure to use peat moss rather than vermiculite.

Notes: Vermiculite is simply air-filled mica granules. Perlite is simply air-filled granules of volcanic sand. Both are sterile and both have great water-holding capacity. You'll find them at garden centers. Sterilized sand is often available at toy stores.

Propagation Pointers

An old-fashioned way of rooting some plants is to place cuttings directly into a jar of water. Fill the jar one-half to two-thirds full of water and drop in a few pieces of activated charcoal (the kind sold for fish tank filters) to keep the water clean. Cover the jar with foil or plastic wrap. Poke small holes in the cover and stick cuttings through the holes. Keep in a warm, light place. Remove the cover every few days and vigorously stir to mix in more air. Check frequently. Soon, white roots will form.

Plant the cuttings in a soilless mix while the roots are still small; otherwise they will have trouble adjusting to the drier environment. Try stem cuttings from plants, like coleus, ivy, and willow. Some plants, like African violets, can form roots from the base of the leaf stalk. Take a leaf with about 2 inches of stalk.

Homemade Grafting Wax

Grafting involves uniting the roots from one plant with a shoot from another and is used especially for plants that are difficult to root. Grafting wax seals the graft union, protects exposed tissue, and discourages disease organisms.

Yield: varies by amount of ingredients chosen

INGREDIENTS

5 parts paraffin wax

3 parts diatomaceous earth

1 part zinc oxide

turpentine (optional)

SUPPLIES

double boiler

rubber work gloves

dust mask

spoon or paddle

sealable container

☛ **BE SAFE.** Wear rubber gloves to protect your hands. Wax and turpentine are flammable. Avoid open flames. Do not smoke. Melt wax in a double boiler; do not melt over direct heat. Wear a dust mask when mixing this formula. Keep zinc oxide powder away from children.

Melt wax in the top part of the double boiler. Turn off heat and, wearing rubber gloves, remove double boiler to a heat-proof surface. Don a dust mask and add diatomaceous earth and zinc oxide. Add a little turpentine, if needed, to soften the mixture. To use, reheat wax in the double boiler and brush onto the graft. Store leftover wax tightly sealed.

➽ **Notes:** Buy paraffin in the canning section of supermarkets and hardware stores. Buy diatomaceous earth at well-stocked garden supply stores and through mail-order garden suppliers. See page 444 for other sources. Buy zinc oxide, also called flowers of zinc, as a powder from your pharmacist.

GOOD IDEA!

To cover a graft union quickly and easily, use rubber strips made from balloons. Simply cut balloons into strips approximately 1/2 inch wide by 6 inches long. Wrap the graft with these strips, being sure to seal the union by overlapping each wrap. Tuck the end of each rubber strip beneath the last wrap to secure it. The balloon strips disintegrate in about two months when exposed to sun and air.

GARDEN PROBLEM SOLVERS

At the top of most gardening wish lists would be a magic potion for every disease or insect that squashes the gardener's dreams and hopes for a perfect garden. The formulas in this section provide realistic solutions—not magic potions. Good gardening practices also prevent problems.

Good gardening practices include: proper site selection, good soil health, diversity of plantings, good air circulation, proper drainage, proper plant spacing, good sanitation (prompt removal of diseased or dying plants), and crop rotation. If you have a recurring insect or disease problem, analyze your gardening practices first. Develop a plan for preventive gardening and, in the meantime, use these formulas to help with the problem at hand.

Anti-Fungal Onion/Garlic Spray

Members of the onion family, including garlic, are known for the ability to suppress disease. In the garden, this spray helps control fungal diseases and discourage insect attacks.

Yield: 1 quart

INGREDIENTS

2 handfuls chopped fresh onion greens or chives or 2 tablespoons dried or 4 cloves garlic, bruised

1 quart boiling water

SUPPLIES

2-quart covered saucepan or casserole

strainer lined with cheesecloth or large coffee filter

garden spray equipment

Place herbs in the saucepan or casserole and pour boiling water over them. Cover and allow to steep for at least 15 minutes, preferably for 24 hours. Strain and use as a spray.

GOOD IDEA!

To inhibit the spread of plant fungal diseases, combine several handfuls of clematis leaves, corn leaves, or papery outer garlic leaves. Place the leaves in a blender and process with enough water to make a slurry. Strain and spray on diseased plants.

Disease Fighters for Organic Gardeners

Sulfur, one of the oldest fungicides known, is mentioned by Homer in the *Iliad* and the *Odyssey*. Though it does give satisfactory control of a number of fungal diseases—including powdery mildew, rust, leaf blight, and various fruit rots—it kills some beneficial insects and can disturb soil microorganisms. Most organic gardeners use it reluctantly, if at all. For best results, apply sulfur as a dust or spray, *before* disease becomes established in the garden. For recurring fungal diseases, reapply every two weeks and after each rain.

Sulfur dust usually controls rose black spot. Apply the dust to infected plants every seven to ten days. Take care to apply this treatment only during early morning or evening hours, when temperatures are lowest. Sulfur will burn leaves if applied when temperatures are above 85°F.

Many common fungal diseases respond to treatment with a commercial **anti-transpirant,** such as Wilt-Pruf. These sprays are biodegradable and work well for preventing powdery mildew on roses, zinnias, and lilacs. For mildew prevention, apply several times during the growing season, at half the standard strength recommended by the manufacturer. For mildew on roses, dilute 3 to 4 teaspoons of anti-transpirant with a gallon of water and apply at monthly intervals, or more often, to protect new growth.

Horticultural oils, such as Safer's Sun Spray, formulated especially for use during the summer growing season, help control insects and some fungal diseases. A 2 percent oil spray controls mildew on lilacs, roses, and horse chestnuts, as well as black spot on roses. Horticultural oils are biodegradable, but since they are also a petroleum product, they may not be acceptable to some organic gardeners.

West German researchers report that **compost tea,** made from a combination of composted manure and vegetable materials, prevents fungal diseases in the garden. (See page 59 for compost tea recipe.) Compost-tea spray helps prevent late blight of tomato and potato, anthracnose and powdery mildew on grapes, and botrytis blight of beans. The spray lasts for only about ten days, however, so it must be reapplied every five to seven days. Compost tea works *only* as a preventive, not as a cure.

Baking soda is helpful in preventing some fungal diseases, notably mildew on some garden crops and black spot on roses. To control mildew on beans, muskmelons, cucumbers, strawberries, and eggplants, combine 2 teaspoons baking soda in 1 gallon water and spray on plants. For mildew on grapes, double the amount of baking soda. For mildew on roses, use 2 tablespoons baking soda in 5 gallons water. To control black spot on roses, dissolve 5 tablespoons baking soda in 5 gallons water. To help the spray adhere to the leaves, add a few drops of insecticidal soap or any mild detergent. Apply the spray to cover both tops and bottoms of leaves and stems.

GOOD IDEA!

When making larger amounts of bordeaux mixture, use the ratio 4-4-50. The first number is copper sulfate in pounds, the second is lime in pounds, and the third is water in gallons.

GOOD IDEA!

To tell whether bordeaux spray is safe to apply to foliage, dip a clean steel knife blade into the spray for a few seconds. If a reddish copper deposit shows on the blade, then more lime is needed to neutralize the acidity of the copper sulfate. A solution not properly buffered with lime may seriously burn foliage. Another point to remember: Bordeaux mixture does not keep well; use it within a day or so of mixing.

Bordeaux Mixture

Bordeaux mixture is an old, tried-and-true spray that was first introduced in 1882. It is used to control fungal diseases on plants, but is not as popular as it once was because of the risk of burning leaves or causing russeting injury on fruit. Bordeaux is used to control leaf spot diseases, blights, and anthracnose; it's also useful as a disinfectant for storage and work areas. With care, you can make your own version from scratch, or you can buy it ready to mix with water from horticultural suppliers.

Yield: about 3 gallons, enough for 2 or 3 trees

INGREDIENTS

2 level tablespoons copper sulfate
2 heaping tablespoons slaked lime
3 gallons water

SUPPLIES

rubber work gloves
goggles, safety glasses, or face shield
1½-gallon plastic bucket
wooden spoon or paddle
4-gallon container (*not* iron or galvanized metal)
strainer lined with cheesecloth or large coffee filter
face mask
garden spray equipment

☛ **BE SAFE.** Wear rubber gloves to protect your hands. This fungicide is a poison. Some states forbid spraying bordeaux without a permit. Check with your county extension agent. Wear protective clothing and a face mask to avoid inhaling the spray. Do not use this formula on fruits and vegetables within a week of harvest. Never use copper-containing sprays on Seibel varieties of grapes. Use copper sprays on peach trees only after fruit has been harvested. To avoid russeting injury, never use on fruit closer than six weeks before harvest. Also, the formula contains copper, a heavy metal that is toxic to the environment when concentrated in the soil. Use this remedy sparingly.

Wearing gloves and goggles, mix copper sulfate crystals into 1 gallon of water in the small bucket and stir until completely dissolved. This mixture can be left overnight to dissolve. In the large container, stir lime into 2 gallons of water until dissolved, then pour the copper solution into the limewater and mix well. Before spraying, strain the mixture to remove undissolved particles.

Use the spray immediately, frequently agitating to keep it well-mixed. Wear gloves, goggles, and a face mask while spraying.

➥ **Notes:** Buy copper sulfate through your local pharmacist. In some areas, crystalline copper sulfate, also known as blue vitriol or blue stone, is available at livestock supply stores. Slaked lime is used in making plaster and is available from building supply stores.

Washing Protective Clothing

When spraying any sort of pest control mixture, you should wear suitable clothing, starting with a long-sleeved shirt and long pants. (A waterproof hat, eye protection, rubber gloves, and rubber boots are also desirable.) Launder your clothing after each day of spraying, or discard heavily contaminated clothing. If possible, pre-rinse the clothes by hosing them off outdoors. Wash protective clothing separately—not with the rest of your family's laundry. Fill the washer with hot water and add ½ cup heavy-duty laundry detergent and ½ cup chlorine bleach. Rinse for two full warm cycles and hang outside to dry. Before doing normal laundry, run the washer through one cycle with water only.

Horsetail Spray for Fungal Diseases

The common field horsetail (*Equisetum arvense*) is a widely distributed, odd-looking plant often found in poor, dry, sandy soil in early summer. The whole plant has an unusually high silica content. After sending up pale brown, unbranched reproductive shoots in the early spring, the plant sends up characteristic slender, green, jointed cylindrical stems with whorls of thin, jointed branches spaced at intervals along the stem. The green parts of the plant are effective against fungal diseases, such as powdery mildew, scab, and damping-off in seedlings. Here's how to use it.

Yield: 1 quart

INGREDIENTS

1 cup chopped horsetail
1 quart water

SUPPLIES

2-quart saucepan
strainer lined with cheesecloth or large coffee filter
garden spray equipment

☛ **BE SAFE.** Horsetail spray is poisonous if ingested. Keep this formula away from children and pets.

In the saucepan, boil horsetail in water for 20 minutes. Cool, strain, and spray as needed to prevent fungal diseases. To prevent damping-off, apply as a soil drench to flats of seedlings.

Alcohol Spray for Houseplants

Ordinary rubbing alcohol controls aphids, whiteflies, mealybugs, soft scale, and thrips. Since alcohol is very toxic to all living things, brief contact with it kills most insects.

Yield: about 1 pint

INGREDIENTS
1 cup rubbing alcohol (70 percent isopropyl)
1 cup water

SUPPLIES
pint container
garden spray equipment

☛ **BE SAFE.** Alcohol sprays are best used on houseplants and tropical foliage plants with thick, waxy cuticles. Don't use alcohol sprays on outdoor ornamentals or on food crops. Don't use alcohol sprays on plants with hairy leaves or on ferns. Always test a single leaf before spraying the entire plant.

Mix alcohol and water in the container and spray directly onto pests; avoid spraying it on any more of the foliage than necessary.

✿ **Variations:** For greater effectiveness, mix an insecticidal soap spray and substitute alcohol for half the water. For more delicate plants, such as wax begonias or impatiens, dilute 1 cup alcohol with 1 quart water. This mixture is generally suitable for plants with thinner cuticles. A fine spray of pure alcohol can be effective on scale or mealybugs. However, this is risky for plants and should be tested on a small part of the plant to see what effect it has on the foliage.

GOOD IDEA!

To quickly rid your **houseplants of mealybug or soft scale infestation,** dip a cotton swab in rubbing alcohol (70 percent isopropyl) and touch it directly to the mealybugs or soft scales. Although this method is time consuming, it is quite effective and worth the effort if only a couple plants are infested. Although insect formulas with oil added to the alcohol have been touted, do not use these on any houseplants. The combination of oil and alcohol damages plant leaves.

GOOD IDEA!

To ensure that you're not collecting beneficial beetles, which may be present in large numbers in your garden, use a photographic insect field guide. While collecting insects, keep a lid on the container to prevent escape, or quickly drop them into a bucket of soapy water as you catch them. Pour off the soapy water before blending the bugs for bug juice spray.

Bug Juice Spray

In the 1960s, people discovered that large numbers of a particular pest collected, ground up, and made into a spray became an effective repellent against the same pest in the field. Many people experimented with the idea and published formulas for making these sprays; however, in 1972 the EPA cautioned against using the sprays because they were not a registered pesticide.

No one knows exactly how the bug juice sprays work. One possible explanation is that in any collection of bugs, some sick ones will be present; by grinding them up, the disease is spread throughout the rest of the population. Insect diseases are common, and some, such as the commercial preparations of *Bacillus thuringiensis,* are sold widely as biological controls. One infected grasshopper alone contains enough spores of the *Nosema* disease to treat 2 to 3 acres of rangeland against grasshoppers. Another explanation is that the odor of crushed bugs alarms other bugs, causing them to leave the area. Alternatively, the odor of dead bugs may attract high populations of predators that eat the pests.

Yield: about 2 cups of concentrate, enough to make 8 to 16 cups of spray

INGREDIENTS

about ½ cup of pest insects (all the same species)
2 cups of water

SUPPLIES

rubber work gloves
old blender, grinder, or mortar and pestle
strainer lined with cheesecloth or large coffee filter
container with lid
goggles, safety glasses, or face shield
dust mask
garden spray equipment

☞ **BE SAFE.** *Wear rubber gloves to protect your hands. Don't use a blender that you use to prepare food. While handling the spray, wear goggles, a dust mask, and protective clothing. Wash sprayed fruits and vegetables well before eating them.*

Wearing rubber gloves, liquefy insects in the blender with water. Strain into the container. To use, dilute ¼ cup of this concentrate with 1 to 2 cups water. Wearing protective clothing, spray plants thoroughly, especially the undersides of leaves, where, shielded from sunlight, insect disease organisms last the longest. Freeze remaining concentrate in labeled containers for up to a year.

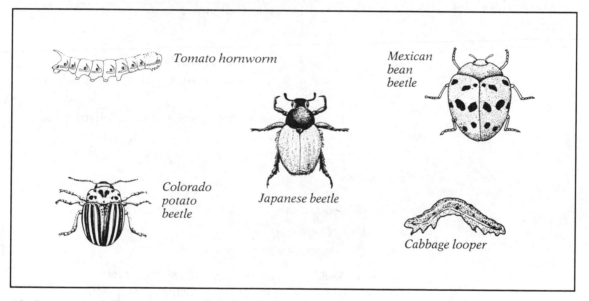

Tomato hornworm

Mexican bean beetle

Colorado potato beetle

Japanese beetle

Cabbage looper

The best targets for bug juice spray are large, slow-moving insects, such as those shown above.

GOOD IDEA!

If there is fish oil in your dormant oil spray, be sure to clean your spray equipment, especially spray nozzles, as soon as you're done. Fish oil dries to a hard, varnishlike coating. It is used in agriculture as a sticker/spreader for other pesticides.

Dormant Oil Spray

Dormant oil as a pest spray dates back to at least the late 1700s. Unlike chemical sprays, dormant oil has never caused the emergence of resistant pests. Basically, dormant oil spray is just a water emulsion of any oil (animal, vegetable, or mineral) that it is sprayed on trees and shrubs while they are dormant. The spray leaves a film of oil on the bark and buds, which suffocates and poisons overwintering pests, such as scales, mealybugs, pear psylla nymphs, aphid and mite eggs, codling moths, fruit moths, and eggs of fruit tree leafrollers.

Yield: about 1½ gallons of concentrate, enough for 12 to 30 trees

INGREDIENTS

1 gallon light grade oil (mineral oil, lemon oil, or fish oil)

1 pound pure oil-based soap, such as olive oil soap (see page 324)

½ gallon water

SUPPLIES

old 8-quart pot

long spoon or paddle

garden spray equipment

☛ **BE SAFE.** Oil is flammable. To avoid accidental burns or fires, use great care in handling such a large quantity of hot oil. Watch the pot at all times until removed from heat.

Pour all ingredients in the pot and heat on medium, stirring constantly until well-blended. When the oil is well-suspended in the water, the solution will look cloudy. Turn off heat and remove pot to a heat-proof surface. Dilute 1 part concentrate in 20 (or more) parts water. Use the spray immediately, frequently agitating to keep the oil well-mixed in the water. Apply 1 to 2½ gallons of spray per tree.

To be effective, dormant oil must evenly and thoroughly coat every part of the bark. The ideal time to apply dormant oil is very early spring before tree buds begin to swell. Wind makes it difficult to apply the oil evenly. So choose a dry, windless day, when temperatures are likely to remain above freezing for a few hours while the spray dries. You can apply spray to wet bark, as long as it dries before rain or before temperatures drop below freezing.

✿ **Variation:** For small orchards, cut the formula. For only 2 or 3 trees, use 1 quart oil, ¼ pound soap, and 1 pint water. Add enough water to make 7½ gallons of spray.

➥ **Note:** Fish oil is used in agriculture as a sticker/spreader for other pesticides. Buy fish oil at farm supply stores, especially dealers offering organic or biodynamic farm supplies. See page 444 for other sources.

Garlic Oil-Water Spray

If you have a small garden, you may find this garlic oil formula more useful than the one above.

Yield: 2 to 4 teaspoons of concentrate, enough to make about 1½ cups of spray

INGREDIENTS
20 to 25 cloves garlic
about 1¼ cups water

SUPPLIES
blender or juice press
strainer lined with cheesecloth
measuring spoons
1-pint bowl
garden spray equipment

Blend or press garlic to extract juice. Strain and measure the amount extracted. Place juice in the bowl and add water in a ratio of 1 part garlic juice to 20 parts water. In diluting the garlic juice, remember that 1 cup equals 16 tablespoons. If you have 1 tablespoon garlic juice, add 20 table-

(continued)

GOOD IDEA!

To control house-plant pests, put a whole clove of garlic in each pot. Garlic is renowned for its pest control properties. If the clove sprouts, cut off the shoot; otherwise it will take root and start to grow.

spoons, or 1¼ cups, water. Spray directly on plants to control leaf diseases such as bean rust, anthracnose and blight. Use immediately; the mixture does not keep.

Garlic Oil-Soap Spray

Garlic not only repels some insects, it also works as an antibiotic and fungicide. Many gardeners control garden pests with garlic, either blended into water or as garlic oil. Garlic oil spray may be effective because of the combined effects of the garlic oil and the soap used with it. Garlic oil sprays seem to be effective against cabbage moths, cabbage loopers, earwigs, leafhoppers, mosquitoes, whiteflies, aphids, squash bugs, tarnished plant bugs, slugs, and hornworms. It does not work well against large, strong insects such as Colorado potato beetles, grasshoppers, ants, sow bugs, and grapeleaf skeletonizers.

Yield: 1 pint of concentrate, enough to make 2 to 4 gallons of spray

INGREDIENTS

20 to 25 unpeeled cloves garlic
 2 teaspoons mineral oil
 2 teaspoons liquid nondetergent soap
 1 pint warm water

SUPPLIES

garlic press or sharp knife
1-cup glass or plastic container
spoon
1-quart plastic, glass, or enamel bowl
strainer lined with cheesecloth or large coffee filter
glass or plastic storage container with lid
garden spray equipment

Crush garlic in the press or chop it finely. Place garlic and mineral oil in the glass or container, stir lightly, and let

---

GOOD IDEA!

Before using garlic oil spray on delicate foliages of flowers and some ornamentals, test spray a few leaves and wait two to three days to make sure the spray causes no leaf injury.

stand for at least 24 hours. Then, in the bowl, place soap, water, and garlic-oil mixture. Mix well and strain the solution into the storage container. Store in the refrigerator for several weeks.

To use, dilute 1 to 2 tablespoons concentrate to 1 pint water and spray on plants, being sure to thoroughly spray the undersides of leaves where pests congregate. The garlic odor does not stay on the plants.

✿ **Variation:** *Substitute garlic powder (not garlic salt) for the fresh garlic. Use 1/8 teaspoon powder for each garlic clove.*

Cedar Spray

Red cedar is a fragrant softwood tree with insect-repellent wood. Cedar wood is traditionally used to make cedar chests to keep moths from stored clothing and linens. Cedar spray works against such pests as Mexican bean beetles, Colorado potato beetles, cucumber beetles, squash bugs, mealybugs, and spider mites.

Yield: 1 gallon

INGREDIENTS

2 to 3 cups cedar sawdust, shavings, chips, or chopped twigs
1 gallon water

SUPPLIES

6- to 8-quart pot
strainer lined with cheesecloth or large coffee filter
garden spray equipment

In the pot, boil cedar in water for a few minutes. Cool, strain, and then spray on plants, being careful to cover the undersides of the leaves.

➼ **Note:** *Buy cedar shavings at pet supply stores.*

GOOD IDEA!

To repel corn earworm moths from laying their eggs, spray cedar tea on cornsilks. A daily application of the tea seems to give the best protection.

Herbal Tea Spray

Homemade teas or infusions of various aromatic herbs have long been popular insect sprays for organic gardeners. Many people swear by these sprays, although a great deal depends on the particular pest to be controlled, because insects and their interactions with plants are all very complex and unique. These sprays are certainly the least invasive way to right the balance of pests and their natural enemies in the garden, and for that reason alone, they're worth trying. Choose the most aromatic plants and follow this basic recipe for making an infusion of any type of fresh or dried plant material.

Yield: 1 gallon

INGREDIENTS

1 gallon water
1 to 2 cups fresh plant material or ½ to 1 cup dried
½ teaspoon liquid nondetergent soap

SUPPLIES

2-gallon bucket or large basin
strainer lined with cheesecloth or large coffee filter
stirrer
garden spray equipment

Place water in the bucket or basin and immerse plant material. Steep overnight. Strain, then gently stir in soap, which helps the spray adhere to the leaves. Spray plants immediately, making sure to thoroughly cover both sides of the leaves. These sprays can be repeated as often as necessary to give control.

Herbal Tea Spray Concentrate

This formula makes an herbal concentrate that you can store and dilute later whenever pests appear.

Yield: about 1 cup of concentrate, enough for about 6 gallons of spray

INGREDIENTS

1 cup fresh aromatic herbs (onions, garlic, chives, hot peppers, mint, thyme, rosemary, or others)
1 cup water
    liquid nondetergent soap

SUPPLIES

blender
strainer lined with cheesecloth or large coffee filter
glass or plastic storage container with lid
garden spray equipment

In the blender, puree herbs and water. Strain and store concentrate tightly covered for up to two weeks in the refrigerator. To use, dilute 1 teaspoon concentrate per pint of water. To make the spray adhere to leaves better, add 1 or 2 drops of liquid soap (no more!) per pint of water. Spray as needed.

GOOD IDEA!

For pest control, use herbs straight from the garden or hang them to dry in a dark, well-ventilated place to preserve them for other times of the year. If you don't have room to hang the herbs, spread them out on a cookie sheet and dry in a 150°F oven for a few hours (until they are crisp). Store the herbs in jars in a cool, dark place.

Lime-Sulfur Spray for Growing-Season Disease Control

Lime-sulfur sprays control various plant diseases as well as some mite and insect pests, including various scales, mildew, anthracnose, leaf spot, and brown rot. Lime-sulfur is usually applied as a dormant or delayed dormant spray on trees because it burns leaves and growing shoots. Commercial lime-sulfur concentrate can also be diluted sufficiently to use during the growing season for such diseases as apple and pear scab, peach leaf curl, brown rot on plums, and black spot and canker on roses.

Yield: varies by amount of ingredients chosen

INGREDIENTS

80 parts water
1 part commercial lime-sulfur concentrate

SUPPLIES

rubber work gloves
goggles, safety glasses, or face shield
plastic or enameled steel mixing container
spoon or paddle
garden spray equipment

☛ **BE SAFE.** Wear rubber gloves to protect your hands. Lime-sulfur spray is caustic. Wear goggles and protective clothing while handling this formula. For accidental splashes, flood skin immediately with water. Lime-sulfur can damage trees and shrubs if improperly used. Do not apply lime-sulfur when the temperature is over 80°F, and do not apply within four weeks before or after a summer oil treatment on foliage. Don't use on fruit trees while they are blossoming. Don't use on cucurbits.

Wearing proper clothing and safety gear, place water in the container. Stir in lime-sulfur concentrate. Mix thoroughly and spray. The typical dilution for home garden applications is, for 5 gallons of spray, mix 1 cup lime-sulfur concentrate with 5 gallons water.

➤ **Note:** Buy lime-sulfur concentrate at garden centers.

Neem-Chinaberry Spray

The seeds of the tropical neem tree (*Azadiracta indica*) contain complex chemicals toxic to insects. Neem oil, which is extracted from the seeds, also repels insects, deters them from feeding, and disrupts their development; yet it seems harmless to humans and other mammals. A neem insecticide for ornamentals is currently available in the United States, and it's possible that within the year, neem-based insecticides will be registered for use on food crops. The neem tree grows in warm, tropical areas and has been planted experimentally in Florida and California. A related tree, the chinaberry tree (*Melia azedarach*), also known as paradise tree or Persian lilac, contains similar compounds, which are not quite as effective against insects as neem. Chinaberry is hardier than neem and is grown widely in the South. This spray controls leafminers, two-spotted spider mites, flea beetles, gypsy moths, Mexican bean beetles, Colorado potato beetles, spotted cucumber beetles, corn earworms, thrips, and oriental fruit flies.

Yield: about 2½ gallons

INGREDIENTS

  1   pound dried neem seeds or chinaberry seeds
2½ gallons water
 ½ teaspoon liquid nondetergent soap

SUPPLIES

cloth bag or old pillowcase
hammer
2½- to 3-gallon bucket
spoon or paddle
garden spray equipment

☛ **BE SAFE.** Chinaberry tree fruit is poisonous. Keep chinaberries, chinaberry seeds, and sprays out of the reach of children.

Place seeds in the bag or pillowcase and pulverize with the hammer. Place 1 gallon water in the bucket and suspend the bag of crushed seeds in it. Leave overnight.

(continued)

GOOD IDEA!

When using pest control sprays, always use clean, properly adjusted, suitable equipment. A good garden sprayer is worth the investment. It sprays the correct amount in the right direction, without dripping. If your sprayer gets clogged, carefully remove the nozzle and rinse it; use a toothpick to clean out the hole. If the nozzle is still clogged, soak it in vinegar for an hour. Rinse before using.

Remove the bag and squeeze out the liquid. Add soap to a quart of water, mix well, and pour into the bucket. Stir to mix. Add remaining water.

Spray on plants, making sure to spray undersides of leaves thoroughly. Reapply as often as needed. To control nematodes and soil stages of some insects, apply around plants as a soil drench. Spray will keep for up to four days in a cool, dark place.

✿ **Variation:** Substitute 2 pounds of fresh neem or chinaberry fruit for the dried seeds in the recipe. Pulverize the fruit in a blender with enough water to make a slurry. Add 2 quarts of water and leave overnight. Strain through a cheesecloth the following day; add soap and water to make a total of 2½ gallons. Since chinaberries are poisonous, you must use a blender that is reserved for yard use and not food preparation.

➤ **Note:** See page 444 for sources of both neem and chinaberry.

Chinch Bug Drench

Chinch bugs are quick-moving red or black bugs with prominent antennae and white markings on their backs. Adults and nymphs damage lawn grasses by sucking the juice from leaves. Large circles of brown and wilted or dead grass are a symptom of chinch bug feeding. For small areas, mix 1 ounce liquid dishwashing detergent in 2 gallons water. Apply with a watering can to treat 1 square yard. For larger areas, dispense the soap through a hose attachment in the correct dilutions. If the hose attachment dispenses concentrates in a ratio of 1:16, mix the soap concentrate at a ratio of 1 ounce of soap per pint of water. This will give a final dilution rate of 1 ounce of soap per gallon (256 fluid ounces) of water. Do not apply the liquid soap without diluting it to 1:256. Incorrectly diluted soap may burn the lawn, causing more damage than the chinch bugs!

Nicotine Tea and Tobacco Dust

The tobacco plant contains nicotine, a potent poison that is extremely toxic to insects (and people!). Gardeners can make a mild insecticide by steeping tobacco leaves in water or a *very toxic* spray from liquid nicotine extract. Both are useful against many species of leaf-eating insects, such as aphids, scales, leafhoppers, thrips, harlequin bugs, leafminers, and pear psylla, as well as against soil-dwelling pests such as fungus gnats and root aphids. Tobacco leaves ground into dust makes a useful insecticide as well. Although liquid nicotine extract (nicotine sulfate) can be substituted for tobacco leaves to make a nicotine tea, it is not a good idea to have this material around your house. It is extremely toxic and can even be absorbed into the body through skin contact.

Yield: about 5 quarts

INGREDIENTS

4 to 5 cups crushed fresh tobacco leaves or 2 cups dried

about 5 quarts water

1 teaspoon liquid nondetergent soap

SUPPLIES

6-quart plastic or glass bowl

strainer lined with cheesecloth or large coffee filter

garden spray equipment

☛ **BE SAFE.** *Nicotine tea is a poison. Keep this formula out of the reach of children. Tobacco also is an alternate host for tobacco mosaic virus, a disease that stunts growth and blossom set on young tomatoes and other solanaceous plants. Don't use nicotine spray near tomato plants that have not yet matured and set blossoms. Tobacco mosaic infection in mature, fruit-bearing tomatoes causes little damage. Do not use nicotine spray on roses; it turns them black.*

Steep tobacco leaves in 2 to 3 quarts water for 24 hours. Strain, add a quart of water in which the soap has

(continued)

GOOD IDEA!

To make your own nicotine sprays, grow a few tobacco plants. Since the seed is very fine, it's best to start the plants in a flat first, then transplant them when they are well-established. Tobacco grows to be 4 to 6 feet tall; plant it where it will not shade other crops. Two or three plants will yield more than enough leaves for a season's worth of spray. Cut the leaves and hang them on the clothesline or in a warm attic to dry. Tobacco grows in almost every part of North America. Even in short growing season areas, you will still be able to harvest a useful amount of leaves from each plant.

been mixed. Add another quart of water (or more if needed) to dilute the tea to a pale brown, weak tea color.

Spray plants, covering all leaves thoroughly, or use the tea as a soil drench by pouring it around the roots of plants attacked by fungus gnats or root aphids. Food sprayed with nicotine tea can be eaten within a few days of spraying, but wash it first to remove spray residue.

✿ **Variation:** Tobacco dust (made by grinding or milling tobacco leaves and stems) makes a good repellent for peachtree borers in young trees. Cut a ring of tin or other flexible metal, 2 to 3 inches high and 4 inches wider in diameter than the trunk of the tree. Place the ring around the base of the tree, and fill the space between the collar and the trunk with tobacco dust. Renew the dust in May for several years until the tree bark is thick and strong.

➥ **Note:** Buy tobacco dust at garden supply centers and through mail-order suppliers for organic gardening.

Remedies for Houseplant Pests

Insect problems on houseplants can be unsightly, but there are several things you can do to control an infestation. The most important step is prevention. Never buy "bugged" plants; remember to check the soil and the underside of leaves for signs of insects. If you set your houseplants outdoors during the summer, thoroughly inspect them for problems before moving them back indoors in the fall. Check all of your houseplants frequently, so you will catch insect problems before they get out of hand. Mist your plants frequently to minimize feeding by spider mites, tiny red creatures that live on the undersides of leaves. For severe infestations, mix flour and buttermilk into a sticky slurry and apply to plants with a soft paintbrush. Aphids are another common houseplant pest; they are small green, red, or black insects that often feed on stem tips. If there are only a few aphids, squash them with your fingers. You can also mist the plant strongly or run it under tepid water to wash off aphids. Scales have small, round, brown shells; mealybugs look like tiny pieces of white cotton. Both insects can appear on stems and the undersides of leaves. Control small numbers by wiping them with a cotton swab dipped in rubbing alcohol (70 percent isopropyl).

Pyrethrum Spray

The dried and powdered flowers of the pretty pyrethrum daisy (*Chrysanthemum cinerariifolium*) have been used as an insecticide since the late 1800s. Most of the active ingredients, called pyrethrins, occur in the flower head seeds and are released when the seeds are crushed. Pyrethrins are contact insecticides, meaning that insects are killed when they come into contact with them. Pyrethrins have a swift paralyzing effect on insects and can be used right up to the day food is harvested because they break down quickly in sunlight and heat. Try this spray against mealybugs, thrips, aphids, and scales. By making your own pyrethrum spray with water you can avoid the additives in commercial formulations.

Yield: about 1 gallon

INGREDIENTS

½ cup powdered pyrethrum flowers (see "Good Idea!")
1 gallon water
3 or 4 drops liquid nondetergent soap

SUPPLIES

dust mask
1-gallon container with lid, such as a milk jug
strainer lined with cheesecloth or large coffee filter
1-gallon bucket
garden spray equipment

☛ **BE SAFE.** *People allergic to ragweed are frequently also allergic to pyrethrum flowers. If you have hay fever, you may have a reaction to these flowers. Avoid breathing pyrethrum dust.*

Wearing a dust mask, pour powdered flowers into the container. Add water and shake to mix flowers and water together. Strain liquid into the bucket, mix in soap, and spray on plants, thoroughly covering both sides of the leaves, to control a variety of chewing and sucking insects.

GOOD IDEA!

To make your own **powdered pyrethrum flowers,** first dry collected flowers in the shade or in an oven on the lowest setting. Seal in a light-proof container and store in a cool place. Make the powder just before you're ready to mix the formula. Simply grind the flowers to a fine powder in a coffee grinder, blender, or mortar and pestle and use immediately in the formula. To avoid inhaling pyrethrum dust, wear a dust mask while you're grinding the flowers.

Pyrethrum Spray Concentrate

This pyrethrum formula makes a concentrate that can be stored and diluted later as needed.

Yield: 2 ounces of concentrate, enough for 3 quarts of spray

INGREDIENTS

1 cup packed pyrethrum flowers
⅛ cup rubbing alcohol (70 percent isopropyl)

SUPPLIES

1-cup glass jar with lid
strainer lined with cheesecloth or a large coffee filter
small storage container with lid
garden spray equipment

☛ **BE SAFE.** People allergic to ragweed are frequently also allergic to pyrethrum flowers. If you have hay fever, you may have a reaction to these flowers. Also, since this formula contains alcohol, test it on a few leaves first to see if it damages the foliage. Do not use this spray on hairy-leaved houseplants, such as African violets or gloxinias.

Pack as many flowers as possible into the glass jar and pour alcohol over the flowers. Cover the jar tightly and allow to soak overnight. Strain the flowers out of the alcohol, and store the alcohol concentrate in a small, well-sealed container.

To make a spray, dilute the alcohol concentrate in a ratio of 1 part concentrate to 48 parts water. For example, to make 1½ quarts of spray, combine 1 fluid ounce of alcohol concentrate with 1½ quarts (48 fluid ounces) water.

Quassia Spray

An infusion from the bark chips and shavings of the Latin American quassia tree makes a mild, safe insecticide for controlling aphids, flies, and, according to one source, leafminers on chrysanthemums. Quassia also is apparently harmless to beneficial insects, such as lady beetles and honeybees.

Yield: about 1 gallon

INGREDIENTS

4 ounces quassia chips and shavings
1 gallon cold water

SUPPLIES

cloth or burlap bag
heavy roller or wooden mallet
1½-gallon bucket
strainer lined with cheesecloth or large coffee filter
garden spray equipment

Put quassia in the cloth or burlap bag and crush with the roller or mallet. Pour chips and water into the bucket and steep for about 12 hours. Strain mixture and spray aphid-infested plants or trees thoroughly, especially the undersides of lower leaves and growing tips—two favorite places for aphids. Repeat sprays as often as necessary to maintain control.

➤ **Note:** Buy quassia bark chips at health food stores and herb shops. When you buy quassia, look for chips that are bright and fresh; old, stale chips are a dull gray color and have lost their potency.

GOOD IDEA!

Whenever possible, **use materials such as quassia spray** that are not known to harm beneficial insects. Reducing pest populations without harming the beneficials gives the "good guys" a chance to control the remaining pests. Other things you can do to encourage beneficials include planting pollen- and nectar-rich plants, such, as dill, catnip, and yarrow. Allow some uncultivated areas in your yard to provide shelter for the good insects. Provide a water source by covering the base of a shallow pan with small rocks and adding enough water to almost cover them. Insects can land on the "islands" and drink without drowning.

Quassia and Larkspur Spray

This spray controls aphids without harming beneficial insects.

Yield: about 2½ quarts

INGREDIENTS

3½ quarts water
3 to 4 ounces quassia chips and shavings
5 teaspoons larkspur seeds

SUPPLIES

1-gallon glass, enameled, or stainless steel saucepan
strainer lined with cheesecloth or large coffee filter
garden spray equipment

Place all ingredients in the saucepan and boil until the liquid is reduced to about 2½ quarts. Cool, strain, and spray plants thoroughly. Repeat as necessary to control aphids.

➜ **Notes:** Buy quassia bark at health food stores and herb shops. When you buy quassia, look for chips that are bright and fresh; old, stale chips are a dull gray color and have lost their potency. Buy larkspur from seed suppliers. Buy untreated seeds.

Quassia Spray for Aphids on Fruit Trees

Place 1½ to 2 quarts water and 8 ounces quassia chips in a 1-gallon glass, enamel, or stainless steel saucepan. Cover, bring to a boil, and simmer for 2 hours. Remove from heat, cool, and strain into a 5-gallon bucket. Mix 5 teaspoons liquid nondetergent soap with 1 to 2 pints hot water, and pour into the quassia water. Add enough water to make 5 gallons; mix well.

Spray plants thoroughly on both sides of the leaves; repeat as often as necessary for control. To avoid soap damage to young leaves, wait at least a week between sprayings. This formula treats 2 or 3 large trees. Double the amount of quassia in the formula to make it more effective. Buy quassia chips that are bright and fresh; dull gray chips are stale and have lost their potency.

All-Purpose Bug-Chaser Spray

Sprays made from a mixture of hot, spicy, or pungent ingredients are often effective against chewing and sucking pests. The following all-purpose spray shows up in similar form throughout the organic gardening literature. Although quantities are given for each ingredient, you can experiment with any combinations and quantities that you have on hand.

Yield: about 1 quart

INGREDIENTS

1 to 3 whole garlic bulbs (several cloves each)
1 small onion
1 tablespoon cayenne pepper
1 quart water
½ teaspoon liquid nondetergent soap

SUPPLIES

blender or food processor
strainer lined with cheesecloth or large coffee filter
stirrer
garden spray equipment
sealable container

☛ **BE SAFE.** *On delicate plants, it is a good idea to rinse the spray residue off the plants several hours after applying the spray. Soap residue may burn some plants, so, if necessary, omit the soap from the formula.*

Puree garlic and onion in the blender or food processor. Add cayenne and water. Allow mixture to steep for 1 to 12 hours. Strain and mix in soap. Spray plants thoroughly, especially undersides of leaves and crevices where pests lurk. This spray will keep for several days if stored tightly sealed in the refrigerator.

GOOD IDEA!

To deal with garden pests, experiment with different controls to see what works best for you. Use whatever formula you have ingredients for at the time if you're in a hurry. Or do a little advance planning and buy the ingredients before the season starts. Record your observations of how each formula works, and write down any variations you make for future reference. There is no one control that will completely eliminate all of the pests 100 percent of the time. And you don't want to kill all the pests, or the beneficial insects will have nothing to eat!

Gardener's All-Purpose Mix

Mix common ingredients to make a strong-smelling spray to repel and confuse leaf-eating pests.

Yield: about 2 quarts of concentrate, enough for 2 gallons of spray

INGREDIENTS

½ to 1 cup fresh mint leaves (any type)
½ to 1 cup green onion tops
½ to 1 cup horseradish root and leaves
½ to 1 cup red hot peppers
2 quarts plus 1 cup water
2 teaspoons liquid nondetergent soap

SUPPLIES

rubber work gloves
goggles, safety glasses, or face shield
blender or food processor
1-gallon bowl or bucket
spoon or paddle
strainer lined with cheesecloth or large coffee filter
3-quart storage container with lid
garden spray equipment

☛ **BE SAFE.** Wear rubber gloves to protect your hands. Use this mixture cautiously in areas where children play. Some people are allergic to hot peppers. Also avoid getting this spray in your eyes or on your skin. Wear goggles when handling this formula. Hot pepper and soap are strong eye irritants.

Wearing rubber gloves and goggles, combine mint leaves, onion tops, horseradish, and peppers with 1 cup water in the blender or food processor and puree. In the bowl or bucket, combine puree with 2 quarts water and stir. Strain into the container and stir in soap. Store concentrate for up to a week in the refrigerator, tightly sealed. To use, mix 1 cup concentrate with a quart of water and spray plants thoroughly to drive away pests.

Rhubarb-Leaf Spray

An old-fashioned aphid spray comes from the leaves of a plant most gardeners have in their backyard—the ubiquitous, prolific rhubarb.

Yield: about 1 gallon

INGREDIENTS

3 pounds rhubarb leaves
1 gallon water
1 ounce laundry soap flakes

SUPPLIES

6-quart glass, enamel, or stainless steel cooking pot
strainer lined with cheesecloth or large coffee filter
garden spray equipment

☞ **BE SAFE.** *Rhubarb leaves are poisonous. Do not tear or chop the leaves on surfaces where you cut food. Thoroughly wash all utensils used in making this formula.*

Tear or chop up rhubarb leaves sufficiently to get them into the pot and add 3 quarts water. Bring the mixture to a boil and simmer for ½ hour. Cool, then strain out the leaves. Dissolve soap in a quart of water, then mix into the rhubarb tea. Spray plants thoroughly to control aphids.

GOOD IDEA!

A **spray made from rhubarb leaves helps control rose black spot** as well as aphids and June bugs on roses. Simply place six chopped rhubarb leaves in a blender. Add 2 to 3 quarts water and process until the leaves and water are a fine slurry. Allow the mixture to stand for several hours, then strain and spray over infected plants. Be sure to cover both tops and bottoms of leaves. Since rhubarb leaves contain high concentrations of oxalic acid, it is best to make this spray in a blender reserved for garden use only. Oxalic acid is poisonous.

GOOD IDEA!

Softened water is an important ingredient for an effective spray. "Hard" water contains minerals that combine with materials in the soap, reducing the soap's effectiveness. To soften small quantities of water, fill a clean pot (with drainage holes) with peat, suspend the pot over a dish, and catch the water that drains through. Or hang a porous bag filled with peat moss in a watering can or bucket overnight.

Soap Spray

Because soap is safe for people and pets, gardeners have used it to control insects pests for more than a century. Soap kills insects on contact by paralyzing them and disrupting their normal cell functions and growth processes. You can choose from several brands of commercial insecticidal soaps on the market, or you can make your own pure olive oil soap. For instructions, see the recipe for "All-Vegetable Soap" on page 324.

Yield: 1 cup

INGREDIENTS

1 teaspoon pure bar soap shavings

⅛ cup boiling softened water

⅞ cup softened water

SUPPLIES

stirrer

garden spray equipment

☛ **BE SAFE.** Before spraying delicate ornamentals, test spray a few leaves first and watch for signs of leaf injury within the next two to three days. To protect delicate plants, wash soap off leaves with clean water a few hours after spraying. To avoid the risk of burning plants, don't apply soap spray to the same plants more than once a week. Soap causes severe damage to ferns and nasturtiums.

Mix soap shavings with ⅛ cup boiling water to dissolve. Add ⅞ cup water to make spray. To make larger quantities, mix soap in a ratio of 1 part soap shavings to 50 parts water. Spray leaves thoroughly, especially the undersides, where most pests hide.

➺ **Note:** Buy pure soap with no additives. Many commercial hand or laundry soaps contain whiteners, perfumes, and dyes that may harm plants.

Starch Spray

An old-fashioned control for cabbage moths is to sprinkle flour on the cabbage heads. The flour gums up the feet and wings of cabbage moths and caterpillars (and makes a mess of the cabbages!), and when it dries, the insects die. Another cabbage moth control is the application of starch in a water spray. Interest in starch as a pest control has stimulated development of a commercial potato starch spray to control aphids, spider mites, thrips, and other small pests. You can make your own starch spray with this recipe.

Yield: about 1 gallon

INGREDIENTS

- 1 cup potato starch
- 1 gallon water
- ½ teaspoon liquid nondetergent soap

SUPPLIES

1- to 2-gallon bucket or bowl
spoon or paddle
garden spray equipment

In the bucket or bowl, combine starch and water and stir well. Wait for 5 minutes to allow starch to soak up water, then add soap and mix well. Spray plants, covering the leaves thoroughly until spray runs off. This spray does not keep; you must make a fresh batch each time you need it. Potato starch spray leaves a translucent, flaky residue which will eventually crack off. If it is unsightly, you can rinse it off with a stream of water the day after spraying.

➡ **Note:** *Potato starch is usually sold as a natural thickener in health food stores.*

GOOD IDEA!

To make starch spray more effective against somewhat larger pests, try using half as much water to make a thicker and stickier spray. Reduce the soap concentration in half as well. Starch is completely nontoxic. You can experiment with any dilution that is still liquid enough to pass through your sprayer. You can also make a spray of cornstarch using ½ to 1 cup starch per pint of water. While spraying, keep agitating the sprayer to keep the solution well-mixed. It settles out very quickly. This spray leaves a powdery residue on plants, which you can rinse off a day or so after spraying.

GOOD IDEA!

To collect tomato leaves without damaging your tomato plants, pick leaves from the lowest part of the plant, below the level of the fruit. Also make spray from shoots and leaves removed during pruning. To help tomato-leaf spray adhere to plants, add a teaspoon of liquid non-detergent soap per quart of spray.

Tomato-Leaf Spray

Tomato leaves contain a range of different water-soluble, toxic compounds, called alkaloids. Sprays made from tomato leaves control aphids. Research has shown that tomato-leaf tea helps control corn earworm by attracting beneficial Trichogramma wasps. These wasps destroy earworm eggs.

Yield: 4 cups

INGREDIENTS

1 to 2 cups tomato leaves
4 cups water

SUPPLIES

1-quart bowl (*not* aluminum)
strainer lined with cheesecloth or large coffee filter
garden spray equipment

Mash or chop tomato leaves in 2 cups water and leave in the bowl to soak overnight. Strain the leaves from the mixture and add 2 more cups water to make a spray. For aphid control, thoroughly spray tips and undersides of leaves, especially lower leaves where aphids are concentrated. To attract Trichogramma wasps to corn, spray the entire plant, especially around the forming ears.

✿ **Variation:** To make a quicker spray, boil tomato leaves in 4 cups water for 30 minutes, strain, and spray.

"Hot" Dust Insect Repellent

Black pepper, chili pepper, paprika, red pepper, powdered dill, and ginger all contain a compound called capsaicin, a chemical that discourages insects from laying their eggs. It is particularly effective against root maggot flies that attack onions, carrots, and cabbage family plants. One research study found that ground cayenne pepper along onion rows in a garden reduced the number of onion fly eggs laid by 90 percent. If your onion or carrot plantings are plagued with root maggots, you can make your own "hot" dust repellent quickly and cheaply.

Yield: 4 ounces, enough to treat a 10- to 12-foot row

INGREDIENTS

Choose any:
finely ground black pepper
finely ground chili pepper
powdered paprika
finely ground cayenne pepper
powdered dill seed
powdered ginger

SUPPLIES

rubber work gloves
goggles, safety glasses, or face shield
dust mask
dust applicator or shaker-topped container

☛ **BE SAFE.** *Wear rubber gloves to protect your hands. Capsaicin is very irritating to sensitive skin and mucous membranes. Keep hot dusts away from your mouth, nasal passages, and eyes. Wear a dust mask and goggles while handling peppers and these dusts.*

Wearing proper safety gear, combine your choice of powders and sprinkle in a 6-inch-wide band along each side of seeded rows of onions, cabbage, or carrots. A fine sprinkling over the surface is sufficient, but the more you use, the more effective it will be. Renew after every rain.

GOOD IDEA!

You can grow hot red peppers, chili peppers, and dill in your garden. Dry them in an airy, warm place and grind to a fine powder in a blender or with a mortar and pestle. Wear protective gloves when handling the dried and powdered "hot" plants.

"Hot" dusts work best in a garden with many different crops. They don't work quite so well in a one-crop planting. One way to keep track of how much hot dust you are applying is to add fine white sand to the mix. The sand will stand out against most dark soils.

GOOD IDEA!

To avoid breathing horticultural dusts, make a long-handled applicator. Use a nail to punch holes in the base of a coffee can; then bolt the side of the can to an old broom handle, so the bottom of the can is about 4 inches from the base of the handle. Put the dust you're using in the can. Apply the dust by tapping the base of the handle on the ground around the plant.

Ashes and Lime Spray

This deters cucumber beetles and sweetens acid soil.

Yield: about 2 gallons

INGREDIENTS

½ cup wood ashes
½ cup horticultural lime
2 gallons water

SUPPLIES

rubber work gloves
goggles, safety glasses, or face shield
two 2-gallon plastic buckets
stiff stirring stick
strainer lined with cheesecloth
garden spray equipment

☞ **BE SAFE.** Wear rubber gloves and goggles when mixing and spraying this formula.

Wearing proper safety gear, mix all ingredients in a bucket. Strain through cheesecloth into the second bucket. Spray on plants, coating both sides of the leaves thoroughly.

➪ **Note:** Buy horticultural lime at garden centers and through mail-order suppliers.

Garden Dusts

Insects have a complex breathing system and a waxy or oily outer coating on their bodies to minimize water loss. Scratching the body coating by applying abrasive dusts around your plants will affect the critical moisture balance, often causing the insect to dehydrate and die. Try dry wood ashes, diatomaceous earth, talc, or lime. Spread the dust generously around the base of the plant, from the stem to the dripline.

Reapply after rain or watering.

These dusts work well against carrot root flies and cabbage root flies. If slugs and snails often are not deterred by dusts, try adding some black, red, or chili pepper to the dusts. Mix ¼ pound diatomaceous earth with 1 teaspoon pure soap and enough water to make a thick slurry. Paint this on the base of trees to repel ants and deter borers from laying eggs.

Dust and Ashes

This formula combines two old standbys of garden pest control, ashes and lime, with other ingredients to repel cabbage flies from laying their eggs around cabbage family plants. The mixture is also a good fertilizer for cabbage and will help suppress club root disease in the soil.

Yield: about 7 quarts, enough to treat 14 to 15 plants

INGREDIENTS

1 gallon wood ashes

1 quart horticultural lime

1 quart rock phosphate

1 quart bonemeal

SUPPLIES

rubber work gloves

dust mask

stiff stirring stick

2- to 3-gallon bucket

☛ **BE SAFE.** *Wear rubber gloves and a dust mask when handling this formula.*

Wearing proper safety gear, mix all ingredients in the bucket. To prevent cabbage flies from laying eggs around the bases of cabbage family plants, pour about 2 cups of the mixture around each plant. Pour close to the stem and extending in a 2-foot radius around the plant. Scratch the dust into the top layer of soil.

✿ **Variations:** *A quart of diatomaceous earth added to the mixture will make it more effective against cabbage flies. To make any other amount of this dust, the correct ratio of ingredients is 4 parts wood ashes to 1 part of each of the other ingredients.*

↝ **Note:** *Buy horticultural lime, rock phosphate, bonemeal, and diatomaceous earth at garden centers and through mail-order suppliers. See page 444 for other sources.*

GOOD IDEA!

If cabbage root flies are a real problem, use paper barriers to protect your crops. These barriers physically prevent the flies from laying eggs at the base of your plants. Cut a 6- to 8-inch square of heavy paper or cardboard and make an X-shaped cut in the center. Plant seedlings through the slit. Fold the edges down, so they fit as close as possible to the stem. Anchor the barrier with pebbles or a little soil. Leave in place all season.

GOOD IDEA!

For complete control of apple maggots, always pick up dropped infected apples. Feed them to livestock or bury them. Don't put maggot-infested apples in your compost pile unless it's a very hot pile.

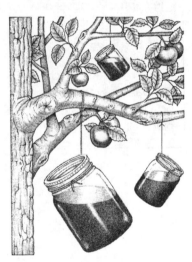

Half-pint jars of fermenting molasses hung in trees

Apple Maggot Fly Traps

Apple maggot flies plague apple growers mostly in the northeastern United States and Canada. The females lay eggs in apples, and when they hatch, the small white maggots tunnel through the apples, usually causing early drop. This old-fashioned recipe attracts apple maggot flies into jar traps; they fall into the gooey bait and can't get out.

Yield: 20 half-pint-size traps

INGREDIENTS

1 pint blackstrap molasses
9 pints water
1 package baking yeast (¼ ounce)

SUPPLIES

1½-gallon bowl or bucket
long-handled spoon or paddle
wire cutters
30 feet of flexible wire
20 half-pint canning jars with canning rings

In the bowl or bucket, mix molasses and water and stir in yeast. Allow to ferment for 48 hours. Fashion wire hangers for the jars by wiring a loop around the bottom part of the jar threads and leaving a long end for hanging. Screw the canning ring down to help hold the wire in place. Divide the fermented molasses mixture equally among the jars.

Hang traps evenly spaced in trees by mid-June, placing them so that there is an open space of 9 to 18 inches around each trap. Once a week, dump out the entire contents of each jar, rinse, and add new bait. In distributing the traps, a good ratio is 1 trap per 100 apples in a tree.

↪ **Note:** Blackstrap molasses is the liquid left after extraction of sugar from sorghum. Buy it at farm supply stores or livestock feed dealers.

Fermented Nettle Spray

Despite the fact that they sting skin on contact, sting-ing nettles are very useful and nutritious plants. People eat them (cooked only!), make them into tea, use them for en-riching fertilizer, and, as in this formula, ferment them to make a spray that repels aphids and suppresses fungal dis-eases of plants.

Yield: 1 gallon of concentrate, enough for 6 gallons of spray

INGREDIENTS
1 pound freshly cut stinging nettles
1 gallon water

SUPPLIES
thick leather gloves

two 2-gallon plastic buckets

large strainer lined with cheesecloth or large coffee
    filter

garden spray equipment

☛ **BE SAFE.** *Stinging nettles applied to bare skin cause an un-pleasant sting. To avoid stings and even possible allergic reac-tions, wear gloves and protective clothing when gathering net-tles. When touched, nettle hairs give off formic acid, the same substance that makes an ant bite memorable.*

Wearing proper clothing and gloves, put nettles in a bucket with water. Set the bucket outside (it will stink) and allow the mixture to ferment for about a week. Remove net-tles by straining concentrate into the second bucket. Make the spray by diluting the concentrate with water in a ratio of 1 part concentrate to 5 parts water. Spray plants, being sure to cover leaves thoroughly on both sides. Fermented nettle spray is also useful as a foliar fertilizer for plants.

GOOD IDEA!

If you're stung by **nettles,** apply yarrow juice for quick pain relief. Simply crush fresh yarrow leaves as hard as you can between your fingers until a small amount of juice is visible. Then press the juice and crushed plant to the net-tle stings. You can also apply a paste of baking soda and water. If noth-ing else is available, spread clean mud on the stings.

GOOD IDEA!

To use insect traps effectively, place the trap at about plant canopy height, for example, at about 2 feet high in tomatoes to catch tomato fruitworm. In fruit trees, place traps as high as the lowest branches. This is easy to manage for dwarf trees, but for standard trees, try hanging the trap from a branch by devising a holder from twine or wire.

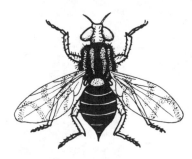

Cherry fruit flies lay eggs on developing fruit found throughout most of the United States. They emerge in early summer.

Cherry Fruit Fly Traps

Cherry fruit flies attack cherries, blueberries, and walnuts. Control these flies by trapping them on sticky traps hung in the branches of orchard trees.

Yield: 8 traps

INGREDIENTS
FOR TRAP LURES

¼ cup ammonia

¼ cup water

SUPPLIES

saw

20 × 24-inch piece of Masonite or thin plywood

drill

wire cutters

10 feet of flexible wire

newspaper

paintbrush

white primer paint

bright yellow paint (Rustoleum brand Federal Safety Yellow No. 659; Day-Glo Corporation brand Saturn Yellow)

petroleum jelly or disposable gloves

3 to 4 ounces trap glue, such as Tanglefoot

glue brush, squeegee, or spatula

1-cup liquid measuring cup

8 small glass or plastic vials (about 1 ounce)

scissors or tin snips

1 square foot fine-mesh window screen

8 rubber bands

string (optional)

Saw Masonite or plywood into eight 10 × 6-inch pieces and drill a hole near one end of each. Cut and loop a 1-foot length of wire through each hole to use as a handle and as a hanger. Put down plenty of newspaper to protect your work surface. Paint each trap on both sides with two coats of white primer, then a double coat of yellow paint.

Before you apply glue, coat your hands with petroleum jelly to make the glue easier to remove, or wear disposable gloves. When painted Masonite is thoroughly dry, apply glue to both sides with a brush, squeegee, or spatula.

When traps are ready to hang, prepare ammonia-scented vials to act as lures. Mix ammonia and water in the measuring cup and half-fill each vial. Cut pieces of window screen large enough to cover the mouth of each vial and secure with a rubber band. Using wire or string, make a loop around each vial to hold it as nearly upright as possible from the hanger wire at the top end of the trap.

Hang one trap in each medium-size tree, 2 traps in a large tree, starting in June and continuing until fruit is harvested. Place traps on the south side of the tree, 6 to 8 feet high among the foliage. Renew the lures weekly and check the stickiness of the glue. After several weeks, scrape off the old glue and spread fresh glue on the traps.

✿ **Variation:** *For western cherry fruit flies, cut a 1-quart plastic soft drink bottle in half and discard the bottom. Paint the top bell-shaped part of the bottle yellow as above, spread glue on the surface, and hang with a wire loop around the neck of the bottle. Hang the ammonia lure inside the bell of the trap.*

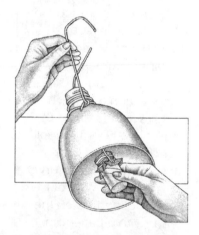

To lure western cherry fruit flies to a trap, use bell-shaped traps

Orchard Sanitation

Keeping the garden clean is your first defense against fruit tree pests. Eliminating hiding places can reduce pest populations significantly. Scrape loose bark from the trees in the spring to cut down on overwintering codling moth larvae. Make a scraper from an old hoe or dull saw blade. Use the tool with smooth, even strokes. You don't want to injure the live bark, or you may have more problems than you started with! Catch the scrapings in an old sheet or tarp spread around the base of the tree; add the scrapings to a fresh compost pile.

When you prune your trees, always use clean, sharp tools. Don't leave stumps, which can rot and provide a perfect habitat for all sorts of pests. Regularly collect dropped fruit during the growing season; use for cooking or add to the compost pile. And in the fall, do a thorough cleanup of any remaining fruit, along with any dropped leaves and branches.

Cutworm Baits

Cutworms cut off seedlings at night and hide in the soil during the day. In this bait, molasses attracts the cutworms to the sawdust and bran, which becomes caked on their bodies and prevents them from burrowing into the soil for protection from the sun or birds.

Yield: about ½ gallon of bait, enough for 35 to 50 transplants

INGREDIENTS

1 pint hardwood sawdust (*not* cedar or pine)
1 pint wheat bran
1 quart molasses
  water

SUPPLIES

3-quart bowl
spoon or paddle

In the bowl, mix sawdust, bran, and molasses, slowly adding cupfuls of water until the sawdust and bran are quite moist and all ingredients are well mixed. Spread a handful of bait around each transplant or spread an even sprinkling along rows of corn seedlings. Destroy any cutworms you see on the ground each morning. Renew the bait after heavy rains.

✿ **Variations:** Add ½ cup of pyrethrum or rotenone to increase the effectiveness of the bait during the first couple of nights. Sunlight gradually reduces the effectiveness of these additives. Or add 2 to 4 tablespoons of commercially prepared Bacillus thuringiensis.

➼ **Note:** Buy pyrethrum, rotenone, or Bacillus thuringiensis at garden centers and through mail-order suppliers for organic gardening. See page 444 for other sources.

Japanese Beetle Trap

Japanese beetles are a common pest on vegetables, flowers, and fruits. The beetles chew holes in the foliage and flowers, while the fat white larvae feed on the roots of the grass, making them a serious lawn pest. Many types of commercial traps are now available. Traps are most useful if a number of traps are set out over a large area, such as the whole neighborhood or community. You can make your own traps from leftover milk, bleach, or fabric softener bottles.

Yield: 1 trap

INGREDIENTS

1   quart fermenting wine or sugar water (½ cup sugar to 1 quart water)
1   or 2 pieces of fruit (preferably fermenting), mashed
1   teaspoon baking yeast

SUPPLIES

heavy scissors or linoleum knife
1-gallon plastic jug
strainer

Cut off most of the top quarter of the jug, leaving the original handle in place to make a convenient handle for the trap. Fill the trap one-third full with the fermenting wine or sugar water. Add fruit and yeast to cause further fermentation. The bait should be quite liquid. The beetles will be attracted to it and drown. Strain the bait daily and burn or bury dead beetles to prevent them from rotting and repelling other beetles from the trap.

Set the trap 1 to 3 feet above the ground in a sunny, open area, well away and downwind from easily infested plants, such as raspberries, cherries, peaches, vegetables, or roses. To trap beetles from a large area, set a trap every 150 to 200 feet around the perimeter of the area.

GOOD IDEA!

If Japanese beetles are "bugging" your plants, try an organic control. If you're not squeamish, handpicking is an effective method. In the morning (while their wings are wet) pick or shake the beetles off your plants into a bucket of soapy water. Or plant flowers such as four-o'clocks and white-flowered geraniums, which are attractive but toxic to the beetles. Or plant a "trap crop." Plants such as borage or soybeans are so attractive to the beetles that the pests are lured away from your good crops.

Snail and Slug Traps

Few garden pests are so widespread or so unanimously troublesome as slugs and snails. Although poison baits are available commercially, they are dangerous to pets and children. These traps are nontoxic.

Yield: 4 traps

INGREDIENTS

2 teaspoons sugar

½ teaspoon baking yeast

2 cups water

SUPPLIES

trowel

four deep saucers or plastic food containers

bowl

Dig shallow depressions in the soil and set the saucers or other containers into the soil with their top edges flush with the surface. In the bowl, dissolve sugar and yeast in water. Pour ½ cup into each saucer. The slugs are attracted to the yeasty or fermenting mixture and drown when they fall in. Add more bait, as necessary, or replace the bait after two days when it begins to lose its effectiveness.

♣ **Variation:** Make a simple slug trap from a gallon plastic milk jug. Cut 1-inch holes, 1 inch up from the bottom, in all four sides of the jug. Bury the the container in the soil up to the bottom edge of the holes, and fill to the same level with the liquid bait.

Wireworm Traps

Wireworms are the immature stage of click beetles; they live in the soil for two to six years before they mature, boring into underground roots, tubers, and corms. Because they have a slow, long lifecycle, it takes time to remove an established population, but once removed, they usually don't reappear in succeeding years. This wireworm trap, described in gardening books as early as 1900, is still useful today.

Yield: varies by amount of ingredients chosen

SUPPLIES

knife
fresh potatoes
8-inch or longer sticks (1 per trap)
bucket of soapy water

Cut potatoes in half and cut out the eyes. Poke a stick into each piece of potato to use as handle. Early in the season, bury the traps 4 to 6 inches deep in the garden or flower bed, before seeds or tubers are planted, to attract wireworms to the potatoes. Every day, pull out the potatoes, using the stick as a handle, and shake off the wireworms into a bucket of soapy water to kill them. Reuse the same potato for a while; replace deteriorated potatoes with new ones. The more traps planted, the better for the garden. A good distribution is one trap for every square yard of soil and more in flower beds where gladioli or begonias will be planted.

GOOD IDEA!

For good **wireworm control,** use traps early in the season and delay planting corn and tubers until the soil is very warm (when the wireworms go deep into the soil for the summer). In the fall, cultivate the garden weekly to expose larvae to birds. Cover crops of alfalfa or clover can repel wireworms. Or try a bug juice spray made by crushing the wireworms and adding some water. Strain and spray the liquid on affected crops.

GOOD IDEA!

If whiteflies are a
problem, try vacuuming
them off your plants with
a small, hand-held vac-
uum cleaner. The gentle
suction should pull off
the whiteflies without
harming the leaves. Pay
special attention to the
undersides of the top
leaves.

Sticky Traps

Bright yellow traps coated with sticky glue attract
whiteflies and fungus gnats in a greenhouse. In the garden,
yellow traps attract imported cabbageworms, onion flies,
cabbage root flies, and carrot rust flies. Other colors attract
different pests (see "Variations" below). Commercial traps
are available, but it's cheaper to make your own.

Yield: varies by amount of ingredients chosen

SUPPLIES

saw or heavy scissors

heavy cardboard, Masonite, or thin plywood

drill or punch

flexible wire or jumbo paper clips

newspaper

paintbrush

white primer paint

bright yellow paint (Rustoleum brand Federal Safety
Yellow No. 659; Day-Glo Corporation brand Saturn
Yellow)

petroleum jelly or disposable gloves

STP oil treatment or trap glue, such as Tanglefoot

glue brush, squeegee, or spatula

Cut the cardboard, Masonite, or plywood into strips 4
inches wide by 1 to 2 feet long. (Scientific research shows
that long rectangles are most attractive to insects.) Drill or
punch a hole in the center of one end of each strip and attach a wire loop or paper clip to act as a holder during
painting and later as a trap hanger. Spread newspaper to
protect the work surface. Paint each trap with two coats of
primer on both sides, then two coats of yellow paint. Before
you apply glue, coat your hands with petroleum jelly to
make the glue easier to remove, or wear disposable gloves.
When the paint is thoroughly dry, spread the STP or glue
on the traps using the brush, squeegee, or spatula.

Hang traps near the top of greenhouse plants to attract whiteflies, using one trap per plant. To catch green-house fungus gnats, attach traps to a stake in each pot or hang near the soil level. In the garden, place traps a couple of feet apart throughout the plantings to catch imported cabbageworm (cabbage white butterflies), onion flies, cabbage root flies, and carrot rust flies.

Renew the STP on the traps weekly; renew less frequently if you're using commercial trap glue. Outdoor traps lose their stickiness faster than those indoors.

✿ **Variations:** Use traps to count insect populations so that you can apply appropriate remedies when populations are at their peak. To count populations of various insects, you may need to change the trap color. For example, bright cobalt blue attracts western flower thrips and white attracts tarnished plant bugs. White also attracts beneficial insects, such as pollinators and aphid predators. In orchards, use white traps only between bud formation and earliest sign of flower opening.

➥ **Note:** Buy STP oil treatment at auto supply stores. Buy trap glue at garden centers and farm supply stores. See page 444 for other sources.

Sticky Trap Pests

Sticky traps are an effective control measure for the pests shown below. Tarnished plant bugs attack a wide variety of garden plants. Keep your garden clean to reduce possible overwintering sites for this pest. Thrips commonly attack flowers, as well as many vegetables and fruits. Besides blue sticky traps, you can try soap spray or a dusting of diatomaceous earth. Whiteflies feed on all sorts of plants. Yellow sticky traps are a good control device. Other methods include knocking the pests off with a blast of water or spraying with a soap solution.

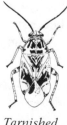

Tarnished plant bug

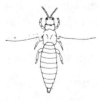

Thrips

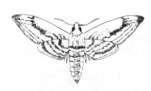

Whitefly

GOOD IDEA!

To enhance the control of corn earworms, apply ¼ to ½ teaspoon mineral oil inside the tip of each ear after the silk begins to dry and turn brown at the tip. If you have a large stand of corn, walk your stand with an oilcan full of mineral oil. To make the treatment more effective, mix a small amount of pyrethrum dust with the oil.

Corn Earworm Bait

The corn earworm is the caterpillar of large, light brown moths that lays eggs on the tips of young corn. The newly hatched caterpillars feed on corn silk, then move into the ear and eventually feed on the corn kernels. The caterpillars drop to the ground to pupate and emerge from the soil as moths in two to three weeks. This formula makes a trap to capture moths as they emerge from the soil thus preventing them from laying eggs for the next generation.

Yield: about 1 quart

INGREDIENTS

3 cups molasses

1 cup warm water

1 cup powdered pyrethrum flowers (see "Good Idea" on page 97)

SUPPLIES

dust mask

2-quart bowl

spoon or paddle

1- to 2-inch wide paintbrush

☛ **BE SAFE.** People allergic to ragweed are frequently also allergic to pyrethrum flowers. If you have hay fever, you may have a reaction to these flowers. When handling and mixing botanical pesticide dusts, always wear a dust mask.

Wearing a dust mask, mix molasses and water in the bowl, then fold in flowers and mix thoroughly. Paint a 4- to 6-inch-wide band of bait around the base of cornstalks and any nearby fence posts. Paint just above the soil line to attract the moths as they emerge.

✿ **Variation:** Substitute ½ cup commercial pyrethrin or rotenone dust for the 1 cup powdered pyrethrum flowers.

↝ **Note:** Buy powdered pyrethrum flowers, commercial pyrethrin, or rotenone at garden centers and through mail-order suppliers for organic gardening. See page 444 for other sources.

Sow Bug Traps

Sow bugs and pill bugs, also called wood lice, are members of a primitive group of animals called isopods. These small, gray creatures, common in damp, dark places, come out at night to nibble at plants. If they're numerous, they can damage or destroy a lot of seedlings. Pill bugs, the ones that roll themselves into a ball when they are disturbed, are particularly damaging. For bothersome pill bugs, try this old-fashioned remedy.

Yield: as many traps as desired

INGREDIENTS

1 part molasses

1 part white sugar

1 part beer

SUPPLIES

scissors

brown craft paper

spoon

bowl

paintbrush

bucket of soapy or boiling water

Cut the paper into long strips, 6 to 8 inches wide by 1 to 1½ feet long. Fold the paper in half lengthwise. Mix all ingredients together in the bowl and brush or smear the bait on the inner surface of the folded papers. Leave the papers overnight in the garden, folded like a pup tent, sticky side down. In the morning, check the traps. The sow bugs will be crowded onto the paper and can be easily shaken off into a bucket of soapy or boiling water.

> ### GOOD IDEA!
>
> **O**ne sow bug control method is garden sanitation. Keep the growing area free of debris and decaying plant material. Try mulching susceptible plants with shredded oak leaves or wood ashes.

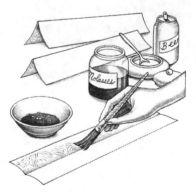

Tent-shaped traps for sow bugs

Cheshunt Compound

Use this formula to make Cheshunt compound, a very old-fashioned fungicide used for fungal diseases on flowers.

Yield: enough compound to make 12 to 13 gallons of spray

INGREDIENTS

1 ounce copper sulfate
5½ ounces ammonium carbonate
water

SUPPLIES

2 squares of heavy paper
kitchen dietary scales or postage scales
rubber work gloves
face mask
goggles, safety glasses, or face shield
8-ounce glass or stoneware jar with tight, nonmetallic stopper
wooden stirring stick
plastic bucket
garden spray equipment (plastic or glass only)

☛ **BE SAFE.** Wear rubber gloves to protect your hands. Ammonium carbonate is a traditional component of smelling salts. It exhudes irritating fumes if heated. Copper sulfate is poisonous. Keep this formula out of the reach of children and pets. Wear gloves, goggles, and a face mask when mixing and spraying this formula.

Fold the squares of heavy paper in half. Place one square on the scales and, wearing gloves and goggles, weigh the copper sulfate. Repeat for the ammonium carbonate. Pour each into the jar. Mix well, then cork the jar tightly, and leave for 24 hours before using.

Wearing gloves, goggles, and face mask, make the fungicide spray. Mix 1 ounce powder into 2 gallons of water in the bucket. *Use the spray immediately; do not store mixed spray for later use.* Do not put the spray into any metal containers or equipment because it will corrode the metal.

⇢ Note: *You can special order small amounts of both copper sulfate and ammonium carbonate from your pharmacist. In some areas, crystalline copper sulfate, also known as blue vitriol or blue stone, is available at livestock supply stores.*

Bordeaux Tree Wound Paint

For tree wounds that need short-term protection, make this inexpensive dressing. This wound dressing doesn't weather well, but it provides good prevention against fungal disease entry at wound sites.

Yield: about 2 pints

INGREDIENTS
1 pound commercial bordeaux powder
1½ pints raw linseed oil

SUPPLIES
rubber work gloves
½-gallon plastic bucket
wooden spoon or paddle
paintbrush

☛ BE SAFE. *Wear rubber gloves to protect your hands when handling this formula.*

Wearing rubber gloves, place bordeaux powder in the bucket and slowly stir in linseed oil until the mixture is thick and creamy. Paint on clean tree wounds.

⇢ Note: *Buy bordeaux powder through garden supply centers and through mail-order suppliers. See page 444 for other sources. Buy linseed oil at paint supply stores.*

G O O D   I D E A !

If the blue-green color of the bordeaux tree wound paint is undesirable, mix in as much lampblack pigment as desired to darken it. Wear gloves to avoid skin contact with the bordeaux powder or the prepared wound paint. Buy lampblack pigment at art supply stores.

GOOD IDEA!

To control fungal disease during wet weather, apply sulfur sprays frequently. Sulfur doesn't actually kill fungal spores. In inhibits the spread of fungi because fungus spores cannot germinate and multiply in a sulfur film. To be most effective, the sulfur film must be on the leaf before spores land. In wet weather, sulfur may be washed away. Reapply frequently for maximum protection.

Sulfur Spray

Sulfur is thought to be the first fungicide ever used (Homer mentions it in the *Iliad* and *Odyssey*). Used as a dust or spray, sulfur is an excellent fungicide for many plant diseases, such as apple scab, black spot on roses, and brown rot on fruit. Sulfur drenches or dust mixed into the soil will acidify it for acid-loving plants, such as azaleas, rhododendrons, and heather.

Yield: 3 gallons

INGREDIENTS

5 teaspoons powdered wettable sulfur (1 ounce)
3 gallons water

SUPPLIES

3- to 5-gallon plastic bucket or barrel
wooden spoon or paddle
garden spray equipment

☛ **BE SAFE.** Never use sulfur on cucumber and melon family plants and never use within four weeks before or after any type of oil spray on foliage. Do not spray sulfur in hot weather (temperatures over 80°F), when it is possible to injure sulfur-sensitive plants, such as viburnum, tomatoes, raspberries, gooseberries, grapes, and blueberries.

Measure sulfur into the bucket and add about a pint of water, mixing well to make a paste. Add remaining water slowly while stirring continuously. Spray on plants and trees at ten-day intervals, as needed, to control fungal diseases. Agitate sprayer during spraying to keep well-mixed.

✿ **Variations:** Slightly higher concentrations (up to 4 ounces sulfur per 3 gallons of water) will control brown rot on fruit. To control black spot and mildew on roses, dust plants with sulfur as soon as buds begin to expand.

➡ **Note:** Buy powdered wettable sulfur at garden centers. See page 444 for other sources.

Protective Tree Paint

This formula protects the bark of young trees from sunscald and wood-boring insects. Protect all young trees from the time they are set out until they are at least five years old.

Yield: about ½ quart

INGREDIENTS

1 teaspoon flax soap or other mild, pure soap
1 cup hot water
¼ pound diatomaceous earth
   water

SUPPLIES

bucket
dust mask
spoon or paddle
wide paintbrush

☛ **BE SAFE.** *Wear a dust mask when mixing this formula.*

Dissolve soap in hot water in the bucket. Wearing a dust mask, mix in diatomaceous earth, adding enough water to make a thick slurry. Paint onto the tree trunks from the soil line up to the first branch. Renew the paint annually or as needed to maintain an unbroken white surface.

➡ **Note:** *Buy diatomaceous earth at well-stocked garden centers and through mail-order suppliers. See page 444 for other sources.*

GOOD IDEA!

Be sure to buy diatomaceous earth sold especially for pest control. Don't buy the type used in swimming pool filters; it doesn't control insects. Filter-grade diatomaceous earth is processed differently than the insecticide grade material and is not appropriate for garden use.

Attack of the Peachtree Borer

Peachtree borers are serious fruit tree pests. The adult is a blue-black, wasplike insect with clear wings. Females lay eggs on tree trunks and branches; as eggs hatch, the developing larvae burrow under the bark. Their feeding eventually girdles and kills the tree. Protective tree paint is one way to control these pests. Or completely encircle each trunk with a metal strip; leave a 2-inch gap all around between the ring and the bark. Tap the circle partially into the ground. Fill this space with tobacco dust in May to make a strong repellent barrier.

GOOD IDEA!

To avoid damaging young tree bark, do not apply tree band glue directly to the bark, especially in hot, sunny weather. It may be damaged when the sun heats up the glue. Instead, wrap a band of burlap or stretchy knit fabric snugly around the bark and cover with a band of plastic wrap or tar paper secured with string. Coat this band with the glue. Just replace the plastic or tar paper when it's time to renew the glue.

Tree Band Glue

Applying a sticky band around tree trunks is a tried-and-true method of preventing pests from climbing on them. Tree bands are excellent barriers against gypsy moth and codling moth caterpillars, ants (who tend aphids on the trees), and beetles.

Yield: about 2¾ pounds

INGREDIENTS

1½ pounds rosin
1 pound linseed oil-based varnish
3 to 4 ounces yellow beeswax

SUPPLIES

double boiler with 2-quart insert
wooden spoon or paddle
rubber spatula or stiff brush

☛ **BE SAFE.** *Ingredients are flammable. Avoid open flames. Do not smoke. Melt ingredients in a double boiler; do not melt over direct heat.*

Melt all ingredients in the top part of the double boiler, heating and mixing until well-blended. Turn off heat and remove double boiler to a heat-proof surface. Allow the mixture to cool to lukewarm and spread in a 3- to 4-inch-wide band around the tree trunks with the spatula or stiff brush. Reapply when glue loses its effectiveness.

✿ **Variation:** *Use canola oil instead of linseed oil to make a glue that remains sticky longer.*

➡ **Notes:** *Buy rosin at dancing or theatrical supply shops. Buy linseed oil-based varnish at well-stocked paint supply stores. Yellow beeswax is simply beeswax that has not been bleached to make candles. Buy it from beekeepers. See page 444 for other sources. Canola oil is available at most supermarkets or specialty food stores. Check labels; you may already have canola oil in your pantry.*

Controlling Animal Pests

A really determined rabbit or deer can effectively de-molish a garden in a single night. Even a sturdy fence is not a fail-safe measure against rabbits, raccoons, groundhogs, and the like. In addition to fencing, try one of these strong-smelling, bad-tasting formulas to discourage animal forag-ing in your garden.

Dried Blood Spray for Deer and Rabbits

Dried blood repels most small animals as well as deer. Though dried blood is fairly expensive when used as a fertil-izer, a 1-pound box purchased just for pest control should last for several years.

Yield: 2 gallons

INGREDIENTS
1 tablespoon dried blood
2 gallons warm water

SUPPLIES
2-gallon bucket
stirrer
garden spray equipment

☛ **BE SAFE.** *Dried blood is rich in nitrogen and may burn plants if applied in overly concentrated doses. Measure carefully when you prepare this spray, and use it somewhat sparingly.*

In the bucket, dissolve dried blood in water. Apply as a spray when needed. Most plants are especially vulnerable to deer and rabbit damage when young.

➡ **Note:** *Buy dried blood at garden centers and through mail-order suppliers. See page 444 for other sources.*

GOOD IDEA!

To repel both deer and rabbits, sprinkle dried blood or dried blood mixed with bonemeal around plants. Dried blood and bonemeal also make ex-cellent soil amendments. Dried blood is a good or-ganic source of nitrogen; bonemeal is a fine source of phosphorus and cal-cium, as well as some ni-trogen.

GOOD IDEA!

If you prepare whole chicken frequently, consider saving the livers in your freezer for later use in a deer repellent spray.

Liver Repellent Spray for Deer and Rabbits

A spray made from raw liver repels deer and rabbits.

Yield: 2 gallons

INGREDIENTS

1 pound raw liver (any type)
2 gallons warm water

SUPPLIES

2-gallon bucket
garden spray equipment

Place liver in the bucket and cover with water. Allow it to soak for ½ hour, then discard liver and use the liquid as a spray.

GOOD IDEA!

For an easy, effective deer repellent, try hanging soap in your garden! Cut a bar of strongly scented deodorant soap in half, put each piece in part of an old stocking, and tie the bundle onto a stake, about 4 feet from the ground. Place the stakes throughout your garden. Experiment with different brands if one kind doesn't work.

Animal Repellent Spray

Hot-pepper sauce is the key ingredient in this repellent formula. This preparation is effective against cats, dogs, and mice, as well as against deer and rabbits.

Yield: 1 gallon

INGREDIENTS

1 tablespoon hot-pepper sauce, such as Tabasco
1 tablespoon commercial sticker/spreader, such as Dragon or Science, or ½ cup nondetergent soap powder
1 gallon water

SUPPLIES

stirrer
2-gallon bucket
garden spray equipment

☛ **BE SAFE.** *Use this mixture cautiously in areas where children play. Some people are allergic to hot peppers. Also avoid getting this spray in your eyes or on your skin. Hot pepper and soap are strong eye irritants. Soap may burn delicate plants. Test a leaf before using.*

Mix ingredients thoroughly in the bucket and apply as a spray, covering the tops and undersides of leaves.

•➤ **Note:** *Buy a commercial agricultural sticker/spreader at garden centers and farm supply stores.*

Cayenne Pepper Repellent Powder

This repellent dust works well for keeping rabbits, groundhogs, and browsing deer away from your garden.

Yield: 1 cup

INGREDIENTS

½ cup talcum powder
½ cup cayenne pepper

SUPPLIES

dust mask
2-cup container
wooden spoon or stick
old sock or cloth bag

☛ **BE SAFE.** *Use this mixture cautiously in areas where children play. Some people are allergic to cayenne pepper. Also avoid getting powder in eyes or on skin. Use a dust mask when applying the powder.*

Wearing a dust mask, mix talcum powder and cayenne together in the container. Pour mixture into the sock or cloth bag and tie shut. Apply the powder by beating the sock with the spoon or stick. The powder adheres best if you apply it early in the morning when plants are still wet with dew. Reapply every few days and after heavy rains.

GOOD IDEA!

Hot pepper can also make an effective dog and cat repellent. Wearing gloves and goggles, grind up 2 or 3 garlic cloves and 3 or 4 hot peppers in a blender. Mix into a bucket of water, add a few drops of liquid dishwashing detergent, and mix well. Sprinkle the solution around the edge of your yard and garden.

GOOD IDEA!

To combat nibbling mice, try this traditional orchardist's trick. Scatter the fall prunings from your fruit trees on the ground around the trees for the duration of the winter. Mice usually prefer the tender bark of branch prunings and will leave the trunks of your trees alone.

Rosin-Based Rabbit Repellent

In the winter, hungry rabbits may nibble the bark of trees and shrubs, sometimes girdling and killing valuable specimens. To prevent this type of winter damage, coat the lower trunks of trees and shrubs with this mixture. Applied in late fall, this repellent is especially helpful in preventing rabbit damage to fruit trees.

Yield: 1 gallon

INGREDIENTS

1 gallon denatured ethyl alcohol
7 pounds finely powdered rosin

SUPPLIES

1-gallon container with lid
paintbrush

☛ **BE SAFE.** Ingredients are flammable. Do not heat the mixture in an effort to dissolve the rosin more quickly. Make only as much repellent as you need so that you won't have flammable materials stored in your work area.

Place alcohol in the container and add rosin. Tightly cover the container and agitate it gently to begin dissolving the rosin. Place the container in a warm, *not hot*, location and shake it gently from time to time over the next 24 hours. At the end of that time, the rosin should be completely dissolved. Paint the mixture on tree trunks and low-lying branches.

Avoid contaminating this formula with water. Water causes formation of a white powder in the solution, making it more difficult to apply and less effective at repelling rabbits. Apply the formula within two to three days of mixing, painting it on dry bark when the temperature is above freezing. Once the repellent is applied, snow or rain will turn it white but will not reduce its effectiveness.

✿ **Variation:** For 1 quart, mix 1¾ pounds powdered rosin with 1 quart denatured ethyl alcohol.

➡ **Notes:** Denatured ethyl alcohol is simply ethyl alcohol with a contaminant added to make it unpalatable for people to drink. Buy denatured alcohol at hardware stores. Powdered rosin is the residue left from distilling turpentine from pine sap. Buy it at dance or theatrical supply stores.

Castor-Oil Mole Repellent

Castor beans, planted around the perimeter of the garden, are a traditional deterrent for moles and shrews. You can substitute this formula for castor bean plants.

Yield: 2 gallons

INGREDIENTS

½ cup castor oil
2 gallons warm water

SUPPLIES

stirrer
2-gallon bucket

Mix oil and water in the bucket and use as a soil drench around the perimeter of your garden. Apply the drench as soon as you see any sign of mole activity. Within three weeks, the garden should be mole-free.

➡ **Note:** Castor oil, an old-fashioned remedy for constipation, is usually available at your pharmacy.

> ### GOOD IDEA!
>
> **T**o keep moles out of your garden, plant a castor bean hedge around it. Castor beans definitely deter moles; however, they are extremely poisonous. Don't plant them in areas frequented by children.
>
> Castor beans (Ricinus communis) are usually grown from seed. Perennials in frost-free garden zones, they are grown as annuals elsewhere. Seeds started indoors in March produce huge, tropical-looking plants by mid-summer.

Mole Control

Moles don't eat plants (although sometimes they munch on tulip bulbs), but they can make unsightly tunnels in your yard and garden. A small windmill or pinwheel set over the tunneled area may create vibrations that deter moles. If you see the tunnels actually being formed, you can try digging out the creature directly. Indirectly, you can control moles by removing their food supply, which includes Japanese beetle grubs. Get rid of the grubs, and you reduce the chances of mole problems. If all else fails, construct a mole-proof fence. Surround your garden with a wire fence buried 1 foot deep.

GOOD IDEA!

To discourage birds from foraging on seedlings, sprinkle lime between the rows. This doesn't always work, but it's worth a try before resorting to more drastic measures, such as tobacco spray. Some seedlings may be too tender to survive heavy applications of tobacco spray. Before spraying an entire row of seedlings, test tobacco spray on a small section first. Wait overnight before spraying an entire row.

Tobacco Bird Repellent

Birds, as they forage for food, help to control problem insects. But to discourage hungry birds that are destroying your seedlings, spray seedlings with the following mixture.

Yield: about 1½ cups of concentrate, enough for 7½ cups of spray

INGREDIENTS

onions
1 cup hot-pepper sauce, such as Tabasco
1 cup cheap pipe tobacco

SUPPLIES

blender or food processor
fine strainer
1-quart container
old nylon stocking
rubber work gloves
garden spray equipment

☛ **BE SAFE.** Avoid getting this mixture in your eyes or on your skin. Wear rubber gloves. Nicotine is a poison. Tobacco also is an alternate host for tobacco mosaic virus, a disease that stunts growth and blossom set on young tomatoes and other solanaceous plants. Don't use tobacco spray near tomato plants that have not yet matured and set blossoms. Tobacco mosaic infection in mature, fruit-bearing tomatoes causes little damage. Use this mixture cautiously in areas where children play. Some people are allergic to hot peppers.

Place enough onions in the blender or food processor to make 1 cup puree. Strain off liquid and combine with hot-pepper sauce in the container. Combine drained onion puree and tobacco and place in the stocking. Suspend the stocking in the onion/hot-pepper sauce liquid. Allow to stand undisturbed for several days. Don rubber gloves and squeeze the stocking to extract remaining juices. To spray, dilute at a rate of 4 parts water to 1 part repellent. Spray sparingly over newly planted rows.

Egg-Based Deer Repellent

Eggs make an effective deer repellent for the garden. At least one commercial deer repellent (Big-Game Repellent) is based entirely on eggs.

Yield: 5 gallons

INGREDIENTS

1½ dozen eggs
5 gallons water

SUPPLIES

electric mixer
large mixing bowl
5-gallon bucket
stiff stirring stick
garden spray equipment

Beat eggs in the bowl, then pour into the bucket. Add water slowly and stir thoroughly. Apply as a spray. Be sure to spray clear water through your spray equipment after you've used this formula. Egg residue left in the nozzle may clog your equipment. To maintain effectiveness, reapply spray after heavy rains.

GOOD IDEA!

If deer are a problem in your area, try planting shrubs and trees that they don't like. Spiny plants, such as hollies (Ilex spp.), barberries (Berberis spp.), and grape hollies (Mahonia spp.), naturally discourage browsing. Japanese pieris (Pieris japonica), boxwoods (Buxus spp.), and drooping leucothoe (Leucothoe fontanesiana) are other plants that seem to be unpopular.

Bird Control Tips

While birds are normally desirable garden residents, sometimes they can cause real problems. Corn is often a favorite target, in both the seedling and mature stages. To deter birds from feeding on seedlings, try spreading lime or a heavy layer of mulch over the planted seeds. Or stretch audiocassette tape between two stakes; wind blowing over the tape causes vibrations than can deter birds. Hang strips of foil or aluminum pie pans around the garden to scare birds away. To protect ripening fruit, the most effective method is plastic netting draped over the plants. Inflatable snakes, owls, or bird-scaring balloons are also effective; vary their use and location to maintain their effectiveness. Or tie one end of a plastic garbage bag to a 5- to 6-foot stake and cut the untied end into strips. The noise and movement of these strips in the wind may deter birds and other small creatures.

GARDEN HELPERS

On the following pages, you'll find a variety of formulas that help with common garden tasks or that will improve your results in many different gardening projects. Included are ways to overwinter tubers of tender plants without rot, a formula with instructions for forcing spring bulbs, and a special soil amendment for rose beds.

Dahlia Storage Method

Dahlia tubers will not tolerate frost and must be lifted from the ground in autumn and stored over the winter. Unfortunately, they are difficult to store. If kept too moist, they rot. If stored completely dry, they desiccate and are hard to revive. This formula uses sulfur dust to inhibit fungal growth and an antidesiccant to prevent dehydration.

Yield: varies by amount of ingredients chosen

INGREDIENTS

1 part Wilt-Pruf
10 parts water
powdered wettable sulfur

SUPPLIES

bucket
stirrer
dust mask
1-gallon sealable plastic bag
old window screen or newspaper
box filled with peat moss

☛ **BE SAFE.** *Wear a dust mask when coating tubers.*

Place Wilt-Pruf in the bucket and dilute with water. To make 5½ cups solution, add ½ cup Wilt-Pruf to 5 cups water. Stir to mix.

Wearing a dust mask, place powdered sulfur in the bag. Place tubers one at a time in the bag, seal, and shake

---

GOOD IDEA!

One way to store dahlia tubers is to coat them with a thin layer of paraffin. Paraffin is flammable; do not melt over direct heat. Melt a pound of paraffin in the top part of a double boiler, turn off the heat, and remove double boiler to a heat-proof surface. Pour paraffin into a bucket of hot water (about 80°F). The paraffin will float. With kitchen tongs, dip carefully cleaned tubers into the wax and draw them slowly out, allowing the wax to cover them completely. Cool, and store in dry peat moss.

gently to coat each tuber. Dip the sulfur-coated tuber in the Wilt-Pruf solution and place it on a screen or layers of newspaper to dry. Store the treated tubers in dry peat moss.

➡ **Notes:** *Wilt-Pruf is a biodegradable antitranspirant spray applied to prevent transplant shock of shrubs and trees. Buy it at garden centers and farm supply stores. Buy powdered wettable sulfur at garden centers. See page 444 for other sources.*

Fertilizer for Bulbs

Research shows that bulbs benefit from more nitrogen than was previously thought. Bonemeal, the standard bulb fertilizer, supplies phosphorus but not enough nitrogen. An autumn application of 16 gallons of compost or dry manure per 100 square feet of bed is recommended. This supplies both nitrogen and phosphorus in ample quantities. Instead of compost or dry manure, you may use this fertilizer.

Yield: enough fertilizer for 100 square feet

INGREDIENTS

2 to 3 pounds bloodmeal

2 to 3 pounds bonemeal

2 to 3 pounds greensand or wood ashes

SUPPLIES

bucket, washtub, or plastic drop cloth

shovel

Mix all ingredients in the bucket or washtub or on the drop cloth. Top-dress bulbs with the mixture every fall.

✿ **Variation:** *In spring, add an additional 2 pounds of bloodmeal or 16 gallons of dried manure per 100 square feet of bed.*

➡ **Note:** *Buy bloodmeal and bonemeal at garden centers and through mail-order suppliers. Buy greensand, a mineral-rich sediment from the ocean through organic gardening suppliers. See page 444 for other sources.*

GOOD IDEA!

If you want garden bulbs to bloom year after year, allow the foliage to ripen completely after flowering. The bulbs use this time to store the food they need for the next blooming season. Plant annuals or strong-growing perennials, like daylilies, around the bulbs to hide the foliage. Or plant bulbs in a groundcover, such as periwinkle or pachysandra.

Soil Mix for Tuberous Begonias

Tuberous begonias are among the showiest shade-loving plants you can grow. They are, however, quite susceptible to rot. Starting them in the right soil and watering them carefully are important for avoiding this problem.

In late winter, start tubers by setting them in pots or deep flats of plain peat moss, sphagnum moss, or vermiculite, covering the tops with only about ½ inch of material. Water quite lightly and place pots in a room kept at about 70°F during the day and 60° to 70°F at night. In a month to six weeks, top growth should appear. When it has reached 2 to 3 inches in height, transplant tubers into the following mix, using 6- to 8-inch pots.

Yield: varies by amount of ingredients chosen

INGREDIENTS

2 parts topsoil
3 parts leaf mold or peat moss
1 part coarse washed sand
¼ part dried manure
bonemeal (2 cups per 8 gallons of mix)

SUPPLIES

5-gallon bucket or other container
shovel
6- to 8-inch pots (1 per tuber)

Combine all ingredients in the bucket or other container and mix thoroughly. Partially fill each pot with mix, plant one sprouted tuber per pot, and cover with more mix. Water just enough to thoroughly moisten the mix. Keep the transplanted tubers indoors in an area with plenty of indirect sunlight. Water sparingly only when the soil surface begins to dry out. Turn regularly for even growth.

When danger of frost is past, move plants outdoors to a partially shaded, well-worked bed prepared with sand and plenty of humus. Plant them exactly level with the soil surface. Fertilize begonias once a month with manure tea, being careful to keep the tea away from direct contact with the tubers. Do not allow soil to dry out, but avoid overwatering these plants during the growing season. Keep water off the foliage as much as possible.

After first frost, dig tubers and remove foliage down to about 1 inch. Soak them in hot water (118°F) for 3 minutes and allow them to dry in the sun. When the stem has withered and dried, store tubers in dry peat moss or vermiculite in a cool, dry basement.

➻ **Note:** Buy bonemeal at garden centers and through mail-order suppliers. See page 444 for other sources.

Wound Dressing for Oak Trees

Research suggests that tree wound dressings for pruning cuts and mechanical damage are usually unnecessary. One exception to this general rule is in the treatment of oaks pruned in the spring. Pruned oak trees are highly susceptible to the destructive oak wilt fungus, and covering pruning wounds appears to help them resist the disease.

Yield: 3 cups

INGREDIENTS

1 cup zinc oxide
2 cups mineral oil

SUPPLIES

wooden spoon or paddle
1-quart container
paintbrush

Stir zinc oxide and oil together in the container and paint over wounds.

➻ **Note:** Buy zinc oxide powder, also called flowers of zinc, through your pharmacist.

GOOD IDEA!

To properly prune large branches from any tree, follow this simple three-step method. Using a saw, make the first cut partially through the underside of the branch, about 6 inches out from the trunk. Next, saw downward from the top of the branch, a few inches out from the first cut; let the branch fall. Finally, remove the stump by cutting downward close to the trunk.

GOOD IDEA!

Brighten dreary winter days with flowering branches. Stems of early-spring-blooming shrubs and trees are often easy to force. In February, cut branches 1 to 2 feet long and bring them indoors. Cut the base of each stem on a long slant, or pound the ends with a hammer, to split the wood and increase water uptake. Arrange the prepared branches in a container with several inches of water in the base. Add a few drops of chlorine bleach to keep the water clean. Set the branches in a warm, humid place. Change the water every five days; mist the branches frequently to prevent drying. Try this method on plants such as forsythia, apple, cherry, pussy willow, or deciduous magnolia.

Soil Mix for Forcing Spring Bulbs

Forced bulb displays bring a breath of spring-to-come during the long, slow days of midwinter. For forcing, buy firm, sturdy bulbs in autumn and plant three to five of each variety in a single pot, using the following mix. Prepare the soil mix in early fall while garden soil is unfrozen.

Yield: varies by amount of ingredients chosen

INGREDIENTS

4 parts topsoil
1 part peat moss
  bonemeal (1 tablespoon per 8-inch pot)
  water

SUPPLIES

wheelbarrow, bucket, or plastic drop cloth
garden spade
8-inch pots for bulbs

In the wheelbarrow or bucket or on the drop cloth, combine topsoil and peat moss. As you fill each pot with soil mix, work in bonemeal. Fill the pots with enough soil mix so that the bulbs rest about 1 inch below pot rims. The tips of the bulbs should barely show at the soil surface. Water thoroughly, allow them to drain, and place them in a cool, dark place where roots can develop. Storage temperature should be 40° to 50°F. Suitable storage places include a shelf in your refrigerator, an unheated garage or basement, or a protected window well on a shady side of your house. Or you can dig a 12- to 15-inch-deep pit outdoors, place pots at the bottom, and cover them with a 6- to 8-inch layer of straw or peat moss. Do not allow bulbs to dry out during their cold period.

After about 8 weeks in storage, check pot drainage holes for evidence of root growth. Beginning top growth also signals roots have developed. Most hardy bulbs require about 8 weeks cold storage for root development; tulips need 10 to 12 weeks. Bring the pots indoors a few at a time, allow them to thaw, and water them well. For the next few days, hold them in a cool, shady part of your house at 50° to 60°F to give them a chance to acclimate. When the new growth is about 3 inches high and green, move them into direct sunlight for continued growth and bloom.

•➤ **Note:** *Buy bonemeal at garden centers and through mail-order suppliers. See page 444 for other sources.*

Super-Rich Organic Fertilizer for the Vegetable Garden

Before embarking on any serious fertilization of your vegetable garden, have your soil tested to determine what your real needs are. This fertilizer is fairly expensive to make. A far cheaper way to add nitrogen and phosphorus is to use composted manure. Wood ash is an equally cheap source of phosphorus.

Yield: varies by amount of ingredients chosen

INGREDIENTS

4 parts dried blood
2 parts bonemeal
1 part kelp meal, greensand, or rock phosphate

SUPPLIES

shovel
bucket or plastic drop cloth

Mix ingredients in the bucket or on the drop cloth and apply to crops that feed heavily, such as asparagus or celery. The optimum application rate is about 3 pounds per 100 square feet of crop.

•➤ **Notes:** *Buy dried blood, bonemeal, and rock phosphate at garden centers and through mail-order suppliers. Kelp meal, which is dried, processed seaweed, and greensand, a mineral-rich sediment from the ocean, are usually available from organic gardening suppliers. See page 444 for other sources.*

GOOD IDEA!

Follow these two simple rules for maximizing sunlight in your vegetable garden: (1) Run all rows east and west. (2) Plant the tallest vegetables, for instance, corn or pole beans, in the northern-most rows of the garden. Next to the tallest vegetables, plant medium-height vegetables—okra, tomatoes, peppers, eggplant. And in the last rows—the south side of the garden—plant the shortest vegetables, such as lettuce, bush beans, onions, and squash.

GOOD IDEA!

Use rose planting as a time to add soil to eroded or damaged garden areas or to your compost heap, since you'll have extra garden soil left from each planting hole. If you have loose, fertile topsoil, sterilize it, and use it in potting mixes. Don't use topsoil alone in houseplant containers; it will compact heavily from frequent watering.

Rose Planting Formula

Roses need extra-rich soil, excellent drainage, and ample nutrients. This formula provides natural sources of phosphorus, magnesium, calcium, and potassium—the elements roses need most to bloom profusely. If you spend the time and effort to get roses off to a good start, they'll reward you with years of dependable bloom.

Yield: enough mix to plant 6 rose bushes

INGREDIENTS

20 pounds rotted cow manure

3 cubic feet peat moss

5 pounds new cat litter (avoid brands that contain deodorizing crystals)

1 tablespoon Epsom salts

1 cup bonemeal

2 cups cottonseed meal

2 cups alfalfa seed meal

2 cups dolomitic lime

SUPPLIES

garden spade

15-cubic-foot garden cart, large wheelbarrow, or large plastic drop cloth

clean plastic garbage bags (optional)

garden hose

☛ **BE SAFE.** Do not include used cat litter in this formula; it may contain disease organisms.

Combine all ingredients in the cart or wheelbarrow or on the drop cloth. Use immediately or store in plastic garbage bags for later use. Using a cart or wheelbarrow for mixing allows you to wheel the filled cart to your garden just as you begin to plant your roses.

To plant roses, excavate a hole 6 inches deeper and 1 foot wider than needed to rest your rose at normal planting level. Mix half of the soil from the planting hole with an equal volume of the rose planting formula. Use this soil/planting formula mixture to fill the planting hole around the rose. Be sure to tamp out air holes as you fill the hole around the rose roots. Leave a 4-inch-high ring of the soil/planting formula mix around the circumference of the planting hole to help retain water for the plant. Immediately after planting, water deeply and watch to see if additional planting formula is needed to completely fill the hole.

➻ **Notes:** Buy Epsom salts at pharmacies. Cottonseed meal and alfalfa seed meal are available at farm supply stores and some garden centers. Buy bonemeal and dolomitic lime at garden centers. See page 444 for other sources.

Controlling Rose Pests

Check your roses regularly to catch insect and disease problems before they get out of hand. Aphids are small pests that feed on leaves and buds. If there are only a few, squash them with your fingers. Or knock them off with a strong spray of water, repeated every day for three to four days. For severe infestations, cover the aphids with a soap spray. Japanese beetles, rose chafers, and rose curculios are also common rose pests. Handpicking is the easiest control method; drop the beetles into a bucket of soapy water. Or try making your own Japanese beetle traps (see page 115). Several types of caterpillars feed on rose leaves and buds. Handpick or try a soap spray. Spider mites cause yellow stippling on the leaves. Spray the plants with water (especially the undersides of the leaves) each day for three to four days. Soap sprays are also effective. Thrips are flower pests; control them by removing spent flowers. Try sprinkling diatomaceous earth on the buds. Make aluminum foil collars for special blooms to repel thrips. Common disease problems include powdery mildew, rust, and black spot. A sulfur spray or dust, such as the one on page 124, is an effective control for these diseases; you can also apply sulfur as a preventive measure. Remove and destroy affected plant parts as soon as you see them. Minimize disease problems by planting resistant cultivars, such as the modern, low-maintenance shrub roses.

Fertilizer for Roses

Roses are fairly heavy feeders and will bloom more prolifically if you fertilize them regularly throughout the growing season. This formula will keep roses blooming all season.

Yield: varies by amount of ingredients chosen

INGREDIENTS

2 parts fishmeal
2 parts dried blood
1 part cottonseed meal
1 part rock phosphate
1 part greensand

SUPPLIES

garden spade
large bucket or wheelbarrow
clean plastic garbage bag or covered container

Thoroughly mix all ingredients together in the bucket or wheelbarrow. Store in a sealed plastic garbage bag or covered container in a cool, dark place. Every month during the growing season, apply 1 to 3 cups of the fertilizer to each rose. Time your last application so that new growth stops well before first frost. In the northern garden zones, this means do not apply fertilizer after August 1; in the middle garden zones, fertilize for the last time around September 1; and in the warmest zones make the last application by October 1.

✿ **Variation:** If soil is very acid, add 1 part wood ashes.

➡ **Notes:** Buy fishmeal at well-stocked garden supply stores and through mail-order suppliers. Buy cottonseed meal at farm supply stores and some garden centers. Buy dried blood and rock phosphate at garden centers and greensand, a mineral-rich sediment from the ocean, at organic gardening suppliers. See page 444 for other sources.

Fruit Tree Fertilizer

Bearing fruit trees require some annual fertilization, especially with nitrogen. Too much nitrogen, however, produces vigorous vegetative growth at the expense of flowers and fruit. A good way to fertilize is to mulch fairly heavily early in the spring with compost or hay that has been fortified with a high-nitrogen organic material like cottonseed meal or manure. Fish emulsion is an excellent source of nitrogen for fruit trees. By following a thrice-yearly fertilization program, you can bring young fruit trees to bearing age without a hitch.

Yield: 5 gallons, enough for 1 application to 1 tree

INGREDIENTS

1 teaspoon fish emulsion
5 gallons water

SUPPLIES

stirring stick
5-gallon bucket

To fertilize newly planted fruit trees, mix fish emulsion and water in the bucket and apply. Soak the feeder root area with all 5 gallons of formula three times, once in early spring while trees are still dormant, once after blossoms fall, and again in early summer.

Every year thereafter, until the trees reach maturity, increase the concentration of fish emulsion by 1 teaspoon. Apply the full 5 gallons to the feeder root area three times per year, just as described above. By the time the tree is full-size, you will probably be using 10 teaspoons of concentrated liquid fish fertilizer with every 5 gallons of water.

To find out how to locate the feeder root area of fruit trees, see "Good Idea!" on page 144.

➼ **Note:** Fish emulsion is a concentrated brown liquid made from fish oils and water. Buy it at well-stocked garden supply stores. See page 444 for other sources.

GOOD IDEA!

For bigger harvests and healthier fruit trees, try removing some of the immature fruit, a process known as thinning. If you allow all the fruit that develops to remain, the resulting harvest will be smaller and possibly less sweet. Heavily laden branches are also prone to breakage. Remove some of the fruit one to two months after full bloom, leaving one fruit per cluster and about 5 inches between the fruit. Use a twisting motion to remove the fruit; don't pull it off.

All-Purpose Tree-Fertilizing Formula

Woodland trees and shrubs receive an annual feeding in autumn, when leaves fall and decompose beneath them, providing a natural mulch of nutrient-rich leaf mold. Plants grown in the landscape rarely receive this form of nourishment, since fallen leaves kill grass. To compensate for the loss of naturally decomposing leaves, fertilize trees and shrubs with compost, which is similar to natural leaf mold. To promote steady growth and disease resistance, fertilize trees with this formula in addition to compost.

Yield: varies by amount of ingredients chosen

INGREDIENTS

3 parts cottonseed meal, soy meal, or bloodmeal

2 parts finely ground rock phosphate or steamed bonemeal

3 parts wood ashes, granite dust, or greensand

1 part calcitic limestone

SUPPLIES

shovel

bucket or plastic drop cloth

Mix ingredients together in the bucket or on the drop cloth. Apply to the soil beneath the tree, starting 6 inches from the trunk and working outward, to about a foot beyond the dripline. Use about 1 pound of fertilizer for every foot in diameter of the crown, as measured at the dripline.

➡ **Note:** You'll find tree-fertilizing supplies at farm supply stores and at some garden centers. For other sources for most of the components, see page 444.

Preservative Formula for Christmas Trees

Maximize the fresh beauty of a Christmas tree or evergreen table decorations by including this formula in the water.

Yield: 1 gallon

INGREDIENTS

¼ cup micronized iron
1 gallon hot water
2 cups light corn syrup
4 teaspoons chlorine bleach

SUPPLIES

2-gallon bucket
long-handled spoon or paddle

☛ **BE SAFE.** This formula will stain some rug fibers. Place a plastic sheet under your tree to avoid the possibility of ruining your rug.

In the bucket, stir micronized iron into water and add corn syrup and bleach. To use as a Christmas tree preservative, first cut an inch of wood from the bottom of the trunk and stand the tree in a 1-gallon capacity container. Fill the container with this solution and add more solution daily as it evaporates from the stand.

➦ **Note:** Buy micronized iron at garden centers and hardware stores.

GOOD IDEA!

Cut flowers benefit from special treatments. When gathering flowers from your own garden, pick them in early morning, when their tissues are full of water. Use a clean, sharp knife or scissors to make a long sloping cut at the base of the stem. Immediately place the stems in tepid water; remove any foliage below the water level. Indoors, condition the flowers by following the directions given for roses in "Good Idea!" on page 142. Add a commercial preservative or try adding 1 part tonic water or lemon-lime soda to 2 parts plain water as a preservative. Change the solution frequently to keep the flowers fresh. Display cut flowers in a cool place, away from fruit. Ripening fruit releases ethylene, which shortens the useful life of your flowers.

General Soil Mix for Houseplants

This light mix, suitable for most tropical foliage plants, won't compact over time.

Yield: varies by amount of ingredients chosen

INGREDIENTS

1 part manure-based compost
1 part topsoil
1 part sand
    bonemeal (1 cup per 8 gallons)
    wood ashes (2 cups per 8 gallons)

SUPPLIES

bucket
shovel
clean plastic garbage bag or covered container
    (optional)

Combine all ingredients in the bucket and mix thoroughly. Use immediately or store in a sealed plastic garbage bag or container in a cool, dark place.

➥ **Note:** Buy bonemeal at garden centers and through mail-order suppliers. See page 444 for other sources.

Repotting and Potting-On

To keep houseplants healthy and vigorous, give them fresh soil from time to time either by repotting or by potting-on. Repotting keeps a plant compact; potting-on produces a larger plant.

For either method, water the plant a day or two before handling. Remove the plant from its pot. Slide one hand, palm down, over the top of the pot, with the plant stem between your first and second fingers. Hold the base of the pot in your other hand. Carefully turn the pot over, and tap the rim on the edge of a solid surface until the rootball separates from the pot.

To repot, gently break old soil from the edges of the rootball. Add fresh soil mix to the old pot, replace the plant, and fill with more fresh soil, pushing it down. Leave about ½ inch of space from the soil mix to the pot rim.

For potting-on, choose a new pot that is 1 to 2 inches larger in diameter. Add fresh mix to the base of the pot, and place the plant in the center. Add more mix to the edges and top; press it down lightly with your fingers. Leave about ½ inch between the mix and the pot rim.

RIGHT SOIL, RIGHT PLANT
Selecting the Best Soil Mix for Potted Plants

Plant Type	Soil Mix	Comments
Cacti and succulents	1 part coarse, washed builder's sand; 1 part roughly screened compost or leaf mold; 1 Tbs. bonemeal per ½ gal. of mix; 1 Tbs. hoof and horn meal per ½ gal. of mix	Only use pots with drainage holes. Do not overwater. Water until water drains from the drain hole. Do not water again until soil has almost completely dried out.
Ferns	4 parts sterilized topsoil; 1 part sand; 1 part well-rotted cow manure; then mix in ½ cup shredded compost or leaf mold per each 6- to 8-inch pot	Ferns flouish in well-drained, humusy soil made acidic by the addition of leaf mold. Ferns also require high humidity. Mist them twice a day with softened water. Occasionally clean fronds by wiping them gently with a solution of 1 Tbs. white vinegar in 1 cup warm water.
African violets	1 part sterilized topsoil; 1 part peat moss; 1 part sand; 1 part shredded compost	Let soil surface dry between waterings. Use tepid water. Avoid overwatering. Plants do well if leaves receive an occasional misting with lukewarm water. Plants bloom best if they are potbound.
Indoor fruit trees	2 parts sterilized topsoil; 1 part shredded compost; 1 part sharp, washed builder's sand; 1 cup bonemeal per 2 gal. of mix	For best results, move indoor fruit trees to a patio or sunny porch during the summer. Citrus, figs, and apricots especially need plenty of sun. During the growing season, top-dress with a high-phosphorus, high-potassium fertilizer.

Fertilizer for Flowering Houseplants

Foliage plants require nitrogen for leaf formation and can be adequately nourished with a high-nitrogen fertilizer like fish emulsion. Flowering houseplants, however, require more potassium and phosphorus. Their needs are best met with a balanced potting soil (see "General Soil Mix for Houseplants" on page 146), plus regular applications of fish emulsion or manure tea. You can also use the following fertilizer, which is high in potassium and phosphorus, with an N-P-K ratio of 5-6-4.

Yield: varies by amount of ingredients chosen

INGREDIENTS

2 parts cottonseed meal
2 parts bonemeal
2 parts wood ashes

SUPPLIES

spoon
bowl

Mix all ingredients together in the bowl. Work into the top soil layer. Apply every six to eight weeks at the rate of 1 teaspoon per 6-inch pot.

➤ **Notes:** Buy cottonseed meal at farm supply stores and some garden centers. Buy bonemeal at garden centers and through mail-order suppliers. See page 444 for other sources.

Soil Mix for Container-Grown Trees and Shrubs

Don't plant potted trees and shrubs in high-humus materials; they decompose over time and aid in soil compaction. The following formula replaces most of the humus in the soil mix with more stable calcined clay and perlite.

Yield: varies by amount of ingredients chosen

INGREDIENTS

45 percent topsoil

10 percent coarse sphagnum peat

25 percent perlite

20 percent calcined clay

SUPPLIES

stirrer

bucket

clean plastic garbage bag (optional)

Combine all ingredients in the bucket and use immediately or store in a plastic garbage bag for later use.

➥ **Notes:** Perlite is simply air-filled granules of volcanic sand. It is sterile and has great water-holding capacity. Buy it at garden centers. Calcined clay is the basis for cat litter. If you use bagged cat litter, be sure to buy plain litter without any additives for odor reduction. Calcined clay is used in turf management at golf courses. Buy it at turf maintenance suppliers.

GOOD IDEA!

Trees and shrubs growing in large containers are difficult to repot. To keep them growing vigorously, try topdressing them at least once a year. Use your fingers or a trowel to scrape off the top 2 or 3 inches of soil mix; replace with fresh mix. Add the old mix to the compost pile.

Trees and Shrubs for Containers

Add a touch of class with a container-grown tree or shrub. Try arborvitae (*Thuja* spp.), azaleas and rhododendrons (*Rhododendron* spp.), bay tree (*Laurus nobilis*), boxwood (*Buxus* spp.), crape myrtle (*Lagerstroemia indica*), dwarf fruit trees, firethorn (*Pyracantha* spp.), Japanese maple (*Acer palmatum*), junipers (*Juniper* spp.), lilacs (*Syringa* cvs.), paperbark maple (*Acer griseum*), and roses (*Rosa* spp.). Some of these plants may not be hardy in your area; check with your local extension agent.

GOOD IDEA!

To provide food for beneficial insects, plant pollen- and nectar-rich flowering plants in your garden. These include yarrow, Queen Anne's lace, daisies, cone-flowers, and many of the herbs, such as dill, fen-nel, parsley, catnip, rose-mary, and thyme.

Beneficial Insect Chow

A well-established method for bringing more benefi-cial insects to your garden is to spray a special food mix-ture onto plants, especially during the times your garden is not completely in bloom. This formula will do the trick.

Yield: about ¾ cup of concentrate, enough for about 1½ gallons of spray

INGREDIENTS

2 tablespoons brewer's yeast

¼ cup sugar

1 tablespoon honey

⅓ cup warm water

SUPPLIES

spoon

small mixing bowl

½-pint storage container with lid

garden spray equipment

☛ **BE SAFE.** Some damage to leaves, especially to grapes, may result from using this spray too frequently. To prevent dam-age, limit spraying to a maximum of two applications, two weeks apart.

Blend all ingredients in the bowl to make a concen-trated paste. You can store the concentrate, tightly covered, for several weeks in the refrigerator.

To make the spray, mix a tablespoon of concentrate with 1 pint water, stirring until completely dissolved. Spray on plants in spring and early summer to bring beneficial in-sects to the garden.

✿ **Variation:** Smear the concentrate on pieces of waxed paper or cardboard and hang them in the garden to attract and feed beneficial insects. Use this technique especially if you have just released purchased green lacewings, ladybugs, or parasitic wasps.

➥ **Note:** Buy brewer's yeast at health food stores.

Houseplant Leaf Polish

Commercial leaf shines or polishes may leave an oily residue that attracts dust. Some aerosol polishes may contain a propellent that actually damages young foliage. One traditional leaf-shine material—plain milk—is safe and certainly inexpensive. You can also make the following leaf-shine formula.

Yield: 5 cups

INGREDIENTS

 5 cups warm water
 1 tablespoon laundry soap flakes
 1 tablespoon wheat-germ oil

SUPPLIES

small funnel
1½- to 2-quart spray bottle
clean, soft cloth

☛ **BE SAFE.** Don't use plant polishes on hair-covered leaves like those of the African violets. The polish damages the leaf hairs. Do not use this polish on bromeliads, cacti, or succulents. The polish damages outer leaf structures necessary for maintaining water balance in these plants.

Pour all ingredients into the spray bottle and shake gently to mix. Spray onto leaves and then wipe with a soft cloth.

➻ **Note:** Buy wheat-germ oil at health food stores.

GOOD IDEA!

The crusty white material that appears on top of potted soil mix is from salt and mineral deposits in your water. Leach these materials out of the soil by thoroughly watering the plant, until water runs out of the drainage holes for several minutes. The soil will obviously be saturated for a while after this treatment; wait to do this until the plant needs watering anyway.

Chapter Four

Beauty

by Trisha Thompson

The summer I turned 11, during one long, rainy week, I took up a new hobby—making lip gloss. At the time, lip gloss was the cosmetic rage among teenagers, including my two older sisters. At about $3 a "pot," the brand-name product I craved seemed outrageously expensive to me.

So, I washed out a few of my sisters' empty lip gloss containers, collected some worn-down tubes of lipstick my mother was about to throw out, scraped the lipstick remnants into the little plastic pots, mixed in some petroleum jelly and made my own. For me, it was the beginning of a life-long fascination with make-it-yourself beauty products.

The beauty of homemade skin-care products, bath treatments, and hair conditioners is that they not only cost less than the store-bought variety, but they also offer the advantage of truly customized skin-care in a way that products labeled "oily," "normal," and "dry" cannot. In addition, natural food- and herb-based concoctions are less likely to cause allergic reactions than commercially made products. (Although, if you have very sensitive skin, it's a good idea to test a little of a homemade product on your wrist or under your chin before applying it all over.)

Many of these formulas originate from the practical experience of New York City skin-care expert Lia Schorr. Although Schorr makes and sells her own line of mail-order skin-care products, she gladly offers suggestions for make-it-yourself skin-care formulas to anyone who'll listen. Schorr feels that homemade products are worthwhile, not only for the attributes already discussed here, but also because she believes that making your own products makes personal skin and hair care more pleasurable and relaxing—like a 10-minute spa trip rather than a hasty scrub and dash out the door. Here's hoping that the ideas contained in this chapter leave your skin smooth, your hair soft, and your spirit pampered. Taking the time to mix them is half the fun.

PUT ON A NATURAL FACE

The foundation of any naturally beautiful face is glowing, healthy skin. The formulas that follow lead you through a good basic skin-care routine that you can adapt to suit your skin type—oily, normal, dry, or mixed.

Facial Steamer

Whether you have oily, normal, or dry skin, you can benefit from a weekly facial steaming. The herbs in this formula can be strained, saved, and reused.

Yield: 1 treatment

INGREDIENTS

¼ cup (or a handful) dried chamomile flowers
    or 3 bags chamomile tea
½ quart boiling water

SUPPLIES

1-quart bowl
2 large towels
teapot

☛ **BE SAFE.** *Never steam your face closer than 1 foot from the bowl.*

Place the bowl on top of a towel-covered surface in a place where you can sit comfortably. Place chamomile in the bowl and pour boiling water over it. Using the second towel as a tent over your head, steam your face about 1 foot from the water. The towel tent traps steam; if it gets too hot, allow some steam to escape. Keep your eyes closed and inhale the herbal scent. Steam your face for about 10 minutes.

➠ **Note:** *Buy dried chamomile flowers at health food stores and herb shops. Buy chamomile tea in the herbal tea section of supermarkets.*

GOOD IDEA!

Steaming your face opens pores so that trapped dirt can be washed away. In an herbal facial steamer, steam does all the work; the herbs add a pleasurable scent—good for the spirit as well as the skin. Good herbs for steaming include dried or fresh mint, lavender, and rosemary. The herbs can be strained, saved, and reused.

Be sure to wash your face and remove makeup before steaming. For extra moisturizing, apply petroleum jelly to your lips.

For best results with any facial mask, first steam your face. Use steam plus a mask treatment about once a week.

Yogurt/Oil Cleansing Routine for All Skin Types

In the morning, use the yogurt alone. In the evening, remove makeup first with the oil, then cleanse with yogurt.

SUPPLIES

cold-pressed vegetable oil such as olive, safflower, or avocado

cotton pads or cotton balls

plain yogurt

Remove makeup by massaging a few drops of oil all over your face and neck and then wiping clean with dampened cotton pads or cotton balls. Repeat until all traces of makeup are gone.

Dampen skin, and massage in enough yogurt to cover your face and neck, concentrating on your forehead, nose, and chin. Rinse thoroughly with warm water.

Cucumber and Milk Cleanser for Dry Skin

You may store this formula in the refrigerator for up to a week. Before cleansing, remove makeup with cold-pressed vegetable oil such as olive, safflower, or avocado.

Yield: about 1 cup, enough for 1 week

INGREDIENTS

1 cucumber, peeled and cut into chunks

¼ to ½ cup whole milk

SUPPLIES

blender or food processor

sieve or cheesecloth

bowl

clean jar or bottle with lid

cotton pads or cotton balls

In the blender or food processor, liquefy cucumber. To remove seeds, pour blended cucumber through the sieve or cheesecloth into the bowl. Mix equal parts cucumber juice and milk in the bottle. Apply to skin with cotton pads or cotton balls and then rinse with cool water. Store, tightly sealed, in the refrigerator.

Sugar Scrub for Oily Skin

The purpose of any facial scrubbing agent is to slough off dead cells that make skin look dull and flaky. For oily skin, the sloughing agent should also help control oil buildup and clogged pores. Although several other gentle abrasives work well, sugar in this formula has an anti-bacterial effect—a plus for acne-prone skin.

Yield: 1 scrub

INGREDIENTS

1 tablespoon white sugar
1 teaspoon tepid water

☛ **BE SAFE.** Don't apply this or any other scrub to acne-inflamed areas—it will only worsen the condition. Don't use any scrub more often than every other day.

With sugar in the palm of your hand, add water drop by drop to make a paste. Using your fingertips, gently massage the scrub over your face and neck, avoiding the eye area. Rinse well with warm and then cool water.

✿ **Variation:** Good substitutes for the sugar include yellow cornmeal, sea salt (not iodized salt), and dry yeast.

GOOD IDEA!

Always make scrubs and masks just before using. When massaging a scrub into your skin, use a lighter touch than you would to apply anything else to your face.

Honey-Almond Scrub/Mask for Normal-to-Dry Skin

The almond meal in this formula very gently removes dead cells while the honey acts as a natural humectant, or moisture trapper.

Yield: 1 scrub/mask

INGREDIENTS

1 tablespoon unsalted, unroasted almonds
1 tablespoon honey
1 egg white

SUPPLIES

blender or food processor
small bowl
spoon

☛ **BE SAFE.** Don't apply this or any other scrub to acne-inflamed areas—it will only worsen the condition. Don't use any scrub more often than every other day.

In the blender or food processor, grind almonds into a fine meal, stopping short of pulverizing them into powder. In the bowl, mix almond meal with honey and egg white. Apply the mixture to your face and neck with your fingertips, massaging gently in circular motions. Let set for 15 minutes, then rinse with warm water.

Banana-Cream Mask for Normal-to-Dry Skin

A rich, deliciously scented mask (and a good use for an overripe banana).

Yield: 1 mask

INGREDIENTS

½ banana
1 tablespoon honey
2 tablespoons sour cream

SUPPLIES

fork
small bowl

Mash banana in the bowl and add honey and sour cream. Blend well. Apply to skin and leave on for 10 minutes. Rinse with warm water.

Cucumber Toner for All Skin Types

The main purpose of a toner is to remove the last traces of cleanser from your face. This toner can be modified for dry or oily skin.

Yield: about ½ cup

INGREDIENTS

½ cucumber, peeled and cut into chunks
¼ cup water

SUPPLIES

blender or food processor
sieve or cheesecloth
small bowl
clean jar or bottle with lid
cotton pads or cotton balls

> **GOOD IDEA!**
>
> **A**vocado makes a **wonderful mask for normal-to-dry skin.** The next time you're peeling an avocado, leave a little of the fruit on the inside of the avocado skin. Then rub the inside of the peel over your face. The gritty texture of the peel sloughs dead skin while the fruit you leave behind moisturizes. Allow the mask to set for 10 minutes. Rinse with cool water.

> **GOOD IDEA!**
>
> **T**ake care when **choosing a skin toner.** A good toner should not be so astringent that it dries skin. Never use straight rubbing alcohol as a toner (not even on oily skin); it's too harsh.

(continued)

In the blender or food processor, liquefy cucumber. To remove seeds, strain blended cucumber through the sieve or cheesecloth into the bowl. Mix cucumber juice with water in the bottle. After cleansing but before applying moisturizer, apply the toner with cotton pads or cotton balls, and don't rinse off. Refrigerate toner for up to a week.

✿ **Variation:** For oily skin, add a few drops of fresh lemon juice; for dry skin, add a few drops of olive oil.

Apple-Cider Vinegar Toner for All Skin Types

Use this toner to remove traces of cleanser before applying moisturizer. The apple-cider vinegar in this toner helps restore skin to its proper pH (acid/alkaline) balance. Use less vinegar for dry skin, and use more vinegar for oily skin.

Yield: 2 cups

INGREDIENTS

½ to 1 teaspoon apple-cider vinegar
2 cups water

SUPPLIES

spoon
clean jar or bottle with lid
cotton pads or cotton balls

Stir vinegar into water in the bottle. After cleansing to remove makeup, saturate cotton pads or cotton balls with toner and wipe your face. You may store this toner in a tightly closed container in the refrigerator.

✿ **Variations:** Substitute vodka for apple-cider vinegar. Witch hazel straight from the bottle also makes a good, gentle toner.

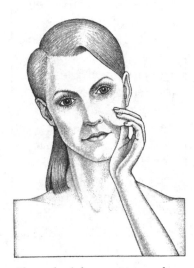

If you don't have cotton pads, use cotton balls. Cotton pads are preferred because they are thicker (fewer are needed), but they are more expensive. If you opt for the cotton balls, try stacking two or three to get the same effect as a pad.

Super-Rich Facial Moisturizer for Dry Skin

The purest, simplest oils make the best moisturizers.

Yield: about ¼ cup

INGREDIENTS

1 tablespoon olive oil
1 tablespoon corn oil
1 teaspoon almond oil
2 teaspoons water

SUPPLIES

stirrer
clean jar with lid

Mix all ingredients in the jar. Refrigerate to solidify. Allow to soften a bit at room temperature before applying with fingertips to dry areas.

Pre-Bath Skin-Moisturizing Treatment

Apply oil before bathing for better moisturizing.

Yield: 1 treatment

INGREDIENTS

sea salt (optional)
2 or 3 drops water (optional)
3 to 4 tablespoons olive oil

☛ **BE SAFE.** *Be careful in the tub—oil makes it slick.*

If desired, make a paste of sea salt and water in the palm of your hand. As bathwater is running, massage the paste into particularly rough and flaky areas of skin. Rinse and pat skin dry. Apply oil to all dry skin areas, like feet and elbows. Soaking will encourage the oil to further penetrate dry skin. Bathe as usual, pat dry, and follow with lotion.

GOOD IDEA!

Dry skin relief is as close as your nearest food store. Pure safflower margarine (available in health food stores), good-quality mayonnaise, and any cold-pressed, pure vegetable oil (olive, safflower, or avocado) all make excellent moisturizers for dry skin. The margarine and olive oil are especially easy for skin to absorb.

GOOD IDEA!

To make your bath special, place herbs in a square of cheesecloth. Tie the cheesecloth like a sachet and toss it into the running water. For a stimulating bath, make the water a little cool (92°F is optimum) and fill the sachet with lemon verbena, mint, or sage. For a relaxing bath, make the water body temperature and fill the sachet with catnip, lavender, or rosemary.

MAKE IT BEAUTIFUL YOURSELF

There's no need to get out your checkbook the next time you're out of moisturizer or cleansing cream. You have everything you need right in your own kitchen or pantry. Use this table to make no-fuss beauty-care products.

PANTRY-WISE BEAUTY CARE How to Make Beauty Products at Home		
Use This Household Item	**To Make This Beauty Product**	**Quick Instructions**
Apple-cider vinegar	Toner	Mix 1 tsp. vinegar and 2 cups water; apply after cleansing and before moisturizing.
Avocado	Facial-moisturizing mask	Rub inside of peel over clean face, leave on 10 minutes, rinse with cool water.
Cucumber	Facial cleanser, toner, moisturizer	For cleanser, mix pureed cucumber with ½ cup milk; for toner, mix with ¼ cup water; for moisturizer, mix with ¼ cup water plus a few drops of olive oil, don't rinse.
Hydrogen peroxide	Bleach for stained nails	Apply with cotton pads to bare nails to bleach polish stains.
Lemon juice	Facial toner, bleach for stained nails	For skin toner, mix 1 Tbs. juice with 2 cups water; apply with cotton pads after cleansing and before moisturizing. For nail bleach, use same as hydrogen peroxide.
Milk of magnesia	Healing and drying agent for acne blemishes	Apply with cotton pads after cleansing; dab lightly on blemishes, let dry, rinse with cool water.
Oatmeal	Exfoliating facial scrub, bath soak	For scrub, mix handful with water to make paste; massage into clean skin; rinse with cool water. For bath soak, add ¼ cup to running bath; shower afterward.
Olive oil	Makeup remover, moisturizer	Massage a few drops into face; wipe with damp cotton pads. For moisturizer, don't rinse.
Plain yogurt	Skin cleanser; also a soother for mild sunburn	Remove makeup with olive oil; massage yogurt into dampened skin, rinse with warm water.
Safflower margarine	Skin moisturizer	Soften at room temperature; after cleansing, massage into skin in a thin layer, don't rinse.
Witch hazel	Mild toner	Apply with cotton pads after cleansing and before moisturizing.

Basic Body Lotion for All Skin Types

If you have very dry skin, this lotion may be useful only during warm weather months when skin is less dry. During winter months, those with very dry skin may need to make frequent use of the "Super-Rich Facial Moisturizer for Dry Skin" and "Pre-Bath Skin-Moisturizing Treatment" on page 159.

Yield: about ¾ cup

INGREDIENTS

1   cucumber, peeled and cut into chunks
¼   cup barely warm chamomile tea
2   tablespoons glycerin

SUPPLIES

blender or food processor
sieve or cheesecloth
small bowl
spoon
clean jar or bottle with lid

In the blender or food processor, liquefy cucumber. To remove seeds, strain through the sieve or cheesecloth into the bowl. Add tea to the cucumber juice along with glycerin, stirring well. When mixture is cool, bottle and refrigerate. Apply to skin after a bath or shower; don't rinse off.

➺ **Note:** *Buy glycerin at most pharmacies.*

GOOD IDEA!

One of the best ways to moisturize dry skin is from the inside out. Be sure to drink plenty of water—six to eight glasses each day is ideal. You can also eat foods with high water content, such as leafy vegetables, salad greens, and fruit.

Another way to battle dry skin is to make sure the environment in your home isn't too dry. You can combat the drying effects of your home's heating system with room humidifiers.

GOOD IDEA!

To nourish hair, break open four to six vitamin E oil capsules and stir into a bottle of store-bought shampoo.

Egg and Oil Hair Conditioner

If your hair is very dry or damaged, repeat this treatment once a week for a month.

Yield: 1 treatment

SUPPLIES

2 tablespoons olive oil

small bowl

whisk

1 egg yolk

shower cap

Using your fingertips, massage oil into the scalp. In a bowl, beat the egg yolk, then apply it to hair working from the ends up but not into the scalp. Put on a shower cap and shower as usual. Then, remove cap and shampoo hair.

Better Hair Care

To get the most out of your hair-cleansing ritual, start by brushing your hair to loosen dirt. But, don't believe the old wives' tale that brushing your hair 100 strokes at bedtime every night is good. Too much brushing can cause brittle hair and split ends.

Hard brushing strips away the outer cells, exposing the soft inner core of the hair shaft. This makes it more susceptible to damage. Remember to use a light touch when brushing your hair; try not to tug or pull at it.

To shampoo after brushing, wet your hair well with warm water. Instead of applying shampoo directly to your head, mix it with an equal amount of water in your hands, then work it through your hair, separating the hair with your fingers as you gently lather. Rinse thoroughly—for at least 1 minute—to avoid dulling effects of shampoo.

When your hair is wet, don't brush it—it stretches easily and readily snaps and breaks. Gentle combing is actually the best method for grooming.

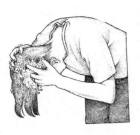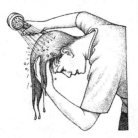

Warm-Oil Scalp Treatment

Many people mistakenly believe that dandruff is the result of oily or dirty hair. Actually, this condition is most often caused by an overly dry scalp.

Yield: 1 treatment

SUPPLIES

2 to 3 tablespoons olive oil or other vegetable oil

small glass measuring cup

saucepan

cotton pads or cotton balls

Place oil in the measuring cup. Fill the saucepan with 1 or 2 inches of hot tap water. Place the measuring cup in the saucepan so that the oil in the cup is heated gently by the surrounding hot water. Place the entire oil treatment apparatus on a low table or counter with a mirror handy. Part your hair in several spots and, using cotton pads or cotton balls, apply a small amount of warm oil to your scalp. Massage lightly into entire scalp. After a few hours, shampoo hair as usual; rinse thoroughly.

GOOD IDEA!

Oil treatments for the scalp should be warm, not hot. Schedule your oil treatment for early evening to allow time for the oil to moisturize the scalp and be shampooed out before bed.

Chapter Five

Health

by Michael Castleman

People got headaches thousands of years before the development of today's popular headache remedies. They became constipated long before the creation of laxatives. They developed hemorrhoids centuries before Preparation H. And they suffered anxiety and insomnia long before tranquilizers.

What did they do? Most grew ingredients and prepared formulas just like the ones used in this chapter. And what did the doctors of yesteryear recommend for most common medical complaints? In many cases, they, too, relied on formulas similar to the ones here. In fact, many doctors maintained medicinal herb gardens right outside their examining rooms, and on trips to visit sick patients, stopped to collect healing plants they encountered along roadsides.

How did city folk do without medicinal herb gardens? They went to their local pharmacists, whose shops looked more like herb shops than modern drug dispensaries. In fact, early pharmacists spent so much time drying and grinding herbs with mortars and pestles that these implements became the universal symbol of pharmacy.

Our great-grandparents used herbal formulas not only because they were the only treatment available but also because *they worked*. Modern scientific studies have lent support to the effectiveness of the herbal remedies in this chapter. In fact, many of our modern-day drugs and foods were originally created from the herbal medicines cited in the following pages.

- The decongestant in Sudafed, pseudoephedrine, is similar to the active ingredient in Chinese ephedra, recommended here for asthma and other respiratory complaints.
- About 150 years ago, German chemists extracted a substance similar to aspirin from white willow bark and meadowsweet. In fact, meadowsweet's old scientific name, *Spirea*, gave us the "spirin" in aspirin.
- Parsley has been used as a breath freshener since ancient history days. Today, we know that parsley is rich in the breath-deodorizing chemical chlorophyll. Chlorophyll is the "clor" in Clorets and one of the active ingredients in Certs.

- Honey was recommended as a wound treatment in the Bible. Recent research has shown that it does, indeed, help prevent wound infections, and some surgeons now cover surgical incisions with a layer of honey.
- Several of today's soft drinks also started out as practical medicinal formulas. During Shakespeare's day, the British drank ginger ale, still widely used today as a home remedy for indigestion.

Unfortunately, most Americans—including the vast majority of physicians—have no idea that many over-the-counter drugs and familiar consumer products began as home remedies similar to the ones presented here. So, some young doctors might blanch if you say you'd rather brew a cup of meadowsweet tea than take two aspirin. But older physicians tend to take a more tolerant view of herbal healing. They still remember the days when bottles of tinctures lined pharmacy shelves and when clove oil was used to ease the pain of a toothache.

How to Use This Chapter

Many of the formulas in this chapter use "hot-water extracts" of healing herbs. Tea is a hot-water extract, but the medicinal formulas here are *not* teas. To make tea, you dunk leaves in hot water for a few moments to flavor it, then drink the resulting beverage. Medicinal hot-water extracts are much stronger and should *not* be considered beverages for casual use.

Although they are not always described as such, the hot-water extracts in this chapter fall into two categories: "infusions" and "decoctions." Both begin with boiling water, but infusions and decoctions are not prepared in exactly the same way.

Infusions are hot-water extracts from the leaves, stems, and flowers of medicinal plants. Unlike teas, which steep for only a few minutes, infusions steep for 10 to 20 minutes—the longer, the stronger. Before drinking, you may prefer to strain the plant material through a tea ball or fine mesh strainer. Since you don't heat an infusion as it steeps, it often cools to room temperature before it's ready. You may reheat it, but don't boil. Boiling causes loss of some medicinal value.

Decoctions are hot-water extracts from the bark and roots of medicinal plants. But unlike infusions, decoctions simmer over low heat during the extraction time. Again, you may strain the plant material before drinking.

Most medicinal infusions and decoctions taste quite bitter and unpleasant. This annoying characteristic is just Mother Nature's way of discouraging people from casual use. Feel free to add honey and/or lemon to taste.

SKIN CARE

Blisters. Burns. Stings. Rashes. Itches. Bites. Our outer armor is prey to more everyday slings and arrows than Hägar the Horrible encounters in an entire year of Viking wars. Before you head off to the drug store for the latest cream, spray, or oil, check the following pages.

Acne Prevention Facial

Use this formula to help keep your face pimple-proof. Goldenseal has some antibacterial properties, and basil has also been shown effective against acne.

Yield: 1 cup

INGREDIENTS

1 cup water
1 teaspoon powdered basil leaves
1 teaspoon powdered goldenseal root

SUPPLIES

saucepan
washcloth

☛ **BE SAFE.** If a rash or any unusual irritation develops, discontinue use. For severe or persistent acne, consult your physician.

Bring water to a boil in the saucepan. Add basil and goldenseal. Turn the heat off and steep for 10 to 20 minutes. To open facial pores, apply a warm washcloth to your face. Then dip the washcloth in the basil/goldenseal infusion and apply generously. After several applications, rinse your face with cool water to close pores.

➥ **Note:** Buy basil and goldenseal from herb shops and health food stores. See page 444 for other sources.

GOOD IDEA!

Combine a facial for acne with a relaxing shower. First prepare a warm infusion and place it on a counter in your bathroom. Since a steamy hot shower will also open your facial pores, you can apply the infusion to your face immediately after you step out of the shower.

Popped Pimple Remedy

Most physicians advise against popping acne pimples because of the risk of scarring and the possibility of spreading bacterial infection to surrounding tissue. But few acne sufferers can resist the temptation to open full whiteheads.

This formula utilizes a tincture, an alcohol extraction that not only carries the herbal oils, but also disinfects the popped pimple. The uva ursi, an astringent, helps close the wound. And the comfrey helps spur the growth of healthy new skin. Since this tincture takes around six weeks to reach its full strength, those with frequent acne outbreaks should make a new tincture before the old one runs out.

Yield: about ½ cup

INGREDIENTS

1 ounce powdered uva ursi leaves

1 ounce powdered comfrey root

5 ounces 100-proof vodka

SUPPLIES

dark-colored glass jar or bottle with lid

clean cloth

☛ **BE SAFE.** If a rash or any unusual irritation develops, discontinue use. For severe or persistent acne, consult your physician.

To make the tincture, add uva ursi and comfrey to vodka in the jar. Seal tightly. Store out of direct sunlight for about six weeks, shaking every few days. The formula reaches its full strength and effectiveness at the end of the storage time.

To use the tincture, wash your hands with soap and water before opening pimples. Apply a tincture-soaked cloth to newly opened pimples.

➥ **Note:** Buy uva ursi and comfrey at most health food stores and herb shops. See page 444 for other sources.

GOOD IDEA!

Prevent alcohol stains on your furniture. Some tincture jars will release alcohol no matter how well you seal them. Don't store tincture-filled jars on valuable furniture.

GOOD IDEA!

To remember the full-strength date of a tincture, label the bottle with the date before your store it. Many tinctures must rest in a cool, dark place for several weeks before they reach their full potential. If stored in a tightly sealed jar, most tinctures will last for several months.

Athlete's Foot Treatment

The term *athlete's foot* is a misnomer. This fungal infection strikes the feet of couch potatoes as well as athletes. The fungus thrives in damp darkness, which is why it loves sweaty feet encased in socks inside shoes. Physicians recommend that athlete's foot sufferers keep their feet dry and use over-the-counter antifungal ointments or powders. This formula uses cornstarch to dry the feet and antifungal herbs applied in a tincture (alcohol solution). Since the tincture takes around two weeks to reach its full strength, make and store a new tincture before the old one runs out.

Yield: about ½ cup

INGREDIENTS

20 to 30 cloves garlic, minced
2 to 4 teaspoons ground cinnamon
2 to 4 teaspoons powdered cloves
5 ounces 100-proof vodka

SUPPLIES

dark-colored glass jar or bottle with lid
cotton balls or clean cloth
cornstarch

☛ **BE SAFE.** If a rash or any unusual irritation develops, discontinue use. If athlete's foot symptoms persist after two weeks of home treatment, consult your physician.

To make the tincture, add garlic, cinnamon, and cloves to vodka in the jar. Seal tightly, store out of direct sunlight for two weeks, shaking to mix every few days. The tincture is ready to use at the end of two weeks.

To treat athlete's foot, use cotton balls or a cloth to apply the tincture to the entire sole of the foot as well as between all the toes. Apply twice a day, morning and night. Let dry, then dust the entire foot with cornstarch.

Boil-Fighting Formula

Boils are bacterial skin infections that may grow quite large and spread. This formula may act to fight infection.

Yield: 1 cup

INGREDIENTS

- 1 cup water
- 2 teaspoons powdered echinacea root
- 10 to 15 cloves garlic, minced
- 1 teaspoon powdered goldenseal root
  honey and/or lemon, to taste

SUPPLIES

saucepan

fine strainer

☛ **BE SAFE.** Pregnant or nursing women should not use this formula without first consulting a physician. Otherwise healthy adults may use up to 3 cups a day. Do not give to children under 2. Older children and those over 65 should use extra water to reduce formula strength. The younger the child, the more dilute the formula should be. Echinacea may cause tingling of the tongue. This is normal and not hazardous. If headache, rash, stomach distress, or other unpleasant effects develop, discontinue use. Use this formula only in consultation with your physician. Do not break boils. Apply warm compresses until the boil breaks naturally. For care of opened boils, see "Honey Treatment for Boils or Burns" on page 170.

Bring water to a boil in the saucepan. Simmer echinacea for 10 to 15 minutes on low heat. Turn the heat off and add garlic and goldenseal. Steep 10 to 20 minutes. Strain. Add honey and/or lemon. Drink cool or reheat.

➔ **Note:** Buy echinacea and goldenseal at health food stores and herb shops. See page 444 for other sources.

GOOD IDEA!

To prevent boils, try antiseptic soap. Boils are usually caused by Staphylococcus bacteria that infect a blocked oil gland or hair follicle. If you're prone to boils, you may be able to lessen their frequency by washing your skin with an antiseptic soap like Betadine.

Boils also occur as the result of infection in a skin cyst. If you have a cyst, don't monkey around with it; you're only courting infection. Leave cysts alone or have them excised by a doctor.

Honey Treatment for Boils or Burns

Treat boils by applying warm compresses until they rupture naturally. When the boil ruptures, it releases the debris of dead cells plus the bacteria that caused the infection. To disinfect opened boils and to prevent the bacteria from spreading, wash the area carefully with soap and water. In addition, apply a honey-based salve made from 2 tablespoons honey mixed with 2 tablespoons aloe vera gel and 1 teaspoon powdered comfrey root.

Honey has been used as a wound treatment since biblical times. Research shows honey acts as an infection-fighting antiseptic. Comfrey and aloe vera gel encourage wound healing. You may also apply the honey salve to the skin to prevent infection in minor burns. (See page 173 for first-aid hints for burns.) In any case, if a honey salve causes a rash or skin irritation, discontinue use and be sure to see a physician.

5-Step Formula for Insect Stings

Ah, summer! Picnics. Ball games. Swimming. The Fourth of July. And all too often, bee, wasp, and yellow jacket stings. If you get stung, this formula will help minimize your pain and suffering.

Yield: 1 treatment

INGREDIENTS

1 cup water
1 teaspoon powdered meadowsweet leaves
2 to 3 teaspoons powdered chamomile flowers
   honey and/or lemon, to taste

SUPPLIES

clean pocketknife or credit card
soap and water
meat tenderizer
ice cubes or commercial gel cold pack
clean cloth
saucepan
fine strainer

☛ **BE SAFE.** Pregnant or nursing women should not use the meadowsweet infusion. Otherwise healthy adults may use up to 3 cups a day. Do not give this infusion to children under 2. Older children and those over 65 should use extra water to reduce formula strength. The younger the child, the more dilute the formula should be. Meadowsweet may cause stomach distress in those with aspirin-sensitive stomachs. If headache, rash, or other unpleasant effects develop, discontinue use. Do not place ice, or commercial ice substitutes, directly on the skin. Always wrap them in cloth. Use this formula only in consultation with your physician. In addition, some people are extremely allergic to insect venom and may develop a potentially fatal reaction (anaphylaxis) within a few minutes after being stung. Symptoms include labored breathing, rapid pulse, and faintness. If any of these develop, go to an emergency room without delay.

Step 1: Remove the stinger. When insects sting, they often leave the stinger and venom sack embedded in the skin. If you attempt to pull it out with fingers or tweezers, you may squeeze more venom into the wound. Instead scrape the stinger out with the pocketknife or credit card.

Step 2: Wash the sting with soap and water to minimize the risk of infection.

Step 3: To hasten the chemical breakdown of venom, generously sprinkle meat tenderizer on the wound.

Step 4: Wrap the ice cubes or gel pack in a cloth and apply to the wound for 20 minutes. Take a 10-minute break before reapplying. Replace the ice cubes as they melt.

Step 5: Sip a meadowsweet/chamomile infusion to reduce pain and inflammation. Bring water to a boil in the saucepan. Add meadowsweet and chamomile and remove from heat. Steep 10 to 20 minutes. Strain. Add honey and/or lemon. Drink cool or reheat.

➾ **Note:** Buy meadowsweet and chamomile at most health food stores and herb shops. See page 444 for other sources.

GOOD IDEA!

To soothe a bee sting quickly, apply fresh papaya to the sting. Meat tenderizer, the traditional sting remedy, contains papaya extract. Fresh papaya works just as well. The enzyme in papaya breaks down the proteins that make up insect venom. For maximum effectiveness, apply this remedy as soon as possible after being stung.

GOOD IDEA!

To prevent and treat dishpan hands, keep your hands out of water as much as possible. Wash one large load of dishes rather than several small ones. Vinyl gloves alone don't help—not even the ones with cotton lining—because once the lining becomes wet from hand perspiration or water, it aggravates the problem.

To heal dishpan hands, many physicians recommend the three-layer approach—petroleum jelly directly on the skin, cotton gloves over both hands, and vinyl gloves over the cotton gloves whenever hands must be immersed in water.

Dishpan-Hands Soother

This formula soothes dishpan hands. The meadowsweet infusion is an herbal aspirin that may help relieve the pain and inflammation of this condition.

Yield: 1 treatment

INGREDIENTS

1 cup water
1 teaspoon powdered meadowsweet leaves and flower tops
honey and/or lemon, to taste

SUPPLIES

petroleum jelly
6 pairs cotton gloves
2 pairs vinyl gloves
saucepan
fine strainer

☛ **BE SAFE.** If skin symptoms do not abate within two weeks, consult your physician. Pregnant or nursing women should not use the meadowsweet infusion. Otherwise healthy adults may use up to 3 cups a day. Do not give this infusion to children under 2. Older children and those over 65 should use extra water to reduce formula strength. The younger the child, the more dilute the formula should be. Meadowsweet may cause stomach distress in those with aspirin-sensitive stomachs. If headache, rash, or other unpleasant effects develop, discontinue use. Use this formula only in consultation with your physician.

Apply a thin layer of petroleum jelly to inflamed hands as often as needed. Cover with cotton gloves and wear all day. Change cotton gloves as soon as they become damp. Before immersing your hands in water, cover the cotton gloves with vinyl gloves. Change vinyl gloves periodically to allow the insides to dry.

To help reduce pain and inflammation of dishpan hands, bring water to a boil in the saucepan and add mead-

owsweet. Remove from heat. Steep 10 to 20 minutes.
Strain. Add honey and/or lemon. Drink cool or reheat.

→ **Note:** *Buy meadowsweet at most health food stores and herb shops. See page 444 for other sources.*

First-Aid for Minor Burns

Physicians classify burns as being first, second, or third degree. First-degree burns cause pain and skin inflammation. Second-degree burns cause greater pain, more inflammation, and blistering. Third-degree burns usually cause no pain because pain-sensing nerves have been destroyed; these burns leave the skin looking charred or white. Third-degree burns are always a medical emergency. Do not attempt home treatment. Also, all facial and genital burns require professional care regardless of the severity of the burn. Seek medical care for any burn that causes severe pain, for any burn that shows signs of infection, and for any burn that doesn't heal in ten days to two weeks. Adults over 60 or infants under 1 year should be seen by a physician for any burn.

In most other cases, small first- and second-degree burns can usually be treated effectively at home, especially if the burn causes only minor discomfort. The best rule of thumb for home treatment is to treat first- and second-degree burns that are no larger than a quarter on a child and no larger than a silver dollar on an adult.

For burn pain relief, apply a few drops of clove oil directly to the burn with a cotton swab. Repeat every 30 minutes, or as needed. Clove oil is poisonous if ingested, so be sure to keep this remedy locked away from children and pets.

In addition, wrap two ice cubes in a clean cloth to make an ice pack. Apply to the burned area and hold it there. As the ice melts, replace it with fresh cubes. Keep the ice pack in place for 20 minutes, remove it for 10 minutes, then reapply it. Repeat this process as long as pain persists. To prevent infection in minor burns, see page 170, "Honey Treatment for Boils and Burns."

After the initial ice-and-clove-oil treatment, you may wish to lightly cover the burn with a gauze pad. Then do nothing for at least 24 hours. Burns should be allowed to begin the healing process on their own. After this 24-hour period, you may wash the injury gently with soap and water or Betadine solution once a day. Two or three days after the injury, break off a piece of fresh aloe and apply the leaf gel directly to the burn. Or squeeze on an over-the-counter aloe cream. Both have an analgesic action that will make your wound feel better. Do not use aloe if you are using blood thinners or have a medical history of heart problems.

When your burn is starting to heal, break open a capsule of vitamin E and rub the liquid into your irritated skin. It will feel good and may prevent scarring. And be sure to leave blisters intact. Those fluid-filled bubbles are nature's own best bandage. If a blister pops, clean the area with soap and water, smooth on a little antibiotic ointment, and cover.

GOOD IDEA!

To prevent sun-fried lips, choose the right lip balm. High sun exposure, no matter whether it's on the ski slope or the beach, damages your lips just as it does the rest of your skin. Treat your lips as carefully as you treat your face. Wear a lipstick or lip balm that contains sunscreen.

Chapped Lips Salve

Dry, cracked lips are often painful and difficult to heal. Most over-the-counter remedies simply use waxes to protect the lips from the drying effects of wind and water. This formula goes further. Aloe vera gel dries to form a protective covering for the lips. And studies show that both comfrey and aloe vera gel help heal injured skin.

Yield: 2 tablespoons

INGREDIENTS

1 teaspoon powdered comfrey root
2 tablespoons aloe vera gel
   honey (optional)

SUPPLIES

spoon
small mixing bowl or cup

☞ **BE SAFE.** If a rash or any unusual irritation develops, discontinue use. Do not swallow aloe vera gel. It tastes extremely bitter, and large amounts taken internally have a powerful laxative effect. Use this formula only in consultation with your physician.

Thoroughly combine comfrey and aloe vera gel in the bowl or cup. Apply a thin coating to the lips. Since aloe tastes very bitter, you may add enough honey to the mixture to make it palatable.

➥ **Notes:** Aloe vera gel works best fresh from the plant. Simply snip off part of a fleshy leaf, cut it open, and scoop out the gel. If you don't have an aloe vera plant, buy aloe vera, as well as comfrey, at health food stores and herb shops. Unprocessed aloe vera gel is more effective than the "stabilized" variety. See page 444 for other sources.

Diaper Rash Reliever

Diaper rash is caused by, among other things, the ammonia in urine coming in contact with baby's skin. In severe cases, the rash becomes complicated by yeast fungus, which grows in the warm, moist creases of the baby's bottom. You can recognize yeast infection by a characteristic baking-bread aroma.

To help keep the skin dry and prevent the growth of yeast, leave your baby diaperless as often as possible. The cornstarch in this formula also helps keep the skin dry, and the powdered chamomile can help control fungus.

Yield: about 4 ounces

INGREDIENTS

¼ cup cornstarch

2 tablespoons finely powdered chamomile flowers

SUPPLIES

hammer

small nail

1 small jar with lid, such as a baby food jar

☛ **BE SAFE.** If the rash becomes worse, or if additional irritation develops, discontinue use. Use this formula only in consultation with your baby's physician.

Add cornstarch and chamomile to the jar, cover, and shake to mix. Remove lid and use the hammer and nail to poke small holes in it. Replace the lid. At every diaper changing, shake the mixture on baby's bottom until evenly dusted with a thin coating.

➡ **Note:** Buy chamomile at health food stores and herb shops. See page 444 for other sources.

GOOD IDEA!

To keep cornstarch in homemade baby powder free flowing, add a few tablespoons of uncooked white rice to the shaker. The rice absorbs moisture from the air and prevents the powder from clumping.

To help fight fungus, add powdered chamomile. Powdered chamomile will keep for several months if stored out of direct sunlight in a tightly sealed container.

GOOD IDEA!

Make an itch-soothing soap substitute with colloidal oatmeal. Simply wrap a handful of colloidal oatmeal in a handkerchief and wrap a rubber band around the top. Dunk the oatmeal-filled handkerchief in water, wring it out, and use as you would a normal washcloth.

You can make your own colloidal oatmeal by grinding dry oatmeal in a coffee grinder or mini-food processor. Any oatmeal will do—slow-cooking, quick-cooking, or instant.

Itch Relief Formula

Mosquito bites. Flea bites. Poison ivy, oak, and sumac. Doctors often recommend antihistamines for itchy skin, but before you pop pills, try this more natural formula. Stinging nettle has antihistamine properties. Baking soda and oatmeal soothe itchy skin.

Yield: 1 cup infusion; 1 skin treatment

INGREDIENTS
FOR INFUSION

1 cup water
1 to 2 teaspoons powdered stinging nettle leaves and stems
  honey and/or lemon, to taste

INGREDIENTS
FOR SKIN TREATMENT

1 teaspoon water
1 tablespoon baking soda
2 to 4 cups colloidal oatmeal

SUPPLIES

saucepan
fine strainer

☛ **BE SAFE.** Pregnant or nursing women should not use the stinging nettle infusion without first consulting a physician. Otherwise healthy adults may use up to 2 cups a day. Do not give to children under 2. Older children and adults over 65 should use extra water to reduce formula strength. The younger the child, the more dilute the formula should be. In large amounts, stinging nettle may cause stomach irritation, burning skin, and urinary suppression. If any of these symptoms develop, discontinue use. If itching persists or becomes worse, or if rash or irritation develops, discontinue use. Use this formula only in consultation with your physician.

To make the stinging nettle infusion, bring water to a boil in the saucepan and add stinging nettle. Remove from heat. Steep 10 to 20 minutes. Strain. Add honey and/or lemon. Drink cool or reheat.

To make the baking soda paste, add water to baking soda in the palm of your hand and spread onto itching area. Allow to dry like calamine lotion. Repeat as needed.

For the oatmeal bath, add oatmeal to bathwater as the tub fills.

✿ **Variations:** For a thicker oatmeal bath, use an extra 1 to 2 cups colloidal oatmeal. You can also add baking soda to your oatmeal bath for additional soothing action.

➵ **Notes:** Buy colloidal oatmeal at pharmacies and health food stores. Buy stinging nettle at health food stores and herb shops. See page 444 for other sources.

Poison Ivy, Oak, and Sumac

Poison ivy grows everywhere in the United States except Nevada, California, and southern Oregon. Eastern poison oak grows in the Southeast from Maryland to east Texas. Western poison oak grows along the West Coast. And poison sumac grows east of the Mississippi. The best way to deal with these plants—and the red, itchy, blistery rash they cause—is to be able to identify them in all seasons and avoid them like the plague they are.

But if one of these pesky plants gets the better of you, temporary relief may be only a hot shower away. As soon as you notice your itch level rising, run hot water on the affected area, as hot as you can stand. "This may seem counterintuitive, as heat increases itching and cold soothes it," says home remedy authority Andrew Weil, M.D., author of *Natural Health, Natural Medicine,* "but trust me. Under hot water, the itching briefly becomes very intense, then it stops for several hours, as if the nerves responsible for conveying the sensation to the brain become overloaded and quit. As soon as itching starts again, use more hot water. If you do this conscientiously, your skin will return to normal much faster than it would otherwise."

And if you can't jump into the shower every few hours, try baking soda or colloidal oatmeal for temporary itch relief. Mix 3 tablespoons baking soda with 1 tablespoon water and cover the rash with a thin layer of the paste. Aveeno, the most popular brand of colloidal oatmeal, is available in many pharmacies and comes with instructions for application.

Sunburn-Soothing Bath

The best way to deal with sunburns is avoid them. Year-round, wear sunscreen whenever you're out in the sun. Sun reflected off snow can give horrendous sunburns. Wear protective clothing, and be extra careful during peak burning hours from 10 A.M. to 3 P.M.

But if you do get burned, this formula may help relieve the sting.

Yield: 1 bath

INGREDIENTS

2 to 4 cups colloidal oatmeal
½ to 1 cup baking soda
1 to 2 cups powdered chamomile flowers

SUPPLIES

cheesecloth (optional)
rubber band (optional)

☛ **BE SAFE.** If a rash or any unusual irritation develops, discontinue use. Use this formula only in consultation with your physician.

As the bathwater runs, add oatmeal, baking soda, and chamomile. Or add just oatmeal and baking soda. With a rubber band, tie chamomile in the cheesecloth and allow the water to run over it. Repeat as needed.

➡ **Notes:** Buy colloidal oatmeal at pharmacies and health food stores. Buy chamomile at health food stores and herb shops. See page 444 for other sources.

Super Sunburn Soother

This formula boosts the skin-soothing action of regular commercial skin moisturizer.

Yield: 1 cup

INGREDIENTS

1 bottle commercial, nonmedicated skin-moisturizing lotion (8 ounces)

5 drops clove oil

5 drops peppermint oil

2 to 4 teaspoons powdered comfrey root

2 to 4 tablespoons aloe vera gel

SUPPLIES

small mixing bowl

stirrer

☛ **BE SAFE.** If a rash or any unusual irritation develops, discontinue use. Never ingest clove or peppermint oils. Small amounts—less than a teaspoon—may cause a possibly fatal poisoning. Use this formula only in consultation with your physician.

Place skin lotion in the bowl. Add remaining ingredients and blend thoroughly. Apply a thin layer to all sunburned areas. Gently rub in. Repeat as needed.

✿ **Variations:** If one ingredient is unavailable, make the formula with the remaining ingredients for similar benefits. Feel free to use more comfrey root and aloe vera gel. However, increasing the amounts of clove and peppermint oils may cause skin irritation.

❧ **Notes:** Aloe vera gel works best fresh from the plant. Simply snip off part of a fleshy leaf, cut it open, and scoop out the gel. If you don't have an aloe vera plant, buy aloe vera gel, as well as comfrey, clove oil, and peppermint oil, at health food stores and herb shops. Or, order clove oil through your pharmacist. Unprocessed aloe vera gel is more effective than the "stabilized" variety. See page 444 for other sources.

GOOD IDEA!

You'll find good sunburn relief in your refrigerator or pantry. Some people get relief on small areas of sunburn by applying thin slices of cold, raw produce. Slices of cucumber, apple, or potato applied directly to the skin seem to work well. Or apply cold, plain yogurt to the sunburned areas. Rinse off in a cool shower, and gently pat the skin dry. To relieve pain and swelling of sunburned eyelids, apply tea bags soaked in cool water.

Hives Remedy

Hives, medically known as urticaria, are itchy, raised, red skin welts that come and go. Hives are a type of allergic reaction, triggered by such things as insect bites, infections, drugs, stress, heat, cold, or certain foods. The first line of defense against hives is to find the trigger and eliminate it.

In hives that cannot be prevented, antihistamines often suppress welts and help itching. This stinging nettle infusion acts as a natural antihistamine, and the oatmeal/chamomile bath provides relief for itching and inflammation.

Yield: 1 cup infusion; 1 skin treatment

INGREDIENTS
FOR INFUSION

1 cup water
1 to 2 teaspoons powdered stinging nettle leaves and stems
   honey and/or lemon, to taste

INGREDIENTS
FOR SKIN TREATMENT

2 to 4 cups colloidal oatmeal
½ to 1 cup baking soda
1 to 2 cups powdered chamomile flowers

SUPPLIES

saucepan
fine strainer
cheesecloth (optional)
rubber band (optional)

☛ **BE SAFE.** Pregnant or nursing women should not use the stinging nettle infusion without first consulting a physician. Otherwise healthy adults may use up to 2 cups a day. Do not give nettle infusion to children under 2. Older children and those over 65 should use extra water to reduce formula strength. The younger the child, the more dilute the formula should be. In *large amounts, stinging nettle may cause stomach irritation, burning skin, and urinary suppression. If any of these symptoms develop, discontinue use. If itching persists or becomes worse, or if rash or irritation develops, discontinue use. Use this formula only in consultation with your physician.*

To make the stinging nettle infusion, bring water to a boil in the saucepan. Add stinging nettle and remove from heat. Steep 10 minutes. Strain. Add honey and/or lemon. Drink cool or reheat.

To make the skin treatment, add oatmeal, baking soda, and chamomile to the bathwater. Or add just oatmeal and baking soda. With a rubber band, tie chamomile in cheesecloth and allow the water to run over it. Repeat as needed.

Notes: Buy colloidal oatmeal at pharmacies and health food stores. Buy stinging nettle and chamomile at health food stores and herb shops. See page 444 for other sources.

Hints for Hives Relief

Hives are the way the skin sometimes reacts to allergies, physical irritation, stress, or emotions. Here are a few things you can do that may relieve the itching or swelling. Like many remedies, what works for some won't work for others. So experimentation is in order.

- Over-the-counter antihistimines provide relief for some people. Look for cold and hay fever medications that contain either diphenhydramine or chlorpheniramine. Caution: Most antihistimines can make you drowsy.
- Cold compresses or baths may provide temporary relief from the swelling of hives. You may also try rubbing an ice cube wrapped in a cloth over the hives. This treatment obviously won't work if your hives develop as an allergic response to cold exposure.
- Astringents applied directly to the hives may soothe the itch and temporarily reduce fluid discharge. Over-the-counter astringents that work include calamine lotion, witch hazel, and zinc oxide.

GOOD IDEA!

Time heals most **warts.** According to one estimate, 40 to 50 percent of all warts eventually disappear on their own, typically within two years. Children, in particular, often lose warts spontaneously.

And while you're waiting for the time to pass, you might want to try applying vitamin A directly to the wart. Dr. Robert Garry, Ph.D., associate professor of microbiology and immunology at Tulane University School of Medicine, recommends using vitamin A capsules containing 25,000 international units of vitamin A. Once a day, simply break open the capsule, squeeze some of the liquid onto the wart, and rub it in. Do not take the vitamin A capsules orally. Large oral doses of vitamin A can be toxic.

Immune-Stimulating Infusion for Warts

Caused by the human papilloma virus, warts are quite common and yet still medically mysterious. This formula combines immune-stimulating and antiviral herbs. Echinacea and ginger may help stimulate the immune system. Garlic has shown scientifically documented effects against many viruses.

Yield: 1 cup

INGREDIENTS

1 cup water
2 teaspoons powdered echinacea root
10 to 15 cloves garlic, minced
2 teaspoons freshly grated or powdered gingerroot
   honey and/or lemon, to taste

SUPPLIES

saucepan
fine strainer

☛ **BE SAFE.** Pregnant or nursing women should not use this formula without first consulting a physician. Adults may use up to 3 cups a day. Do not give to children under 2. Older children and those over 65 should use extra water to reduce formula strength. The younger the child, the more dilute the formula should be. Echinacea may cause tingling of the tongue. This is normal and not hazardous. If headache, rash, stomach distress, or other unpleasant effects develop, discontinue use. Use this formula only in consultation with your physician.

Bring water to a boil in the saucepan. Add echinacea, garlic, and ginger. Remove from heat. Steep 10 minutes. Strain. Add honey and/or lemon. Drink cool or reheat.

➡ **Note:** Buy echinacea at health food stores and herb shops. See page 444 for other sources.

INFECTION FIGHTERS

Chronic infection (whether bacterial, viral, or fungal) usually means chronic misery. Chronic infections can range from merely annoying (athlete's foot fungus) to imminently life threatening (tuberculosis bacilli that spread to vital organs).

The formulas in this section may help stimulate your body's natural immune system. If you have a chronic infection, first follow your doctor's advice. Use these formulas as a supplement to good professional care.

Garden-Variety Infections

When it comes to minor injuries, gardening is a risky business. Most green thumbs eventually get cut, scraped, stung, bitten, or gouged. And although most gardening injuries aren't deep, they're prone to infection because they're usually dirty.

Believe it or not, you will probably find infection-fighting help for a gardening injury right in your own backyard. Pick clean leaves of apple, lemon balm, bay laurel, marjoram, peppermint, rosemary, sage, tarragon, thyme, or yarrow. Crush the leaves and press the mass into the wound. To stop bleeding, continue pressing the crushed leaves into the wound until you are able to wash it.

Wash the wound thoroughly with soap and water. If bleeding persists, press the wound firmly with a clean cloth or gauze pad until bleeding stops. Apply an over-the-counter antibiotic salve or a homemade salve made with 2 tablespoons honey, 2 tablespoons aloe vera gel, and 1 teaspoon powdered comfrey root.

After applying a salve, you may leave small wounds open to the air. For larger wounds, cover with an adhesive bandage or sterile gauze. Check the wound once or twice a day for any sign of infection. Reapply the salve and rebandage if necessary. Consult your doctor promptly if any wound becomes painful, red, swollen, or pus-filled.

GOOD IDEA!

Use these tricks to soothe canker sores. One of the problems in treating canker sores is that it's difficult to get the remedy to stick to the slippery sore. Solve that problem by applying a wet, black tea bag directly to the sore. Black tea contains tannin, a pain-relieving astringent.

Or try milk of magnesia swished around in the mouth to protectively coat the sore. This old-fashioned remedy not only soothes and protects, it may also have some antibacterial effect.

Avoid the foods that usually make canker sores even worse. Coffee, spices, citrus fruits, nuts high in the amino acid arginine (especially walnuts), chocolate, and strawberries irritate canker sores and can even cause them in some people.

Canker Sore Formula

Canker sores, small ulcers in the mouth lining, usually heal within a week or two, but stress or a suppressed immune system may cause chronic canker sores. Try this immune-stimulating formula.

Yield: 1 cup

INGREDIENTS

1 cup water
2 teaspoons powdered echinacea root
2 teaspoons powdered chamomile flowers
1 teaspoon ground cinnamon
10 to 15 cloves garlic, minced
1 teaspoon powdered goldenseal root
   honey and/or lemon, to taste

SUPPLIES

saucepan
fine strainer

☛ **BE SAFE.** Pregnant or nursing women should not use this formula without consulting a physician. Otherwise healthy adults may use up to 3 cups a day. Do not give to children under 2. Older children and adults over 65 should use extra water to reduce formula strength. The younger the child, the more dilute the formula should be. Echinacea may cause tingling of the tongue. This is normal and not hazardous. If headache, rash, stomach distress, or other unpleasant effects develop, discontinue use. Use this formula only in consultation with your physician.

Boil water in the saucepan. Add echinacea and simmer for 10 to 15 minutes. Add chamomile, cinnamon, garlic, and goldenseal. Remove from heat. Steep 10 to 20 minutes. Strain. Add honey and/or lemon. Drink cool or reheat.

↠ **Note:** Buy echinacea, chamomile, and goldenseal at most health food stores and herb shops. See page 444 for other sources.

Toenail Infection Formula

If your toenails become thickened and disfigured and turn brownish or white, you may have a fungal toenail infection. Consult your physician to rule out other possibilities. Doctors prescribe an antifungal drug (griseofulvin) derived from penicillin, but this is a powerful medication. If you'd like to try a more natural approach, garlic offers antifungal effects, and some scientific studies show that echinacea may enhance the immune system's response to fungal infections. You may see new, healthy-looking nail growing from the cuticle within a month.

Yield: 1 cup

INGREDIENTS

1 cup water

2 teaspoons powdered echinacea root

10 to 15 cloves garlic, minced

    honey and/or lemon, to taste

SUPPLIES

saucepan

fine strainer

☛ **BE SAFE.** *Pregnant or nursing women should not use this formula without first consulting a physician. Adults may use up to 3 cups a day. Do not give to children under 2. Older children and adults over 65 should use extra water to reduce formula strength. The younger the child, the more dilute the formula should be. Echinacea may cause tingling of the tongue. This is normal and not hazardous. If headache, rash, stomach distress, or other unpleasant effects develop, discontinue use. Use this formula only in consultation with your physician.*

Bring water to a boil in the saucepan. Add echinacea and simmer for 10 to 15 minutes. Add garlic and remove from heat. Steep 10 to 20 minutes. Strain. Add honey and/or lemon. Drink cool or reheat. To eliminate toenail fungus, you will need to use this formula daily for as long

(continued)

GOOD IDEA!

Stock up on breath fresheners before you treat your foot. Since some formulas use large quantities of garlic over a period of weeks or months, you'll stay more popular with your friends if you use breath fresheners regularly. Also, if you find the garlic flavor too strong, dilute the final brewed formula with half water and drink it in two separate doses.

as it takes for a new nail to grow from the cuticle. For the nail of the big toe, this may take several months.

➥ **Note:** Purchase echinacea at most health food stores and herb shops. See page 444 for other sources.

Coping with Urinary Tract Infections

Urinary tract infections (also called UTIs, cystitis, and bladder infections) cause burning on urination, frequent urge to urinate with little production, and often fever, chills, bloody urine, and an overall feeling of being ill.

UTIs develop when bacteria—usually intestinal bacteria from the anal area—climb up the urine tube (urethra) and infect the bladder. The bacterial invasion may result from any of a host of causes, including: careless lovemaking practices, improper personal hygiene, habitually ignoring the urge to urinate, or the use of perfumed toilet tissue or vaginal products.

Women get UTIs more often than men because the female urethra is shorter, giving infectious bacteria a shorter route to the bladder.

If you suffer from frequent UTIs, ask your doctor about what personal habits and precautions you might adopt to avoid future infection. Some chronic cases of UTI clear up when women stop using diaphragms and tampons. For a number of reasons, both diaphragms and tampons are sometimes associated with the introduction of bacteria into the urethra.

And to resist recurrent UTIs, try drinking plenty of cranberry juice, a traditional UTI preventive. A recent study in the *Journal of the American Medical Association* showed that it helps prevent UTIs by keeping bacteria from attaching to the bladder wall.

Urinary Tract Infection Fighter

If you're suffering from a urinary tract infection (UTI), consult your doctor and try this formula. Cranberry juice is a traditional UTI preventive. Goldenseal may help kill the bacteria associated with UTIs, and echinacea may help boost your immune system.

Yield: 1 cup

INGREDIENTS

8   ounces cranberry juice cocktail

2   teaspoons powdered echinacea root

1   teaspoon powdered goldenseal root

    honey and/or lemon, to taste

SUPPLIES

saucepan

fine strainer

☛ **BE SAFE.** *Pregnant or nursing women should not use this formula without first consulting a physician. Otherwise healthy adults may use up to 3 glasses a day. Do not give to children under 2. Older children and adults over 65 should use extra water to reduce formula strength. The younger the child, the more dilute the formula should be. Echinacea may cause tingling of the tongue. This is normal and not hazardous. If headache, rash, stomach distress, or other unpleasant effects develop, discontinue use. Use this formula only in consultation with your physician.*

Bring cranberry juice to a boil in the saucepan. Reduce heat and simmer echinacea for 15 minutes. Remove from heat and add goldenseal. Steep 10 to 20 minutes. Strain. Add honey and/or lemon. Drink cool, iced, or reheated.

➼ **Notes:** *Pure cranberry juice is tart. Cranberry juice cocktail, available at supermarkets and health food stores, includes sugar for palatability and works fine for this formula. Buy echinacea and goldenseal at health food stores and herb shops. See page 444 for other sources.*

GOOD IDEA!

Drink copious amounts of fluid to soothe the pain of a urinary tract infection (UTI). Women suffering from UTIs often experience painful burning upon urination. Many of these sufferers come to the erroneous conclusion that the best cure is to drink less so that voiding is unneccessary. Nothing could be further from the truth.

The reason: The longer <u>any</u> amount of urine stays in the bladder, the more bacteria there are in it. E. coli (a primary cause of UTI) doubles its population about every 20 minutes. The higher the bacteria count, the greater the pain.

To fight the burning sensation, drink plenty of fluids to flush out the bacteria that are causing the inflammation. A rule of thumb: If your urine is clear, you're drinking enough. If it's colored, you're not.

Herpes Formula

The echinacea infusion is an immune stimulant that may help the body fight herpes outbreaks and prevent re-currences. The salve may aid the healing of herpes sores.

Yield: 1 cup infusion; ¼ cup salve

INGREDIENT
FOR INFUSION

1 cup water
1 teaspoon powdered echinacea root
   honey and/or lemon, to taste

INGREDIENTS
FOR SALVE

1 teaspoon honey
1 teaspoon aloe vera gel
1 teaspoon powdered comfrey root

SUPPLIES

saucepan
fine strainer
small mixing bowl or cup
spoon
cotton balls or cotton swabs

☛ **BE SAFE.** Genital herpes can cause serious complications in newborns. Pregnant women with a history of genital herpes should inform their obstetricians. Active herpes sores at term may require delivery by cesarean section. Use the salve as needed on the lips and genitals, but do not use it for cold sores inside the mouth. It tastes extremely bitter. If rash or skin irrita-tion develops, discontinue use. Pregnant or nursing women shold not use the echinacea infusion without first consulting a physician. Otherwise healthy adults may use up to 3 cups a day. Do not give echinacea to children under 2. Older children and those over 65 should use extra water to reduce formula strength. The younger the child, the more dilute the formula should be. Echinacea may cause tingling of the tongue. This is *normal and not hazardous. If headache, rash, stomach distress, or other unpleasant effects develop, discontinue use. Use this formula only in consultation with your physician.*

For the infusion, bring water to a boil in the saucepan. Add echinacea and simmer 10 to 15 minutes on low heat. Strain. Add honey and/or lemon. Drink cool or reheat.

For the salve, place all ingredients in the bowl or cup and mix thoroughly. Using cotton balls or cotton swabs, cover the affected area with a thin layer of the mixture. Repeat as needed.

Notes: *Aloe vera gel works best fresh from the plant. Simply snip off part of a fleshy leaf, cut it open, and scoop out the gel. If you don't have an aloe vera plant, buy aloe vera gel, as well as echinacea and comfrey, at health food stores and herb shops. Unprocessed aloe vera gel works better than the "stabilized" variety.* *See page 444 for other sources.*

Help for Herpes Simplex

Genital herpes and its related illness, cold sores around the mouth, are both caused by the herpes simplex virus. Both conditions cause painful, blisterlike sores.

The virus spreads by direct contact with someone with an active sore or contact with skin about to erupt into a sore. Initial outbreaks typically cause painful, open, red blisters and often fever and generalized illness. Initial sores take up to two weeks to heal.

After the sores heal, the virus remains in the body. Whenever the immune system is overwhelmed with other health problems, herpes sores may recur. An estimated 50 to 75 percent of herpes sufferers experience recurrences. In people with chronic medical problems, outbreaks may continue for years. But in most people, recurrences subside as the immune system eventually gets the better of the infection.

During a herpes outbreak, either genital or around the mouth, use care not to spread the virus to other parts of your body. Avoid touching the sores. Touching an open genital sore and then bringing your fingers in contact with your mouth or eyes may cause an outbreak in a new location. If you scratch at night, cover your sores with gauze.

To avoid spreading mouth sores, discard your toothbrush. Toothbrushes may harbor herpes viruses for many days after an initial outbreak of cold sores. To protect yourself against reinfection, throw your toothbrush away when you notice you're getting this virus. If you still develop a cold sore, throw it away after the blister develops. When your sore heals completely, replace your toothbrush again.

COLD AND FLU REMEDIES

Rare is the year that we don't experience at least one whopper of a cold or one bone-shaking case of the flu. These home remedies won't do a thing to actually kill the virus of the hour, but they may help stimulate your own immune system to fight back a little harder. Also, all these formulas offer real symptom relief—respite from the fever, coughing, raw throat, and other assorted aches that make you so miserable you can't sleep.

Cold and Flu Formula

Colds and flu are by far humanity's leading infectious diseases. Authorities estimate that over a lifetime, the average person spends more days sick with these viral upper respiratory infections than with all other infectious diseases combined.

There's an old saying that if you ignore a cold, it clears up in a week, but that if you seek medical attention, you can get rid of it in just seven days. This formula is no miracle cure, but some scientific studies show that both echinacea and ginger may have immune stimulating properties similar to those of one of the body's own antiviral chemicals, interferon. Chinese ephedra contains ephedrine, a powerful decongestant. Slippery elm bark and honey help soothe the throat. And lemon juice is high in cold-fighting vitamin C.

Yield: 1 cup

INGREDIENTS

1 cup water
2 teaspoons powdered echinacea root
1 teaspoon powdered Chinese ephedra (*ma huang*)
2 teaspoons powdered slippery elm bark
2 teaspoons freshly grated or powdered gingerroot
   honey and/or lemon, to taste

GOOD IDEA!

To knock out cold congestion, get the right herb. Be sure to use Chinese ephedra, known botanically as Ephedra sinica. American ephedra is a different plant and has much less decongestant action.

SUPPLIES

saucepan

fine strainer

☞ **BE SAFE.** Pregnant or nursing women should not use this formula without first consulting a physician. Otherwise healthy adults may use up to 2 cups a day. Do not give to children under 2. Older children and adults over 65 should use extra water to reduce formula strength. The younger the child, the more dilute the formula should be. Echinacea may cause tingling of the tongue. This is normal and not hazardous. If headache, rash, stomach distress, or other unpleasant effects develop, discontinue use. Chinese ephedra is a stimulant that may cause insomnia, nervousness, irritability, and increased blood pressure. Those with insomnia, high blood pressure, diabetes, glaucoma, or heart disease should not use this formula. This formula should be used only in consultation with your physician. Consult your physician promptly if: (1) Fever develops or recurs toward the end of a cold or flu; (2) Chest pain or difficulty breathing develops at any time; or (3) Red or rust-colored sputum appears at any time.

Bring water to a boil in the saucepan. Add echinacea, Chinese ephedra, and slippery elm bark and simmer 10 to 15 minutes on low heat. Add remaining ingredients and remove from heat. Steep 10 to 20 minutes. Strain. Reheat before drinking.

✿ **Variation:** During the initial stage of a cold, when sore throat is the main symptom and congestion has not yet developed, make this formula without the decongestant Chinese ephedra. If taken without ephedra, adults may increase use to 3 cups a day.

➻ **Note:** Buy echinacea, Chinese ephedra, and slippery elm bark at health food stores and herb shops. See page 444 for other sources.

GOOD IDEA!

Zap your cold with zinc. Researchers in Great Britain and the United States have discovered that sucking on zinc lozenges can cut colds short by an average of seven days. The down side is that zinc has an unpleasant taste. There are, however, lozenges on the market that contain honey and/or citrus that are more palatable. Follow your doctor's advice on proper dosage. Zinc taken in large doses can be toxic.

Goldie Sackner's Cold-Relieving Chicken Soup

In 1978, Goldie's son, Marvin Sackner, M.D., a pulmonologist (lung doctor) at Mt. Sinai Medical Center in Miami Beach, Florida, showed that chicken soup, an 800-year-old Jewish remedy, actually helps relieve symptoms of the common cold. Dr. Sackner's research team gave cold sufferers various fluids and measured how quickly mucus cleared from their noses. Chicken soup worked best. The study turned Dr. Sackner into an instant media celebrity. His mother, Goldie, felt quite proud, of course, but one thing bothered her. Her son had used chicken soup purchased at a deli near Mt. Sinai, and not her infinitely more therapeutic recipe, which she subsequently released as a public service. Here it is.

Yield: about 1 quart

INGREDIENTS

1   quart water
1   whole chicken (preferably kosher), skinned, boned, and cut up
2   carrots, chopped
2   celery stalks, chopped
1   large onion, chopped
large bunch chard (or other soup greens), chopped
parsley, dill, salt, and pepper, to taste

SUPPLIES

4-quart soup pot

Bring water to a boil in the pot. Add chicken and simmer covered for 45 minutes. Add remaining ingredients. Simmer 15 minutes covered. Serve very hot.

✿ **Variations:** Substitute defatted chicken broth for part of the water. Add more carrots, celery, onions, and other vegetables, to taste.

Decongestant Inhalant

The highly aromatic herbs in this formula mostly relieve nasal congestion, but partial relief of chest congestion is also possible.

Yield: 1 cup

INGREDIENTS

1 cup water

2 teaspoons powdered eucalyptus leaves

2 teaspoons powdered pennyroyal leaves and flower tops

2 teaspoons powdered rosemary leaves

SUPPLIES

saucepan

☛ **BE SAFE.** As an inhalant, use as needed, being careful not to scald yourself with the steamy vapors. Children and adults over 65 are especially sensitive to high temperatures. You may also drink this infusion. Pregnant or nursing women should consult a physician before drinking. Otherwise healthy adults may drink up to 2 cups a day. Do not give the infusion to children under 2. Older children and adults over 65 should use extra water to reduce formula strength. The younger the child, the more dilute the formula should be. Pennyroyal oil is highly toxic if taken internally. It is also associated with spontaneous abortion. But pennyroyal leaves are considered safe when used as part of the inhalant/infusion recommended here. If headache, rash, or other unpleasant effects develop, discontinue use. Use this formula only in consultation with your physician.

Bring water to a boil in the saucepan. Add herbs and simmer on low heat. Turn off heat and remove pan to a heat-proof surface. Inhale the vapors deeply.

↦ **Note:** Buy eucalyptus and pennyroyal at health food stores and herb shops. See page 444 for other sources.

GOOD IDEA!

Sip hot tea for bedtime cold relief. A hot herbal tea taken at bedtime may help relieve nasal stuffiness as well as aid sleep. Teas made from hops or valerian are particularly helpful in bringing on drowsiness. Or try Celestial Seasonings Sleepytime tea. Add a teaspoon of honey, a simple carbohydrate that may have a mild sedative effect.

GOOD IDEA!

Take over-the-counter drugs at night. Many cold remedies, such as Nyquil or Contac, treat a number of different symptoms with a combination of drugs, plus even alcohol sometimes. Some of these combination drugs, however, cause drowsiness or nausea. If you take your over-the-counter remedy only at night, you probably won't feel the side effects while you're sleeping. Of course, for prescription drugs, take exactly as directed by your doctor.

Decongestant Cough Formula

Ephedra is one of the world's oldest medicines. The Chinese began using it to treat asthma and chest congestion about 5,000 years ago, and we're still using it today. Ephedra's pharmaceutical equivalent, pseudoephedrine, is the decongestant in many over-the-counter cold and allergy medications. Licorice root has scientifically verified cough-suppressing properties. And highly aromatic pennyroyal adds to the decongestant action of this formula.

Yield: 1 cup

INGREDIENTS

1 cup water
1 teaspoon powdered Chinese ephedra (*ma huang*)
½ teaspoon powdered licorice root
1 teaspoon powdered pennyroyal leaves and flower tops
   honey and/or lemon, to taste

SUPPLIES

saucepan
fine strainer

☛ **BE SAFE.** Pregnant or nursing women should not use this formula without first consulting a physician. Otherwise healthy adults may use up to 2 cups a day while congestion persists. Do not give to children under 2. Older children and those over 65 should use extra water to reduce formula strength. The younger the child, the more dilute the formula should be. Chinese ephedra is a stimulant that may cause insomnia, nervousness, irritability, and increased blood pressure. Those with insomnia, high blood pressure, diabetes, glaucoma, or heart disease should not use this formula. If headache, rash, stomach distress, or other unpleasant effects develop, discontinue use. In very large quantities taken for unusually long periods, licorice may cause pseudoaldosteronism, a serious hormonal disorder. Pennyroyal oil is highly toxic if taken internally. It is also associated with spontaneous abortion. But pennyroyal leaves are considered *safe in the amount recommended here. Use this formula only in consultation with your physician.*

Bring water to a boil in the saucepan. Add ephedra and licorice and simmer for 10 to 15 minutes on low heat. Add pennyroyal and remove from heat. Steep for 10 to 20 minutes. Strain. Add honey and/or lemon. Reheat before drinking.

➡ **Note:** *Buy herbs at health food stores and herb shops. See page 444 for other sources.*

Quieting Croup

Croup, a common infant and early childhood illness, is a throat infection usually caused by a virus, but sometimes caused by bacteria as well. It commonly strikes children from 3 months to 3 years old and often begins with the child waking suddenly in the middle of the night feeling very frightened. Symptoms include hoarseness and a shrill barking cough that sounds somewhat like crowing.

When croup strikes, call your physician immediately. Most croup cases can be treated at home, but occasionally croup symptoms indicate epiglottitis, inflammation of the windpipe valve, a true medical emergency.

If your child's physician diagnoses croup, he or she will most likely recommend steam and over-the-counter cough suppressants. You can make an effective cough suppressant at home by combining ¼ teaspoon licorice root and a teaspoon of honey with a cup of water. Just bring the water to a boil, add the licorice root and honey, and simmer on low heat for 10 minutes.

To begin home treatment, hold the child to relieve the anxiety associated with croup. Take the child into the bathroom and turn the shower on hot. Allow the room to fill with steam. Give the warm licorice cough suppressant to the child 1 tablespoon at a time until the cough subsides.

Call the child's physician immediately if: (1) the cough doesn't show significant improvement after 1 hour of home treatment, (2) the child appears to have difficulty breathing, (3) the child's lips start to turn blue, (4) the child develops any unusual symptoms in addition to the barking cough.

GOOD IDEA!

Flood fevers with fluid. When you're hot, your body perspires to cool you down. But if you're sweating a lot with a fever, your body may turn off the normal sweating mechanism to forestall dehydration. That means you've lost one important coping mechanism that helps keep fever in bounds.

The moral is: Drink plenty of fluids to keep your body sweating and coping with the problem at hand. Plain water is fine, but fruit and vegetable juices are also a good choice. If you feel too nauseated to drink, suck on ice or on frozen fruit juice cubes prepared in an ice-cube tray. To entice a feverish child, embed a grape or strawberry in each cube.

First-Aid for Fever

Fever may be a symptom of many different illnesses. This formula may reduce fever related to minor illnesses. Most illnesses that involve fever require professional care.

Yield: 1 cup

INGREDIENTS

  1 cup water
  2 teaspoons powdered echinacea root
  1 to 2 teaspoons powdered meadowsweet leaves
10 to 15 cloves garlic, minced
  1 teaspoon powdered goldenseal root
     honey and/or lemon, to taste

SUPPLIES

saucepan
fine strainer

☛ **BE SAFE.** Pregnant or nursing women should not use this formula. Otherwise healthy adults may use up to 3 cups a day. Do not give to children under 2. Older children and those over 65 should use extra water to reduce formula strength. The younger the child, the more dilute the formula should be. Echinacea may cause tingling of the tongue. This is normal and not hazardous. Meadowsweet may cause stomach distress in those with aspirin-sensitive stomachs. If headache, rash, stomach distress, or other unpleasant effects develop, discontinue use. Use this formula only in consultation with your physician. Fevers that rise or last longer than 24 hours despite home treatment require professional care.

Bring water to a boil in the saucepan. Add echinacea and simmer 10 to 15 minutes on low heat. Add meadowsweet, garlic, and goldenseal and remove from heat. Steep 10 minutes. Strain. Add honey and/or lemon. Drink cool or reheat.

➻ **Note:** Buy herbs at health food stores and herb shops. See page 444 for other sources.

Sore Throat Soother

Both herbal ingredients in this formula contain a substance called mucilage, which absorbs water and swells to form a throat-soothing, slippery (hence the "slippery" in slippery elm), gelatin-like beverage. The honey in this formula is another traditional sore-throat remedy.

Yield: 1 cup

INGREDIENTS

1 to 3 teaspoons powdered slippery elm bark

1 cup water

1 to 2 teaspoons powdered mullein leaves, flowers, or roots

honey and/or lemon, to taste

SUPPLIES

saucepan

fine strainer

☛ **BE SAFE.** *Pregnant or nursing women should not use this formula without first consulting a physician. Otherwise healthy adults may use up to 3 cups a day. Do not give to children under 2. Older children and those over 65 should use extra water to reduce formula strength. The younger the child, the more dilute the formula should be. If headache, rash, stomach distress, or other unpleasant effects develop, discontinue use. Use this formula only in consultation with your physician.*

Blend the slippery elm with ¼ cup of the water in the saucepan until it's smooth. Add the rest of the water and boil. Simmer 15 minutes on low heat. Add mullein and remove from heat. Steep 10 to 20 minutes. Strain. Reheat before drinking. Add honey and/or lemon.

➡ **Note:** *Buy slippery elm bark and mullein at health food stores and herb shops. See page 444 for other sources.*

GOOD IDEA!

At the first sign of a sore throat, throw away your toothbrush. Believe it or not, bacteria that lurk in your toothbrush may perpetuate an existing throat infection. Bacteria collect in the bristles as you brush, and any injury to the gums during brushing gives these bad bugs a new point of entry into your system.

As soon as you feel a sore throat coming on, replace your toothbrush with a new one. Sometimes that's enough to stop a developing sore throat in its tracks. And if you do come down with a full-fledged infection, replace your toothbrush again after you recover.

Rx FOR WOMEN

In the more leisurely past, women helped each other—they exchanged remedies and offered caring support for common lifecycle passages ranging from birthing to the onset of menopause. This tradition of mutual support continues today in birthing centers and women's medical centers that offer counseling and midwifery services.

These formulas spring from the tradition of women helping each other. But they're meant to cope with annoying symptoms, not real illnesses. For symptoms that disrupt your daily routine or interfere with your enjoyment of life, see your doctor. The formulas that follow may be a useful addition to traditional medical care, or they may be totally inadequate for your problem. You can only make an informed decision with the help of your physician.

Menopause Symptom Relief

This formula is a natural alternative to estrogen replacement therapy (ERT). While the formula is *not* as potent as medically supervised ERT, it might provide some relief for women with mild menopausal discomforts.

Yield: 1 cup

INGREDIENTS

1 cup water
2 teaspoons bruised anise seeds
2 teaspoons bruised fennel seeds
3 teaspoons powdered red clover flower tops
   honey and/or lemon, to taste

SUPPLIES

saucepan
fine strainer

☞ **BE SAFE.** Because these herbs are estrogenic, women with a history of estrogen-dependent breast cancer should not use them. Menopausal women at significant risk of endometrial

---

GOOD IDEA!

To keep hot flashes from getting you down during your normal working day, dress in layers. That way, you can peel off a layer when a hot flash threatens and add a layer if you feel chilled afterward. And since natural fibers, such as wool or cotton, wick perspiration away, stay away from heat-trapping synthetics.

cancer should not use this formula; ask your physician about hormonal approaches to endometrial cancer prevention. Otherwise healthy menopausal women may use up to 3 cups a day. If headache, rash, stomach distress, or other unpleasant effects develop, discontinue use. Use this formula only in consultation with your physician.

Bring water to a boil in the saucepan. Add seeds and clover and remove from heat. Steep 10 to 20 minutes. Strain. Add honey and/or lemon. Drink cool or reheat.

✿ **Variation:** All the herbs in this formula have mild estrogenic effects. If one or more are not available, use a total of 7 teaspoons of any combination of the herbs for a similar effect.

➥ **Note:** These herbs are available at supermarkets, health food stores, and herb shops. See page 444 for other sources.

Help for Menopause Symptoms

As menopause occurs, women in their fifties produce less and less estrogen, which may cause vaginal dryness and hot flashes—sudden episodes of heat in the face, neck, and upper chest followed by sweating and a slight chill. Physicians treat menopausal symptoms with estrogen replacement therapy (ERT). ERT also decreases risk of osteoporosis, though it may increase risk of endometrial (uterine) cancer. To make an informed decision about ERT, you may want to undergo a complete evaluation by a physician experienced in this type of therapy.

Your physician may also recommend other coping strategies that help keep menopause symptoms under control. Many women find that avoiding caffeine and alcohol reduces the frequency of hot flashes. Eating five or six small meals a day instead of the normal three also seems to help regulate the body temperature mechanism. And don't forget to drink lots of fluids, especially after exercising. Good fluid balance helps keep body temperature in check.

GOOD IDEA!

Take a spa break for cramps. Since warmth increases blood flow and relaxes pelvic muscles, many women find that a warm, relaxing bath relieves cramps. As you run the bathwater, you may want to add a cup of sea salt or some relaxing herbs, such as chamomile flowers or valerian root. To increase the warmth reaching your abdominal region, sip a cup of herbal tea or hot lemonade as you relax in the tub.

Menstrual Cramp Relief

Menstrual cramps are caused by the uterine contractions that accompany menstrual flow. The force of these contractions—and the pain of cramps—is related to chemicals the body produces, called prostaglandins. Aspirin and its herbal counterpart, meadowsweet, both may calm menstrual cramps by decreasing prostaglandin levels. Fifty years ago, a now-famous British study showed that raspberry leaves relax the uterus. It's been used in herbal remedies for menstrual discomfort ever since.

Yield: 1 cup

INGREDIENTS

1 cup water
1 to 2 teaspoons powdered raspberry leaves
1 teaspoon powdered meadowsweet leaves
   honey and/or lemon, to taste

SUPPLIES

saucepan

☛ **BE SAFE.** Pregnant or nursing women should not use this formula. Otherwise healthy women may use up to 3 cups a day. Meadowsweet may cause stomach distress in those with aspirin-sensitive stomachs. If headache, rash, stomach distress, or other unpleasant effects develop, discontinue use. Use this formula only in consultation with your physician.

Bring water to a boil in the suacepan. Add raspberry and meadowsweet. Remove from heat. Steep 10 to 20 minutes. Strain. Add honey and/or lemon. Drink cool or reheat.

➼ **Note:** Buy raspberry leaves and meadowsweet at health food stores and herb shops. See page 444 for other sources.

Relief from Premenstrual Bloating

This formula contains natural diuretics—substances that promote urination and help eliminate extra fluid.

Yield: 1 cup

INGREDIENTS

1 cup water
1 teaspoon powdered sarsaparilla root
1 teaspoon powdered *buchu* leaves
1 teaspoon powdered dandelion root
1 teaspoon bruised juniper berries
2 teaspoons dried parsley leaves
   honey and/or lemon, to taste

SUPPLIES

saucepan
fine strainer

☞ **BE SAFE.** Use up to 3 cups a day while bloating persists. Do not use to promote weight loss. Extended use may deplete potassium stores; increase potassium intake by eating bananas and fresh vegetables. Those with a history of kidney problems should not use juniper. Do not use juniper for extended periods of time. Large amounts of sarsaparilla may cause a burning sensation in the mouth, throat, and stomach. If headache, rash, stomach distress, or other unpleasant effects develop, discontinue use. Use this formula only in consultation with your physician.

Bring water to a boil in the saucepan. Add sarsaparilla and simmer 10 to 15 minutes on low heat. Add buchu, dandelion, juniper, and parsley and remove from heat. Steep 10 to 20 minutes. Strain. Add honey and/or lemon. Drink cool or reheat.

↝ **Note:** Buy herbs at health food stores and herb shops. See page 444 for other sources.

GOOD IDEA!

To minimize premenstrual bloating, stay away from salt for seven to ten days before the onset of your menstrual period. A low-sodium diet may help alleviate the fluid retention brought on by premenstrual hormone changes. In addition, eliminate caffeine—including chocolate and cola as well as tea and coffee. Caffeine has been shown to contribute to the painful breast tenderness that so often accompanies premenstrual bloating.

Yeast Infection Relief

Vaginal yeast infections cause intense itching, reddening of vaginal tissue, and a "cheesy" discharge. The discharge arises from the yeast *Candida albicans*.

Yeasts normally inhabit the healthy vagina, but when the vaginal environment becomes unbalanced, they multiply and cause infection. Birth control pills, moisture, and heat all encourage the growth of yeast. Synthetic fabric underpants or leotards encourage the buildup of body heat and moisture and often contribute to recurring yeast infections.

To prevent recurrent yeast infections, use a contraceptive other than the Pill, wear cotton or cotton-lined underwear, keep the vaginal area cool and dry, and use this formula. In a study at New York's Long Island Jewish Medical Center, *Lactobacillus acidophilus* yogurt was shown to be effective against vaginal yeast infection. Studies show that cinnamon also may thwart the growth of Candida.

Yield: 1 cup

INGREDIENTS

1 cup yogurt, Columbo's or any brand with live *Lactobacillus acidophilus* bacterial culture

1 to 2 teaspoons ground cinnamon

SUPPLIES

spoon
small mixing bowl
clean bulb-type poultry baster

☛ **BE SAFE.** If headache, rash, stomach distress, or other unpleasant effects develop, discontinue use. Do not treat children with signs of yeast infection; consult a physician.

Mix cinnamon and yogurt thoroughly in the bowl. Insert using the baster. Use daily.

➽ **Note:** Acidophilus yogurt is available at some supermarkets and most health food stores. You can make your own using acidophilus milk.

Treatment for Vaginal Yeast Infections

This formula uses a garlic suppository and a goldenseal/echinacea infusion to treat yeast infections.

Yield: 1 suppository; 1 cup infusion

INGREDIENTS

1 cup water
2 teaspoons powdered echinacea root
1 teaspoon powdered goldenseal root
honey and/or lemon, to taste

SUPPLIES

garlic clove, carefully peeled without nicking
sterile gauze
saucepan
fine strainer

☛ **BE SAFE.** *Any woman may use the suppository. Pregnant or nursing women should not use the echinacea infusion without first consulting a physician. Otherwise healthy women may drink up to 3 cups a day for up to two weeks. Echinacea may cause harmless tingling of the tongue. If headache, rash, stomach distress, or other unpleasant effects develop, discontinue use. Do not treat children with signs of yeast infection; consult a physician. Adults over 65 should use extra water to reduce formual strength. Use this formula only in consultation with your physician.*

For the suppository, wrap garlic clove in the gauze. Insert and leave in place 12 hours. Repeat as needed.

To make the infusion, bring water to a boil in the saucepan. Add echinacea and simmer 15 minutes on low heat. Add goldenseal. Remove from heat. Steep 10 minutes. Strain. Add honey and/or lemon. Drink cool or reheat.

➹ **Note:** *Buy echinacea and goldenseal at health food stores and herb shops. See page 444 for other sources.*

GOOD IDEA!

Fight yeast with vinegar. Vinegar has approximately the same acidity as a normal healthy vagina. Some doctors suggest that a vagina with a correct acid balance is less likely to grow excess yeast. If you feel a yeast infection coming on with the beginnings of the telltale itch and "cheesy" discharge, you may be able to stop the yeast overgrowth by douching with a vinegar solution made from 1 pint warm water mixed with 4 teaspoons white vinegar.

TUMMY TROUBLES

Too much cotton candy at the circus. Queasy remembrance of your last bumpy airplane flight. Wishing for the constipation relief that seems to take its own sweet time. Heartburning regret that you ate three tacos topped with "the works." We all have a stream of consciousness that seems to revolve around our sensitive, never-tell-a-lie tummy troubles. The formulas here work as well as most over-the-counter indigestion and constipation remedies, and in some cases, even better.

Infant Colic Formula

Infant indigestion makes both babies and parents miserable. Both dill and savory are stomach soothing and mild enough for infants and young children.

Yield: 6 ounces

INGREDIENTS

6 ounces water or infant formula

1 teaspoon bruised dill seed

1 teaspoon powdered savory

SUPPLIES

saucepan

dairy or candy thermometer

fine strainer

☛ **BE SAFE.** Use this formula only in consultation with your infant's physician. Prolonged crying in an infant warrants a doctor visit.

In the saucepan, heat water or formula to about 100°F. Add dill and savory. Let sit 10 minutes. Strain. To use immediately, reheat to 100°F; it should be warm, *not* hot. If you plan to use the formula later, refrigerate immediately for up to a few hours. Discard unused formula more than several hours old.

GOOD IDEA!

Calm colic with a milk-free diet. Many child-care specialists believe that colic in breast-fed infants is sometimes caused when an element of cow's milk is transmitted to the infant through breast milk. Mothers can try eliminating milk from their diets to see what happens. If that doesn't end the colic, try cutting back on other dairy products.

Occasionally, other foods may cause colic in breast-fed infants. Potential troublemakers include caffeine-containing drinks, chocolate, bananas, oranges, strawberries, and spicy foods.

Indigestion-Soothing Dessert

Today, "dessert" implies something sweet. Centuries ago, people had nothing against topping off a meal with sweets, but dessert was also meant to soothe the stomach and prevent indigestion. Some scientific studies suggest that the papaya and peppermint in this stomach-soothing dessert may help calm the gastrointestinal tract and possibly ward off indigestion. The yogurt may help combat the bacteria often responsible for infectious (traveler's) diarrhea.

Yield: 2 servings

INGREDIENTS

2 to 4 teaspoons powdered peppermint leaves and flower tops

4 to 8 tablespoons plain yogurt

1 ripe papaya, halved and seeded

SUPPLIES

small mixing bowl

spoon

Stir almost all the peppermint into the yogurt. Divide yogurt in half and fill each papaya half with the mixture. Sprinkle with remaining peppermint.

✿ **Variation:** Substitute other stomach-soothing herbs, either ginger or cinnamon, for the peppermint.

➺ **Note:** Buy peppermint at health food stores and herb shops. See page 444 for other sources.

GOOD IDEA!

To choose a ripe papaya, think peaches. Any dessert made from papayas tastes best if the papayas are perfectly ripe. To choose papaya at its peak, look for a smooth, somewhat yellow skin. When you press the fruit gently, it should feel soft, but not mushy, to the touch—like a ripe peach.

GOOD IDEA!

Psyllium with ice is nice. Although psyllium seed is tasteless, it imparts a gritty texture some people find unpleasant to drink. To help psyllium-laced coffee go down smoothly, mix it with crushed ice and drink it down quickly. Also, some people find coffee alone sufficient to deal with occasional minor constipation. And some people use psyllium alone in water or fruit juice.

Gentle Java Laxative

Coffee is a mild laxative. Psyllium, when mixed with liquid, swells in the digestive tract, adds bulk to stool, and helps stimulate natural colonic contractions. As an added benefit, recent studies show that psyllium helps reduce cholesterol.

Yield: 1 cup

INGREDIENTS

1 cup cold coffee (*not* decaffeinated)
1 to 2 teaspoons psyllium seeds
   crushed ice

☛ **BE SAFE.** Pregnant or nursing women should not use this formula without first consulting a physician. Otherwise healthy adults may use up to 3 cups a day. Do not give to children under 2. Older children and adults over 65 should use extra water to reduce formula strength. The younger the child, the more dilute the formula should be. If headache, rash, stomach distress, or other unpleasant effects develop, discontinue use. Persons suffering from insomnia, high blood pressure, diabetes, glaucoma, high cholesterol, or heart disease, should not use this formula. Use this formula only in consultation with your physician. Inhaling dust from psyllium seeds may trigger allergic reaction. A person who is sensitive to psyllium could later experience allergy symptoms from ingesting it. Severe allergic reactions are extremely rare, but if you have breathing difficulties after ingesting psyllium, seek emergency help immediately.

Stir psyllium seeds into the cup of coffee. Add crushed ice and drink at once.

↦ **Note:** Buy psyllium seeds at pharmacies, health food stores, and herb shops. See page 444 for other sources.

Overnight Laxative

Try exercise, fluids, whole grains, fruits and vegetables, and the formula on the opposite page. If that doesn't provide sufficient relief from constipation, try this laxative.

Yield: 3 cups

INGREDIENTS

3 cups water

1 teaspoon powdered cascara sagrada

3 to 6 teaspoons dried chamomile flowers

    honey and/or lemon, to taste

SUPPLIES

saucepan

fine strainer

sealable container

☛ **BE SAFE.** *Pregnant or nursing women should not use this formula without first consulting a physician. Otherwise healthy adults may use up to 2 cups a day. Do not give to children under 2. Older children and adults over 65 should use extra water to reduce formula strength. The younger the child, the more dilute the formula should be. Use this formula only occasionally. Prolonged use can cause a form of constipation called lazy bowel syndrome, an inability to defecate without chemically stimulating the colon. Large doses of cascara sagrada may cause severe intestinal cramps. Allergic reactions are rare, but possible. If headache, rash, stomach distress, cramps, or other unpleasant effects develop, discontinue use. Use this formula only in consultation with your physician.*

Bring water to a boil in the saucepan. Add cascara sagrada and simmer 30 minutes on low heat. Add chamomile and remove from heat. Steep 10 to 20 minutes. Strain. Add honey and/or lemon. Drink warm or cool. For morning relief, drink before bedtime. This formula keeps for up to a week if refrigerated in a tightly sealed container.

➡ **Note:** *Buy cascara sagrada and chamomile at health food stores and herb shops. See page 444 for other sources.*

GOOD IDEA!

Outwit constipation with a bran mash snack. You don't need to pay the premium price of psyllium-based laxatives. Buy psyllium seed and flax seed at health food stores. Combine 2 parts ground psyllium, 1 part ground flax, and 1 part oat bran. Mix these ingredients with enough water to make a mash and eat a little before bedtime.

GOOD IDEA!

To soothe a touchy stomach, eat smaller meals and eat slowly. Gastroenterologists recommend the small meal approach as a way to prevent the stomach acid reflux that causes heartburn. If you notice that your heartburn worsens at night, plan to have dinner early in the evening (at least 3 hours before bedtime). Allowing your stomach to empty before you go to sleep will reduce the pressure on your lower esophogeal sphincter, the muscle that controls the reflux of acid into your esophagus.

Indigestion-Soothing Tea

This formula includes ginger, a stomach-soothing remedy used by the ancient Greeks. In fact, Greek bakers invented gingerbread as a remedy for an overloaded stomach.

Yield: 1 cup

INGREDIENTS

1 cup water
1 teaspoon powdered peppermint leaves
1 teaspoon freshly grated or powdered gingerroot
2 to 3 teaspoons powdered chamomile flowers
    honey and/or lemon, to taste

SUPPLIES

saucepan
fine strainer

☛ **BE SAFE.** Some authorities recommend these herbs to relieve the morning sickness of pregnancy. Pregnant or nursing women should not use without first consulting a physician. Otherwise healthy adults may use up to 3 cups a day. Do not give to children under 2. Older children and those over 65 should use extra water to reduce formula strength. The younger the child, the more dilute the formula should be. If headache, rash, stomach distress, or other unpleasant effects develop, discontinue use. If you suffer from frequent indigestion, see your physician. Use this formula only in consultation with your physician.

Bring water to a boil in the saucepan. Add peppermint, ginger, and chamomile and remove from heat. Steep 10 to 20 minutes. Strain. Add honey and/or lemon. Drink cool or reheat.

➠ **Note:** Buy herbs at health food stores and herb shops. See page 444 for other sources.

Nausea Relief Formula

For nausea relief, try this ginger/peppermint infusion. Both herbs have been used to calm stomach upsets for centuries. This formula may also soothe morning sickness in pregnant women. Physicians advise against taking drugs to treat the discomforts of pregnancy because they might harm the fetus. But the amounts of ginger and peppermint in this formula have never been associated with fetal harm.

Yield: 1 cup

INGREDIENTS

1 cup water

1 teaspoon freshly grated or powdered gingerroot

1 teaspoon powdered peppermint leaves and flower tops

honey and/or lemon, to taste

SUPPLIES

saucepan

fine strainer

☛ **BE SAFE.** Use up to 3 cups a day, but no more. In very large doses (30 cups a day), ginger may promote miscarriage. Pregnant and nursing women should not use this formula without first consulting a physician. Do not give to children under 2. Older children and those over 65 should use extra water to reduce formula strength. The younger the child, the more dilute the formula should be. If headache, rash, stomach distress, or other unpleasant effects develop, discontinue use. Use this formula only in consultation with your physician.

Bring water to a boil in the saucepan. Add ginger and peppermint. Remove from heat. Steep 10 to 20 minutes. Strain. Add honey and/or lemon. Drink cool or reheat.

•• **Note:** Buy these herbs at health food stores and herb shops. See page 444 for other sources.

GOOD IDEA!

To combat motion sickness, try ginger capsules. Whether it happens in a boat, car, or plane, motion sickness feels the same—sudden dizziness, nausea, vomiting, and misery while traveling. A scientific study at Brigham Young University showed that ginger is as effective in relieving motion sickness as the standard over-the-counter drug Dramamine.

If you're traveling, the most convenient way to take ginger is to swallow ginger capsules 30 minutes before your departure. Adults may take up to three 550-milligram capsules. Older children may take one capsule, and adults over 65 may take two. Ginger capsules are not appropriate for children under 2. Buy ginger capsules in health food stores and some pharmacies.

HELP FOR TENSION AND STRESS

We live in a stressful world, so no wonder we feel anxious. The formulas that follow offer simple, low-risk ways for coping with stress-related symptoms like tension headaches and insomnia.

Anxiety Soother

All the herbs in this formula have tranquilizing properties. But unlike Valium, nothing in this formula is addictive.

Yield: 1 cup

INGREDIENTS

1 cup water
1 teaspoon powdered chamomile flowers
1 teaspoon powdered hop leaves
1 teaspoon powdered passionflower leaves
1 teaspoon powdered skullcap leaves

SUPPLIES

saucepan
fine strainer

☛ **BE SAFE.** Pregnant or nursing women should not use this formula without first consulting a physician. Otherwise healthy adults may drink up to 3 cups per day. Do not give to children under 2. Older children and adults over 65 should use extra water to reduce formula strength. The younger the child, the more dilute the formula should be. If headache, rash, stomach distress, or other unpleasant effects develop, discontinue use. Use this formula only in consultation with your physician.

Bring water to a boil in the saucepan, add all ingredients, remove from heat, and steep 10 to 20 minutes. Strain. Drink hot or cold.

➮ **Note:** Buy herbs at health food stores, and herb shops. See page 444 for other sources.

See page 444 for other sources.

GOOD IDEA!

Before you tranquilize, try exercise. Tranquilizers often impair driving ability and other skills, and if used for long periods, they're potentially addictive. Instead of medication for anxiety, try these ideas for anxiety relief.

- Exercise—try going for a 20- to 60-minute walk or bike ride at least three times a week
- A hot bath
- Yoga
- Meditation
- Visiting or calling close friends or family members
- Laughing—try renting a comedy video

Tension Headache Soother

The meadowsweet in this formula contains salicin, an aspirinlike chemical that helps relieve headaches.

Yield: 1 cup

INGREDIENTS

1 cup water
1 teaspoon powdered meadowsweet leaves and
   flower tops
   honey and/or lemon, to taste

SUPPLIES

ice cubes or commercial gel cold pack

clean cloth

saucepan

fine strainer

☛ **BE SAFE.** *Pregnant or nursing women should not use meadowsweet. Otherwise healthy adults may use up to 3 cups a day. Do not give meadowsweet to children under 2. Older children and adults over 65 should use extra water to reduce formula strength. The younger the child, the more dilute the formula should be. Meadowsweet may cause stomach distress in those with aspirin-sensitive stomachs. If headache persists, or if rash, stomach distress, or other unpleasant effects develop, discontinue use. Do not place ice or commercial ice substitutes directly on the skin. Always wrap them in a cloth. Use this formula only in consultation with your physician. Severe or chronic headaches require professional care.*

Wrap a few ice cubes or the gel pack in a cloth, place across your forehead, and hold there for 20 minutes. Remove ice pack for 10 minutes. Repeat as needed.

For the infusion, bring water to a boil in the saucepan. Add meadowsweet and remove from heat. Steep 10 minutes. Strain. Add honey and/or lemon. Drink cool or reheat.

➠ **Note:** *Buy meadowsweet at health food stores and herb shops. See page 444 for other sources.*

GOOD IDEA!

Wipe out your headache with white willow bark. Soak a teaspoon of powdered white willow bark in a cup of water for 8 hours. Strain and drink the infusion cool or reheat and drink warm. White willow bark is the herbal equivalent of aspirin. People with an aspirin-sensitive stomach may find it causes stomach upset. If you choose to use this remedy, follow the "Be Safe" note at left.

Many people find that the application of a cold pack alone relieves headache without aspirin. For occasional headaches, keep a forehead-size commercial gel pack in your freezer. You may get acceptable relief by taking a ½-hour nap while you apply a cold gel pack to your head.

Good Night's Sleep Formula

If you have problems falling asleep, try this herbal formula.

Yield: 2 cups

INGREDIENTS

2 cups water
2 teaspoons powdered hop flowers
1 teaspoon powdered passionflower leaves
2 teaspoons powdered valerian root
    honey and/or lemon, to taste

SUPPLIES

saucepan
fine strainer

☛ **BE SAFE.** Pregnant or nursing women should not use this formula without first consulting a physician. Otherwise healthy adults may drink up to 2 cups before bedtime. Do not give to children under 2. Older children and those over 65 should use extra water to reduce formula strength. The younger the child, the more dilute the formula should be. If headache, rash, stom-ach distress, or other unpleasant effects develop, discontinue use. Use this formula only in consultation with your physician.

Bring water to a boil in the saucepan. Add hop flow-ers, passionflower, and valerian root. Remove from heat. Steep 10 to 20 minutes. Strain. Add honey and/or lemon. Drink warm.

✿ **Variation:** All the herbs in this formula have sedative proper-ties. If one or more are not available, use a total of 5 teaspoons of any combination of the herbs for a similar effect.

➜ **Note:** Buy herbs at health food stores and herb shops. See page 444 for other sources.

PAIN-SOOTHING REMEDIES

The formulas that follow relieve pain associated with a few specific injuries or minor health problems. You'll find help for a tooth that can't be fixed until next Monday and for an arthritic knee that kicks up whenever the weather changes. While none of these formulas are for pain caused by serious illness or injury, you'll find they provide safe, inexpensive alternatives to over-the-counter painkillers.

Toothache First-Aid

Before dentists had modern painkillers, they rubbed aching teeth with anesthetic herb oils. Dentists still use clove oil today, and it's included in some dental first-aid kits for temporary relief of toothache pain.

SUPPLIES

clove oil

cotton swabs

☛ **BE SAFE.** Do not swallow clove oil. Do not use this formula for children of any age. Small amounts—less than a teaspoon— can cause possibly fatal poisoning. Clove oil provides only temporary relief of toothache pain. Toothaches require professional dental care.

Dip a swab into clove oil. Rub the oil-filled swab on the painful tooth.

➟ **Note:** Buy clove oil at health food stores and herb shops. Or, order it through your pharmacist. See page 444 for other sources.

GOOD IDEA!

Massage your toothache away. When you have an achy tooth, rub an ice cube into the V-shaped area where the bones of the thumb and forefinger meet. Gently push the ice over the area for 5 to 7 minutes. Reasearch has shown that ice massage may ease the pain of a toothache by 50 percent. It's possible that this technique works by flooding the pain-carrying nerves with sensation from the cold ice rubbing on the skin.

GOOD IDEA!

Cool away hemorrhoid pain. Prepare a large quantity of salve using ½ cup honey, ½ cup comfrey root, and 4 teaspoons aloe vera gel. Store it in your refrigerator and apply as needed.

If you use over-the-counter remedies, most doctors recommend that you choose hemorrhoid creams over suppositories. Even for internal hemorrhoids, suppositories tend to make poor contact with the hemorrhoidal tissue.

Hemorrhoids are frequently associated with constipation, obesity, or pregnancy. To help prevent hemorrhoids, maintain your recommended weight and prevent constipation by eating a high-fiber diet, drinking plenty of fluids, and exercising regularly.

Soothing Wipe for Hemorrhoids

This formula helps reduce hemorrhoid discomfort and aids healing.

Yield: ¼ cup of salve

INGREDIENTS

- 2 tablespoons honey
- 1 teaspoon powdered comfrey root
- 2 tablespoons aloe vera gel
- witch hazel

SUPPLIES

spoon
small mixing bowl or cup
cotton balls

☞ **BE SAFE.** If rash or any unusual irritation develops, discontinue use. Use this formula only in consultation with your physician. If hemmorhoids bleed frequently, seek professional care.

To make the salve, thoroughly combine honey comfrey, and aloe vera gel in the bowl.

Using cotton balls, apply witch hazel liberally to the affected area. Using fresh cotton balls, cover the affected area with a thin layer of salve. Repeat as needed.

➡ **Notes:** Aloe vera gel works best fresh from the plant. Simply snip off part of a fleshy leaf, cut it open, and scoop out the gel. If you don't have an aloe vera plant, buy aloe vera, as well as comfrey, at health food stores and herb shops. Unprocessed aloe vera gel is more effective than the "stabilized" variety. See page 444 for other sources. Purchase witch hazel at pharmacies and supermarkets.

Swimmer's Ear Remedy

When the ear canal is repeatedly exposed to moisture, its protective wax may be stripped away, allowing bacteria to cause infection in the canal lining. Symptoms progress from itching to considerable pain and sometimes discharge. Painful cases of swimmer's ear should be treated by a physician, who will probably prescribe antibiotic ear drops. But for mild cases involving only itching and mild discomfort, this formula is appropriate. Both alcohol and vinegar are antiseptics that can kill swimmer's ear bacteria. If you know swimming frequently gives you an ear infection, drop this swimmer's ear formula into your ears *before* you swim and after you finish.

Yield: ¼ cup

INGREDIENTS

⅛ cup rubbing alcohol (70 percent isopropyl)
⅛ cup white vinegar

SUPPLIES

small saucepan
dairy or candy thermometer
eyedropper
washcloth
sealable container

☛ **BE SAFE.** *If ear pain increases or if symptoms do not abate within one week, consult your physician.*

Combine alcohol and vinegar in the saucepan and heat to about 100°F. The solution should be comfortably warm, *not* hot. Lie on your side. Using the eyedropper, fill the ear canal with the warm solution. Wait 5 minutes before rising. Drain into the washcloth. Repeat several times a day. Refrigerate tightly sealed for one to two weeks.

GOOD IDEA!

If you wear a hearing aid, be extra careful. Those who wear hearing aids can get swimmer's ear without going near the water. Hearing aids tend to trap moisture in the ear canal, and trapped moisture makes a prime breeding spot for infection. To avoid swimmmer's ear associated with a hearing aid, remove your hearing aid as often as possible to give your ear a chance to dry out.

Arthritis Pain Reliever

Physicians usually treat common osteoarthritis with either aspirin or aspirin-like nonsteroidal anti-inflammatory drugs (NSAIDs). Meadowsweet is an herbal aspirin.

Yield: 1 cup

INGREDIENTS

1 cup water
2 teaspoons powdered echinacea root
3 teaspoons powdered chamomile flowers
2 teaspoons freshly grated or powdered gingerroot
1 teaspoon powdered meadowsweet leaves and flower tops
honey and/or lemon, to taste

SUPPLIES

saucepan

fine strainer

☛ **BE SAFE.** Pregnant or nursing women should not use this formula. Do not give to children under 2. Otherwise healthy adults may use up to 3 cups a day. Older children and those over 65 should add extra water to reduce formula strength. The younger the child, the more dilute the formula should be. Echinacea may cause tingling of the tongue. This is normal and not hazardous. Meadowsweet may cause stomach distress in those with aspirin-sensitive stomachs. If headache, rash, stomach distress, or other unpleasant effects develop, discontinue use. This formula should be used only in consultation with your physician.

Bring water to a boil in the saucepan. Add echinacea and simmer 10 to 15 minutes on low heat. Add chamomile, ginger, and meadowsweet. Remove from heat and steep for 10 to 20 minutes. Strain. Add honey and/or lemon. Drink cool or reheat.

➥ **Note:** Buy herbs at health food stores and herb shops. See page 444 for other sources.

Deep Heat Relief for Muscle Aches

For centuries, people have rubbed red pepper into sore muscles and cold feet for warmth and relief of soreness. In fact, the hot chemical in red pepper, capsaicin, is used in several over-the-counter ointments and linaments for sore muscles. But why hobble off to a drug store when you can get the same benefits at lower cost, simply by mixing up this formula?

Yield: 2 tablespoons

INGREDIENTS

2 teaspoons cayenne pepper
2 tablespoon vegetable oil

SUPPLIES

small saucepan or glass measuring cup
clean cloth

☛ **BE SAFE.** *Use as needed, but do not rub into skin injured by burns, cuts, or other wounds. If a rash or any unusual irritation develops, discontinue use. Use this formula only in consultation with your physician.*

Stir cayenne thoroughly into oil in the saucepan or cup. Heat the pan on the stovetop or the glass cup in the microwave until it's just warm, *not* hot. Dip the cloth into the mixture and rub into the sore area.

GOOD IDEA!

Give your muscles a break. Every time you exercise, your muscles are injured. Soreness means real damage. You should stop exercising when you feel sore. How much you should rest depends on the severity of the injury and the situation. If you're noticeably sore after increasing your jogging mileage by 10 percent, that's a signal you may be trying to increase your mileage too fast. You may want to rest a few days and drop back to your earlier level of exercise. Overall, never underestimate the value of rest in healing sore muscles. Your body needs time to repair the damage.

Chapter Six

Home Repair and Remodeling

by Walter Jowers

If I were to get three wishes tomorrow from some kind of modern quartz-halogen-lamp genie, one wish would be that all my house-fixing jobs could be done by following a simple formula. When I got ready to build that stair in the seriously out-of-square upstairs hall, the plan would be revealed to me, in ten easy steps. If I needed to match the pattern of some overpriced, special-order, nonreturnable wallpaper on walls as wavy as funhouse mirrors, I'd have a formula: do this, then do that, and everything would work out perfectly. Unfortunately, things are not that simple.

I live in a house that's seventy-something years old—a house that was much abused by earlier occupants. Something here always needs fixing, and nothing is as easy as it looks. Like the fabric of space-time, the fabric of my battered house is curved and full of curious places like black holes, where every law but Murphy's breaks down on a regular basis.

When I got a chance to write this chapter of house-fixing formulas, I had to do it. Formulas, yes sir. Formulas are neat and tidy. A pinch of this and a dab of that. No—exactly ½ ounce of this and 0.769 of an ounce of that. Something scientific that people can measure precisely and repeat as many times as they want with predictable results. No guesswork. Well, maybe just a little guesswork . . .

These are house-fixing formulas, after all. Even the most orderly ones have a little slip built in, like the automatic transmissions in old Corvairs. Some of the concrete formulas are figured by weight—as laboratory accurate as you can get, right? Well, not exactly. You might have to adjust some of the ingredients up or down a little bit to allow for the ambient humidity or the dampness of the sand or the coarseness of the gravel. It's a little bit of an art. Many of these formulas take a little eyeballing, a little holding something up to the light, a little head scratching and chin rubbing to get just the right results. As they say here in Tennessee, to get it to work, you have to hold your mouth right.

You have to use sensible precautions with these formulas, too. There's not a thing in this chapter that you can drink or take a bath in without getting into serious trouble. Vinegar and toothpaste are probably the only ingredients here that you'd want to put in your mouth. So, before you start, read *all* of the instructions, including the part that tells you how to stay out of trouble.

If you decide to try some of the fancier formulas—like wall glazing, false wood graining, or marbleizing—practice. And use good tools. The quickest way I know to conjure up Murphy's Law is to start on a serious job with little preparation and cheap, awkward tools bought off a rack next to the shoe polish at a convenience store.

If you're careful with the hazardous stuff and practice the hard stuff, these formulas will help you with lots of common house-fixing jobs. And even if you use only a few of these formulas, this chapter provides lots of secret-formula trivia—like how to make whitewash or how to strip paint with fireplace ashes. You'll even find out how to make one of those expensive furniture "finish revivers" as advertised on TV.

The fun never stops. Did you know that ketchup makes a good brass polish? The vinegar and acid in the tomatoes make it work. Ketchup brass polish isn't in this chapter, because I couldn't think of a way to make it into a formula. My mission here is to tell you how to brew up stuff that'll help you keep your house repaired, not stuff that's equally good on tea kettles and home fries.

CONCRETE AND MORTAR

Mixing concrete, making colored patio pavers, tuckpointing an old brick wall, fixing broken stucco—all these jobs are well within the abilities of most ambitious do-it-yourselfers. These formulas provide all the directions needed to get the job done right. As with all concrete formulas, you may have to adjust the ingredient amounts up or down to deal with on-site variables, such as temperature, humidity, and the moisture content of the sand.

Hand-Mixed Concrete

One cubic foot of concrete is about the maximum amount you can mix by hand. Mixing a larger volume usually requires a power mixer. A proper mix is just wet enough to allow the concrete to be worked with a float or a trowel. Weighing the ingredients gives the best results.

Yield: 1 cubic foot

INGREDIENTS

11 pounds drinkable water
53 pounds concrete sand
27 pounds Type I portland cement
55 pounds ½-inch gravel

SUPPLIES

two 5-gallon buckets
bathroom scales
wheelbarrow or mortar box
goggles, safety glasses, or face shield
waterproof gloves
dust mask
shovel
mixing hoe

☛ **BE SAFE.** Both cement and newly mixed concrete are caustic and will irritate or burn skin and eyes. Wear goggles, protec-

---

GOOD IDEA!

To speed mixing of later concrete batches, mark lines on the buckets during the first weighing of each ingredient. You won't have to weigh the ingredients of subsequent batches. Use wet sand—sand that forms a ball when squeezed and leaves your palm relatively dry. If the sand is only damp (crumbles when you squeeze it), decrease the quantity of sand by 1 pound and increase the water by 1 pound. If the sand is very wet (exudes noticeable moisture when squeezed), increase the quantity of sand by 1 pound, and decrease the water by 1 pound.

tive clothing, and waterproof gloves during the mixing and application of concrete. Wear a dust mask when opening and emptying bags of cement.

To assure accurate weighing, the actual weight of the
empty bucket must be allowed for. Place one empty bucket
on the scales and note the weight of the bucket. Then weigh
the necessary amount of water (adding the weight of the
empty bucket to the needed amount). Set aside. Repeat the
procedure for weighing the sand. Spread sand out evenly in
the wheelbarrow or mortar box. Wearing proper clothing
and safety gear, weigh cement the same way. Dump cement
evenly on top of the sand, and mix thoroughly. Weigh and
add in gravel and mix all three ingredients thoroughly, turning the final mix over at least three times. Form a hollow in
the middle of the dry mix and slowly add most of the water.
Using the hoe, turn all ingredients toward the center and
continue mixing while gradually adding remaining water.
Mix until all ingredients are thoroughly combined.

✿ **Variation:** You can change the gravel size, but the amounts
of other ingredients must change as well. For 1-inch gravel, the
mix would be 10 pounds drinkable water, 45 pounds concrete
sand, 24 pounds Type I portland cement, and 70 pounds 1-inch
gravel.

➟ **Notes:** Buy portland cement at building supply stores. Type
I portland cement is a general-purpose cement, useful for pavement and buildings. It typically comes in 94-pound bags,
enough for 3 to 4 cubic feet of concrete. Concrete sand varies
by region. In some places, river bottom sand is cheap and plentiful and is usually sold by the ton. In other areas, bagged manufactured sand is the only material available. Building supply
stores often sell gravel by the bag.

> **GOOD IDEA!**
>
> **F**or best results
> when mixing con-
> crete, be sure to buy a
> gravel mix suitable to the
> thickness of your con-
> crete slab. Each grade of
> gravel mix contains a
> range of gravel sizes. The
> size of the largest gravel
> pieces should measure
> no more than one-third
> the thickness of the slab
> you're pouring. For exam-
> ple, if you're pouring a
> slab 3 inches thick, the
> size of the largest gravel
> pieces should be no
> greater than 1 inch in di-
> ameter.

Concrete Mixed by Volume

Mixing concrete by weight yields the most consistent results and allows for easier adjustments of ingredient amounts. If you use a power concrete mixer, measuring by volume allows you to set up an "assembly line" with helpers.

Yield: about ⅔ the combined volume of all ingredients

INGREDIENTS

    2 parts ½-inch gravel
    ½ part drinkable water
    1 part Type I portland cement
 2½ parts concrete sand

SUPPLIES

four 5-gallon buckets
goggles, safety glasses, or face shield
waterproof gloves
dust mask
shovel
power concrete mixer

☛ **BE SAFE.** Both cement and newly mixed concrete are caustic and will irritate or burn skin and eyes. Wear goggles, protective clothing, and waterproof gloves during the mixing and application of concrete. Wear a dust mask when opening and emptying bags of cement.

Mark each bucket at 1-gallon intervals. Wearing proper clothing and safety gear, measure the correct volumes of each ingredient. Begin with the mixer power OFF. Pour in all the gravel and half the water. Then start the mixer. As it turns, add cement and sand, then the remaining water. Continue running the mixer for at least another 3 minutes, or until all the materials are thoroughly mixed and the concrete has a uniform color.

✿ **Variation:** You can mix this concrete formula by hand in a wheelbarrow or mortar box, using a shovel and mixing hoe. First, spread the sand out evenly in the wheelbarrow, then the cement. Mix thoroughly. Mix in gravel, turning final mix at least three times. Add most of the water in a well formed in the center of the dry mix. Use the hoe to turn and mix the ingredients, while adding the rest of the water, until all ingredients are thoroughly combined.

➼ **Notes:** Buy portland cement at building supply stores. Type I portland cement is a general-purpose cement, useful for pavement and buildings. It typically comes in 94-pound bags. Concrete sand varies by region. In some places, river bottom sand is cheap and plentiful and is usually sold by the ton. In other areas, bagged manufactured sand is the only material available. Building supply stores often sell gravel by the bag.

Colored Concrete

To color concrete, add mineral pigments to the concrete mix. For best results, use a power mixer and white portland cement. Weigh the ingredients and repeat the weights exactly for each batch. Make test batches using different amounts of pigment, keeping careful records of each. Let cure for two to three days; the color will be close to the finished color. The weight of pigment needed depends on the color and type of pigment. You may need as little as 1½ pounds or as much as 9 pounds of pigment per 94 pounds of cement. The maximum pigment weight is 10 percent of the cement weight. Never add more than this.

COLORFUL PATIOS Tinting Concrete with Mineral Pigments	
To Get This Color	**Use This Pigment**
White	White portland cement and white sand
Brown	Burnt umber or brown iron oxide
Buff	Yellow ocher or yellow iron oxide
Green	Chromium oxide
Pink	Small amount of red iron oxide
Rose	Red iron oxide
Cream	Yellow iron oxide

GOOD IDEA!

To get the best mortar compaction, buy a tuckpointing trowel that is slightly narrower than the joints to be pointed. Mix only as much material as you can use in 1½ hours—generally between ½ gallon and 1 gallon of mortar. To perfect your technique, tuckpoint an inconspicuous area first. Some tuckpointing jobs are just too difficult for the average do-it-yourselfer. Ask for professional help if your home features highly textured brick, colored mortar, textured mortar, or unique joint profiles.

Mortar for Tuckpointing

Sooner or later, every brick house needs some tuckpointing. Cracks or erosion in the original mortar allow water penetration, which leads to even more damage. Even the best modern mortars will need touching up eventually. If your house was built before 1900, the mortar may be a high-lime mortar, which you should duplicate. New, harder mortars may damage pre-twentieth-century houses. For most houses built in this century and for just about every house built since World War II, this mortar formula is fine for tuckpointing aboveground-level walls.

Yield: varies by amount of ingredients chosen

INGREDIENTS

1 part Type N masonry cement
3 parts damp, loose masonry sand
   water

SUPPLIES

cold chisel or old screwdriver
wire brush or shop vacuum
goggles, safety glasses, or face shield
waterproof gloves
dust mask
5-gallon bucket
trowel
spray bottle
mortarboard, hawk, or clean scrap of plywood
tuckpointing trowel
sponge
rags

☛ **BE SAFE.** Cement is caustic and will irritate or burn skin and eyes. Wear goggles, protective clothing, and waterproof gloves during the mixing and application of concrete. Wear a dust mask when opening and emptying bags of cement.

To prepare the joints for tuckpointing, use the chisel or screwdriver to chip out the loose mortar to a depth of at least ½ inch, or until you reach sound mortar. With the wire brush or vacuum, remove all loose debris in the joints.

Wearing proper clothing and safety gear, combine cement and sand in the bucket. Mix until color is uniform. Add enough water to make a damp mix that holds its shape if you squeeze it in your hand. Mix for about 5 minutes, or until the mix is uniformly damp. To control shrinkage, let the damp mortar stand for about an hour. Finally, add enough water to get a workable mix and stir for another 5 minutes. Good tuckpointing mortar should be a little dryer than mortar used to lay bricks. If the unused mortar seems to dry out as you work, add a little more water. Discard any mortar that is more than 2½ hours old.

Before beginning to tuckpoint, dampen the joints with a spray of water. Keep the joints damp, but not saturated, while you work. Dump the mortar onto the mortarboard, hawk, or plywood. With the tuckpointing trowel, push the mortar from the board into the joints, packing it firmly. Then, strike off the packed mortar to match the original joint profile. Remove excess mortar from bricks with a wet sponge. If mortar haze remains on bricks, wipe it off with a rag.

➡ **Notes:** Type N masonry cement is a mixture of portland cement and lime. Masonry sand contains a much higher percentage of fine particles than cement sand. Buy masonry sand and masonry cement at well-stocked building supply stores and through professional masonry suppliers.

GOOD IDEA!

If you're tuckpointing to make a brick wall weathertight, keep in mind this advice from the Portland Cement Association. Before beginning the job, make a thorough inspection of flashings, lintels, sills, and caulked joints. If it is obvious that water is leaking through only one crack, you can tuckpoint only the mortar joints in the vicinity of the crack. Otherwise, it is best to tuckpoint all the mortar joints in the wall so that minute cracks aren't overlooked.

PAINTS AND SEALERS

In this section, you'll find formulas and complete instructions for many finishes that you just can't buy in a paint store. From a fancy, decorative wall glaze to an inexpensive but practical basement wall coating, the formulas here offer a host of paint and sealer options—both for saving money and for creating special effects.

2-Color Wall Glazing

Wall glazing is a fancy interior finish popular during the Victorian era. To glaze a wall, apply two or more layers of translucent colors and then finish off with varnish. The appearance is somewhat like rich leather or a semiprecious stone. The directions here explain how to apply a two-layered wall glaze. Note that you must mix the glazing coat ingredients twice, using two different Japan colors.

Yield: about 2 quarts

INGREDIENTS
FOR ONE GLAZING COAT
(mix twice)

1   quart Penetrol
1   quart high- or low-gloss varnish
1   pint paint thinner
    Japan color

SUPPLIES

two 1-gallon buckets
paint stirrers
rubber work gloves
2 natural sponges
1 to 2 gallons varnish
China bristle paintbrush

☛ **BE SAFE.** Wear rubber gloves to protect your hands. All ingredients are flammable. Avoid open flames. Do not smoke. Make sure the room is well-ventilated.

GOOD IDEA!

To get perfect results with wall glazing, practice first in a closet or on a piece of drywall. Carefully mask woodwork and any other areas you don't want to glaze. Clean brushes and containers with paint thinner.

GOOD IDEA!

To get spectacular results for any wood finishing, buy the best brushes you can afford. Cheap brushes will not give a good finish. A good-quality, 2-inch China bristle paintbrush may cost as much as $20, but the extra expense will pay off in a professional-looking job.

Pour all ingredients for one color into a bucket and stir well. Mix the second color the same way.

Wearing rubber gloves, apply the colored glazing coats, using the following technique. Apply the first color by stippling (dabbing) it on the wall with a natural sponge in a 2-foot-wide strip from floor to ceiling. Work quickly to reach the ceiling before the paint has begun to dry. Then apply the second color the same way, making sure that the stippled edges of the second color overlap the edges of the first color.

To get a proper glazing job, you must keep a *wet edge*. That is, after you apply the first colored stippling, you must return to the bottom of the strip where you started and apply the second color before the first color begins to dry. The color combinations you choose will give unique effects. For instance, if you want green walls, apply a blue coat and then a yellow one.

After you've applied both color coats to the entire room, allow the paint to dry thoroughly. Then, apply one to three finish coats of varnish to achieve a high-gloss surface that appears to have depth.

✿ **Variation:** You can use more than two colors of glazing. Use a new bucket for each new color.

➡ **Notes:** Penetrol, manufactured by the Flood Company, is a conditioner for improving the flow and coverage of oil-based paints. Japan colors are pigments available in 3- or 4-ounce tubes. A single tube supplies enough color to glaze an entire room. Buy glazing supplies at well-stocked paint supply stores that deal with professional decorators and at art supply stores. See page 444 for other sources.

GOOD IDEA!

There's more than one way to apply wall glazing. Experiment with different glazing effects by applying glaze with wads of paper, a comb, the end of a paintbrush—the possibilities are endless. Experiment in an inconspicuous place, like the walls leading downstairs into your basement.

GOOD IDEA!

Use color to "correct" a room's dimensions. Light colors "open up" a small room, making it seem larger. Dark colors help "shrink" large rooms. Low ceilings can be "raised" by painting them a lighter shade than the walls, while high ceilings can be "lowered" by painting them the same shade as the walls.

GOOD IDEA!

Practice false grain-
ing on a throwaway
workpiece, such as a
drywall scrap or a dis-
carded piece of furniture,
before trying the real
thing. It helps to have a
piece of real wood
nearby to use as a model
for the grain you wish to
duplicate. If you're applying a false grain to a
wood project you've
made, practice the grain-
ing on the larger pieces
of your leftover scrap
wood.

False Wood Graining

False graining is a useful technique for touching up filled areas in furniture or woodwork. It also makes a good decorative finish for doors, woodwork, or cabinets. This false grain mimics the look of walnut.

Yield: about 1½ quarts

INGREDIENTS

1 cup boiled linseed oil
2 cups satin-finish, oil-based varnish
  (*not* polyurethane)
3 cups mineral spirits
½ teaspoon Japan drier
3 tablespoons burnt umber Japan color
2 tablespoons raw umber Japan color

SUPPLIES

wood filler
#220-grit sandpaper
China bristle paintbrushes
white, high gloss, oil-based paint tinted with raw
  sienna Japan color for base coat
tack rag
rubber work gloves
2-quart container for mixing, such as a coffee can
paint stirrer
clean, lint-free rags

☛ **BE SAFE.** Wear rubber gloves to protect your hands. All ingredients are flammable. Avoid open flames. Do not smoke.
Work in a well-ventilated area.

To prepare a wood piece for false wood graining, carefully fill any holes and sand. Apply a base coat to the entire
piece. After the paint dries, sand the piece and wipe the surface with a tack rag.

Wearing rubber gloves, place all ingredients in the container and stir thoroughly. Brush a moderate coating of this

over the base-coated piece. Then, with a dry brush, pull the topcoat into long, curving lines to simulate wood grain. If the grain doesn't look right, simply remove the fresh topcoat with a clean, lint-free rag and try again.

✿ **Variations:** Use different techniques for applying the topcoat. Pat the topcoat on, rotate the brush in your hand as you paint, shake your hand from side to side. The options, like real woodgrain patterns, are nearly endless. Use pencil erasers, combs, feathers, or other small tools to pull the topcoat along the piece. Each of these devices will give a different effect.

➡ **Notes:** Buy most of the ingredients at well-stocked paint supply stores. Japan colors are pigments available in 3- or 4-ounce tubes. Buy them at well-stocked paint supply stores that deal with professional decorators and at art supply stores. See page 444 for another source. Japan drier is a clear, colorless liquid that hastens the drying time of normally slow-drying linseed oil. Buy it at art supply stores and well-stocked hardware stores.

Practice Makes Perfect

The key to a professional-looking wood finish is practice. Whether you're painting, varnishing, or staining, never apply your finish directly to the wood unless you're an experienced wood finisher. You'll want to experiment with techniques, colors, and materials on scrap wood first until you achieve the look you want. The best way to get duplicable results is to practice on the same type of wood that you will be putting your final finish on. Remember that light, both artificial and natural, will have an effect on the way your paint or stain will look on, say, kitchen cabinets. So before you settle on a color or technique, if possible, bring your practice wood into the same room as the wood you'll be finishing so you can see the full effect.

GOOD IDEA!

For a convincing marbleized finish, buy three different colors of interior, high-gloss paint. Use one color as the base coat. Feather in the two remaining colors as the marbleizing coats. The color combination that most closely resembles real marble is a white base coat, followed by pink and then gray featherwork. As with all decorative painted finishes, it's best to practice on a throw-away piece before working on the real thing.

Marbleizing Finish

This finish looks like marble. Try it on tabletops, tiles, counters, walls, or floors.

Yield: varies by amount of ingredients chosen

INGREDIENTS
FOR MARBLEIZING

3 colors of interior, high-gloss, oil-based paint thinned with mineral spirits

INGREDIENTS
FOR GLAZE

1 part boiled linseed oil

6 parts mineral spirits

SUPPLIES

wood filler (if working on wood)

#220-grit sandpaper

shellac

tack rag

China bristle paintbrush

#0000 steel wool

rubber work gloves

paint stirrers

containers for thinning paint and mixing glaze

roll of cotton

turkey feather

paper towels

clean, lint-free cloth

☛ **BE SAFE.** Wear rubber gloves to protect your hands. Ingredients are flammable. Avoid open flames. Do not smoke. Make sure the room is well-ventilated.

To prepare the base coat: Fill any holes and sand. Seal unpainted wood with shellac. When dry, wipe with a tack rag. Apply four very thin coats of the lightest color paint. After the second and fourth coats, sand and wipe with a tack rag. After the fourth coat is dry, apply two coats of shellac. When the last shellac coat is dry, rub with steel wool and wipe with a tack rag.

To marbleize the piece: Wearing rubber gloves, mix glaze ingredients in a container. Thin the two remaining paints with enough mineral spirits so that they flow smoothly off the turkey feather.

Dip a wad of cotton into the glaze mixture. Squeeze out excess glaze and apply a thin film to a small area—1 to 2 square feet.

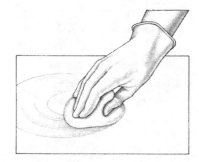
Glazing with cotton

Dip the turkey feather into one of the thinned paints; tap off excess onto a paper towel. Using the edge of the feather, paint in veins, always starting at an edge of the piece. Continually turn your hand at the wrist and the feather with your fingers. Veins will look more natural if you change the pressure you apply to the feather. Also, use different parts of the feather—tip, edge, or broadside—to change the shape of the vein. If you make a mistake, remove it with a dry cloth and start over. Before the first veins dry, apply the second thinned paint in the same manner.

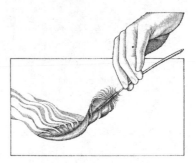
Turkey feather application

Then dip a piece of cotton in the glaze; squeeze out excess. Dab the glaze-moistened cotton on the newly applied veins and on unveined areas. This step feathers the vein edges and distributes small amounts of vein colors into unveined areas. Change the cotton when the distinction between the two colors blurs.

Repeat marbleizing steps over an adjacent 1- to 2-square-foot area. Vary the spacing and location of the dabbing to imitate the random pattern of colors found in nature.

When you're satisfied with the marbleized surface, let it dry thoroughly. Then, apply a coat of shellac.

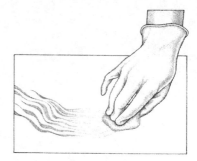
Feathering the edges

⚫ Notes: Buy marbleizing supplies at well-stocked paint supply stores. See page 444 for a turkey feather source.

GOOD IDEA!

You can mix paint quickly with a paddle mixer attachment for an electric drill. To keep the paint from spattering, place the paint can or bucket in a large paper shopping bag while mixing. The bag does a good job of containing the paint spatters. When you're done mixing, simply throw away the bag.

Orange Peel Paint

This paint will disguise minor flaws such as hairline cracks in plaster ceilings. It gives a slightly irregular surface—enough to break up light—and fills in small cracks. It's also washable.

Yield: 1 gallon

INGREDIENTS

1 gallon high-quality, interior, flat latex paint
1 quart drywall joint compound

SUPPLIES

2-gallon bucket
stirring attachment on an electric drill or a stiff stirring stick
lamb's-wool or high-quality paint roller suitable for rough surfaces

Pour paint into the bucket. Add joint compound and mix thoroughly with the drill attachment or stirring stick. If you mix several batches, be sure to use the same proportions each time. For best results, apply with the roller and apply two coats.

✿ **Variation:** To get consistent results for a larger area or multiple areas, mix up a little less than 5 gallons of paint in a 5-gallon bucket. This will cover the ceilings of at least two average-size rooms. Mixing one big batch allows you to vary the amount of drywall joint compound or paint to get just the right consistency.

➥ **Note:** Drywall joint compound is a thick, plasterlike material used normally to apply drywall tape. Buy it at hardware stores, home centers, and paint supply stores.

Sand Paint

Sand paint is a good choice for crazed or slightly cracked plaster walls or ceilings. The textured surface helps hide cracks. It's also attractive in any area where you want an unusual texture. Sand paint was quite popular from the late 1800s through the turn of the century.

Yield: 1 gallon

INGREDIENTS

2 to 3 cups fine white sand
1 gallon interior latex paint

SUPPLIES

window screen
2-gallon bucket
paint stirrer
paintbrush

First, sift sand through a piece of ordinary window screen. Sand that won't go through the screen is too coarse to give good results. Pour paint into the bucket, add sand, and mix thoroughly. Be sure to record the exact amount of sand you added so you can duplicate the effect with subsequent cans of paint. Apply the paint in short, choppy strokes or in half-circle strokes to create an attractive pattern.

➥ **Note:** You can use any type of fine, clean sand—except beach sand. Play sand, usually available at garden supply stores, toy stores, and home centers, gives good results. Do not clean brushes and other supplies inside. You do not want sand in your plumbing.

GOOD IDEA!

Before tackling a whole room with sand paint, practice on a new piece of drywall to perfect your technique. Once the job is done, clean your brushes outside with a garden hose—you don't want sand in your plumbing. Keep in mind that sand paint is not a good choice for walls that must be scrubbed often, such as those in kitchens and bathrooms.

GOOD IDEA!

For a true "country" **look,** distress the piece by lightly banging it with a stone or brick, especially around areas that would normally get more use—handles, corners, and legs. Then apply the pickled finish. The lighter paint will show up in the distressed areas.

GOOD IDEA!

A pickled finish **looks great with a topcoat of varnish,** but be sure to buy a varnish that's compatible with the paint you're using. Satin varnish reduces the sheen of the pickled finish, and high gloss adds shine. It usually takes three or four coats of varnish to get a good finish.

Pickled Finish

Pickling is not only attractive on country-style furnishings, it's also at home on a slick modern piece.

Yield: varies by amount of ingredients chosen

INGREDIENTS

oil-based, dark-colored, high-gloss paint
oil-based, white or light-colored, high-gloss paint
paint thinner

SUPPLIES

rubber work gloves
2 clean containers, such as coffee cans
paint stirrers
China bristle paintbrushes
clean, lint-free cloths

☞ **BE SAFE.** *Wear rubber gloves to protect your hands. Paint thinner is highly flammable. Avoid open flames. Do not smoke. Make sure the room is well-ventilated. Rags soaked with oil-based paint are subject to spontaneous combustion. Soak used rags in water and dispose of them outside.*

Pour dark-colored paint into a container. Fill the container only about one-quarter full. Gradually add paint thinner to dilute the paint as much as possible without losing the color you want. Your final mix will be anywhere from one-tenth to one-third paint thinner. Be sure not to thin the paint more than the manufacturer's recommendations. Apply the paint to the piece and let dry thoroughly.

Apply a coat of unthinned or very slightly thinned white or light-colored paint to a small portion of the piece. While it's wet, wipe the wood with a cloth. The idea is to leave the light-colored paint only in the pores and pronounced grain of the wood. Experiment as you like. It's easy to apply more light paint and wipe it off. When you get the look you want, repeat the process all over the piece and allow to dry.

Whitewash

Feel like playing Tom Sawyer? Here's how to make your own whitewash. Maybe you can hornswoggle somebody else into painting your fence or barn.

Yield: 3 gallons

INGREDIENTS

water

hydrated masonry lime

1/3 cup table salt

SUPPLIES

goggles, safety glasses, or face shield

long rubber gloves

1-gallon plastic milk jug for measuring lime and water

5-gallon plastic bucket

stirring attachment on an electric drill or a stiff stirring stick

whitewash brush

☛ **BE SAFE.** *Lime is caustic and will irritate or burn skin and eyes. Wear goggles, protective clothing, and long rubber gloves while working with it. Keep clean water and some vinegar nearby to wash off and neutralize skin.*

Cut the top off the 1-gallon milk jug leaving the handle intact. Measure 1 jugful of water into the bucket. Wearing proper safety gear, add 2 jugfuls of lime. Add salt. The idea is to make a lime slurry that's roughly the consistency of thin cake icing. If necessary, add a little more or less lime or water to reach the desired consistency.

Whitewash is a cheap and effective way to brighten up dingy basement walls and whiten the insides of barns and chicken coops. Apply with a whitewash brush.

↠ **Note:** *Hydrated masonry lime typically comes in 40-pound bags, which makes enough whitewash to paint about 150 square feet. Buy masonry lime at lumber yards, well-stocked building supply stores, and masonry supply stores.*

GOOD IDEA!

For a semi-opaque wash, use more water than called for in milk paint recipes. Apply the wash with a cloth and let dry. This finish can be sealed with a thin shellac.

Milk Paint

During colonial days, milk paint was the traditional wood finish for farm furniture. It was popular because it was durable and attractive, and it used a cheap, abundant resource—cow's milk. Milk paint soaks into wood and produces a finish that resembles stain more than paint.

Yield: about 1 quart

INGREDIENTS

about 1 quart water
1 box nonfat dry milk (9.6 ounces)
universal tinting color for latex paint

SUPPLIES

old 2-quart saucepan

paint stirrer

clean, lint-free cloths

☞ **BE SAFE.** Paint tints may be toxic. Don't cook in utensils that have been used to mix tinted milk paint.

Place water in the saucepan and heat until just below boiling. Stirring continuously, add dry milk. Simmer, stirring constantly, until the mixture resembles a thick soup. Gradually add tinting color, stirring until the color is uniform and is the color you want. If the color is too strong, add water; if it's too weak, add pigment.

With a clean cloth, wipe the warm paint onto the wood. Keep the paint warm as you work. As the paint dries, rub the wood with a damp cloth. This technique gives an antique-looking finish.

➻ **Note:** Buy universal tinting colors for latex paint at well-stocked paint supply stores.

Basement Wall Coating

It's hard to get ordinary paint to adhere to damp cinder blocks or stone. Although this coating won't cure a severe basement water problem, it will spruce up basement walls that are merely damp and unsightly.

Yield: 1 gallon

INGREDIENTS

1 gallon exterior latex paint
portland cement

SUPPLIES

goggles, safety glasses, or face shield
waterproof gloves
dust mask
5-gallon bucket
stirring attachment on an electric drill or a stiff stirring stick
stiff, wide paintbrush

☛ **BE SAFE.** Cement is caustic and will irritate or burn skin and eyes. Wear goggles, protective clothing, and waterproof gloves when you're mixing the formula. Wear a dust mask when opening and emptying bags of cement. Wear eye goggles and gloves while painting.

Wearing proper clothing and safety gear, place paint in the bucket and add cement, 1 cupful at a time, stirring vigorously after each cup. Add just enough cement to give the paint the consistency of spreadable cake frosting. The amount of cement needed to get the right consistency will vary with the brand and color of paint. Apply the paint with a wide brush. If appearance is important, apply paint with a repetitive motion of short strokes or arcs to achieve a stuccolike finish.

➾ **Note:** Buy portland cement, typically sold in 94-pound bags, at building supply stores.

GOOD IDEA!

To prepare your already-painted basement walls for a new wall coating (if they are mildewed or are chalking), start by washing them with a trisodium phosphate (TSP) and bleach solution. Mix 1 cup TSP, 3 quarts warm water, and 1 quart chlorine bleach. Wear rubber work gloves to protect your hands and cover the basement floor with a tarp to prevent any dicoloration from bleach spills. Liberally apply the solution with a brush. Allow to dry for 24 hours, then scrape off the old paint. Brush off any dust, then apply the new wall coating.

PLASTER AND STUCCO

Designed especially for the novice plasterer, these formulas should give nearly foolproof results. Before beginning a plaster or stucco project, first read all the instructions completely. And since plaster is only workable for a short time after the initial mixing, assemble all supplies and tools *before* you begin to mix the formulas.

Old-Fashioned Finish Plaster

If you need to patch a spot on a plaster wall where the old finish coat (the top $1/16$ to $1/8$ inch) has failed, this formula will do it. It gives a much harder and smoother finish than drywall joint compound. For an authentic plaster finish, you can use this as a topcoat on a plaster patch.

Yield: a quantity about the size of a football

INGREDIENTS

cold water

finish lime, such as U.S. Gypsum's Ivory

gauging plaster

SUPPLIES

goggles, safety glasses, or face shield

waterproof gloves

dust mask

5-gallon plastic bucket

stirring attachment on an electric drill or pointing
    trowel

mortarboard, hawk, or clean scrap of plywood

margin trowel

plasterer's trowel

☛ **BE SAFE.** Lime is caustic and will irritate or burn skin and eyes. Wear goggles, protective clothing, and long rubber gloves while working with it. Keep clean water and some vinegar nearby to wash off and neutralize skin.

GOOD IDEA

Don't paint finish plaster until it has cured for at least a week. Before painting, prime the plaster with shellac or Kilz, available at paint supply stores and home centers.

Wearing proper clothing and safety gear, pour ½ gallon water into the bucket, then add in finish lime until it starts to float. Mix thoroughly with the drill attachment or pointing trowel. If needed, adjust the mix by adding a little water or lime until the final mix (lime putty) resembles cream cheese with no lumps or standing water.

Place some of the lime putty on the mortarboard, hawk, or plywood and form it into a ring with the margin trowel. Fill the center about two-thirds full with cold water. Slowly sprinkle in gauging plaster until the water can't hold any more. Mix these together until you get a mix slightly stiffer than the lime putty. Then, fold in the lime putty and mix all ingredients thoroughly. The ideal final mix should be 1 part gauging plaster to 3 parts lime putty.

With the plasterer's trowel, pull the plaster onto the board and apply a chunk of it to the surface in an arc; work it smooth with the trowel. It will level and stiffen as you work. Discard unused, unworkable plaster after 20 minutes. Adjust future batches so that they can be used in 20 minutes.

➡ **Note:** Buy plastering supplies at stores that deal with the plastering trade; they are hard to find at hardware stores.

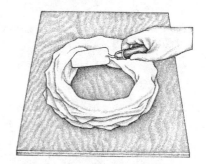

Forming a lime putty ring

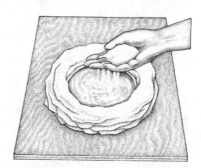

Mixing gauging plaster

Repairing Holes in Drywall

Repair small holes and cracks in drywall with joint or spackling compound applied with a wide putty knife. Holes up to 6 inches square call for another technique.

First, cut a rectangle out of a clean piece of drywall. The rectangle should be large enough to encompass the hole you will patch. Place the piece of drywall over the hole and trace around it. Using a keyhole saw, cut out the rectangle on the wall. This produces a clean regular opening to repair and a drywall patch that fits it exactly.

Cut a 1 × 2-inch board about 4 inches wider than the rectangular opening. Apply construction adhesive to the ends of the board. Insert the board into the opening, position it horizontally in the middle of the hole, and press it against the wall's inside surface until the adhesive holds. This 1 × 2 board will serve as additional support for the new piece of drywall. To completely secure the 1 × 2, drill pilot holes through the drywall and drive a drywall screw through the drywall and into each end of the 1 × 2-inch board.

To help hold the drywall patch in place, apply construction adhesive to the middle of the board. Gently tap the drywall patch into place and press it against the board. Cover the patch seams with mesh drywall tape and joint compound. Apply several successive coats of joint compound, sanding smooth after each coat.

Plaster Wall Repair

Fixing a hole in a plaster wall is a little different from patching a hole in modern drywall. This method works for relatively small holes, such as a hole left after the removal of a wall outlet or ceiling fixture. For bigger holes, you either need a fair amount of plastering experience or you need a plastering contractor.

Yield: varies by amount of ingredients chosen

INGREDIENTS

water

perlite gypsum plaster, such as U.S. Gypsum's
    Structolite

drywall joint compound

SUPPLIES

goggles, safety glasses, or face shield

dust mask

wire brush or shop vacuum

tin snips

wire lath (or chicken wire, in a pinch)

18-gauge tie wire

needlenose pliers

keyhole saw (optional)

drywall nails (optional)

mud pan

6-inch drywall taping knife

#100-grit sandpaper

☛ **BE SAFE.** *Wear goggles and a dust mask when chipping out old plaster. Wear a dust mask when mixing plaster. Wear goggles when working with plaster.*

Wearing proper safety gear, remove all loose plaster, and brush or vacuum out loose debris. Cut a piece of wire lath to fit over exposed existing lath. Secure the new lath with tie wire, using needlenose pliers to twist together loose ends and push them into the wall cavity. If there is no existing lath, use a keyhole saw to cut the existing hole back to two studs. Using drywall nails, mount new wire lath between the two newly exposed studs.

In the mud pan, slowly add water to plaster until the plaster is just wet, but not runny. With the drywall knife, spread a thin coat of plaster onto the wire lath, applying just enough plaster to fill the gaps in the lath, but no more. After the first coat has cured, mix a second batch of plaster and apply it to the first coat. This coat should finish flush with the wall.

After the second coat has cured, use the drywall knife to apply a coat of joint compound over the patch. Don't worry about making this coat smooth. When the first coat of drywall joint compound cures, knock off any ridges with the drywall knife and apply a second coat of drywall joint compound, feathering the edges to meet the wall surface. When this coat cures, sand the patch smooth. The patch is now ready to prime and paint.

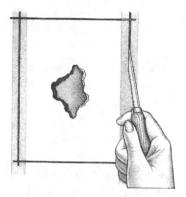

Cutting plaster hole with a key-hole saw

➥ **Notes:** Drywall joint compound is a thick, plasterlike material used normally to apply drywall tape. Buy it at hardware stores, home centers, and paint supply stores. Plastering supplies are available at stores that deal with the plastering trade; they are typically hard to find at hardware stores.

Stucco Formulas

These formulas represent three periods in American building. High-lime stucco is typical of the nineteenth century, lime-portland cement stucco might have been used in the transitional period at the turn of this century, and the third is a modern formula. If you're patching stucco, use a formula that matches the original closely: It should look, weather, and expand and contract the same. If in doubt, ask a mason to help you identify the stucco.

Yield: varies by amount of ingredients chosen

INGREDIENTS
FOR HIGH-LIME STUCCO

3 cubic feet sand matched to original

1 shovelful white portland cement

1 bag hydrated masonry lime

   coarse aggregate matched to original, not to exceed 15 percent of the total volume of hydrated lime

   water

INGREDIENTS
FOR LIME-PORTLAND CEMENT STUCCO

5 to 6 cubic feet masonry sand

1 bag portland cement

1 to 1½ bags hydrated masonry lime

   coarse aggregate matched to original, not to exceed 15 percent of the total volume of hydrated lime

   water

INGREDIENTS
FOR MODERN STUCCO

6 cubic feet masonry sand

1 bag portland cement

½ bag hydrated masonry lime

   coarse aggregate matched to original, not to exceed 15 percent of the total volume of hydrated lime

   water

SUPPLIES

waterproof gloves
goggles, safety glasses, or face shield
dust mask
mortar box
shovel
mixing hoe

☛ **BE SAFE.** Both cement and lime are caustic and will irritate or burn skin and eyes. Wear goggles, protective clothing, and waterproof gloves when mixing these formulas. Wear a dust mask when opening and emptying bags of cement or lime.

Wear proper clothing and safety gear. To mix these formulas, place half the sand in one end of the mortar box. Spread cement and lime over the sand. Then, pour the rest of the sand over top of the cement-lime layer. Place the coarse aggregate on top of the sand. Start at the empty end of the box and pull the hoe toward you through the materials. Repeat until the material is thoroughly mixed and assembled at one end of the box.

Pour some water into the empty end of the box, and pull the dry material into the water with the hoe, making sure the hoe cuts to the bottom of the box. Continue to add water until the mix is a soft, pliable mass. Keep chopping with the hoe until the material is uniformly wet and all in one end of the box. Then change direction and pull the mortar to the other end of the box. The mortar is ready when it is a uniform color.

➾ **Notes:** Buy portland cement, typically sold in 94-pound bags, enough for 3 to 4 cubic feet of stucco, at building supply stores. Masonry sand contains a much higher percentage of fine particles than cement sand. Buy masonry sand at well-stocked building supply stores and through professional masonry suppliers. Hydrated masonry lime typically comes in 40-pound bags. Buy it at lumber yards, well-stocked building supply stores, and masonry supply stores.

GOOD IDEA!

To properly restore old, high-lime stucco on pre-1900 homes, you must match the sand and gravel (aggregate) used in the original stucco. To examine the original sand and aggregate, dissolve a piece of the old stucco in a dilute solution of muriatic acid, which is available at hardware stores. Sift out the original sand and aggregate and take them to a local supply yard. There, you may be able to find a good match.

GOOD IDEA!

Don't make up more parge than you can use in about an hour. For a first project, the maximum volume of parge you should make in one batch is around 5 gallons. Try to apply all of the parge within a half hour to an hour. Discard parge that begins to set-up before you are finished.

It's easy to make colored parge. Simply add the mineral pigments used for coloring cement. See the table "Colorful Patios" on page 223.

Parge Coating for Foundation Walls

Parge is a thin, mortarlike coating for stone or concrete block walls. It helps prevent water penetration and it improves the appearance of dissimilar materials.

Yield: varies by amount of ingredients chosen

INGREDIENTS

1 part hydrated masonry lime
1 part portland cement
3 parts masonry sand
½ part drinkable water

SUPPLIES

goggles, safety glasses, or face shield

waterproof gloves

dust mask

wheelbarrow or mortar box

shovel

mixing hoe

wire brush or shop vacuum

spray bottle

mortarboard, hawk, or clean scrap of plywood

trowel

☛ **BE SAFE.** *Both cement and lime are caustic and will irritate or burn skin and eyes. Wear goggles, protective clothing, and waterproof gloves when mixing this formula. Wear a dust mask when opening and emptying bags of cement or lime.*

Wearing proper clothing and safety gear, place all dry ingredients in the wheelbarrow or mortar box and mix until ingredients are a uniform color. Add about ⅔ of the water and mix thoroughly. Add remaining water and mix again.

Brush or vacuum all loose debris from the work surface. Dampen the surface with a spray of water. Place the mix on the mortarboard, hawk, or plywood and trowel a ¼- to ⅜-inch coat of parge onto the damp surface. Before the parge sets, crosshatch it with a corner of the trowel to create a "tooth" for the second coat. Wait at least 24 hours, then dampen the surface with a spray of water and apply a second coat. Keep the parge damp for at least 48 hours to assure proper curing.

➻ **Notes:** Buy portland cement, typically sold in 94-pound bags, at building supply stores. Masonry sand contains a much higher percentage of fine particles than cement sand. Buy masonry sand at well-stocked building supply stores and through professional masonry suppliers. Hydrated masonry lime typically comes in 40-pound bags. Buy it at lumber yards, well-stocked building supply stores, and masonry supply stores.

WOOD FORMULAS

These formulas will help with stripping old wood as well as finishing new projects. But before stripping an old piece, try a wood finish reviver. Afterward, you may find your old furniture looks fine without refinishing.

Tack Rag

Tack rags pick up the dust, dirt, and lint that accumulates on a piece as it's being finished.

SUPPLIES

rubber work gloves

cotton cheesecloth or soft linen

oil-based varnish (*not* polyurethane)

airtight container

☞ **BE SAFE.** Wear rubber gloves to protect your hands. Rags soaked with varnish may spontaneously ignite. Store tack rags in a cool place in an airtight container. Soak used rags in water and dispose of them in an airtight container outside.

Wearing rubber gloves, dampen a piece of cloth with varnish. Squeeze out excess and work varnish through the rag until it is damp and sticky all over.

GOOD IDEA!

Tack rags should be made only of cotton cheesecloth or linen. Do not use synthetics or any fabric with stitching. Add more oil-based varnish, as necessary, to keep the tack rag usable.

GOOD IDEA!

To get the best-looking results when applying sealers, choose paintbrushes appropriate for the job. Use angled sash brushes for window sashes and straight brushes for flat surfaces. When you're done for the day, clean the brushes with paint thinner.

Weather-Resistant Wood Sealer

This simple formula applied to old exterior wood provides excellent protection against further weathering. It also prepares weathered wood surfaces for a new paint job and is particularly useful for window sashes, sills, fence boards, and the like.

Yield: varies by amount of ingredients chosen

INGREDIENTS

1 part boiled linseed oil
1 part paint thinner

SUPPLIES

rubber work gloves
paint scraper
wire brush
stirrer
container, such as a coffee can
paintbrushes

☛ **BE SAFE.** Wear rubber gloves to protect your hands. Ingredients are flammable. Avoid open flames. Do not smoke. Make sure the area is well-ventilated.

To prepare the wood surface, scrape off loose or flaking paint. Use a wire brush to remove loose paint from pores or checks in the wood.

To make the sealer, mix equal parts linseed oil and paint thinner in the container. Stir thoroughly. Apply a heavy coat of the sealer to the wood, letting it soak into the grain. Let the sealer dry for 24 hours, then repeat the treatment. If the wood is severely weathered, apply a third coat in the same way.

Allow the surface to dry completely. This may take several days because linseed oil dries very slowly. When the surface is completely dry, finish with any latex or oil-based primer plus the paint of your choice.

➡ **Note:** Buy linseed oil at paint supply stores.

Water Repellent for Wood

This nontoxic water repellent was developed by the U.S. Forest Products Laboratory, which is the wood research branch of the U.S. Forest Service. It's not only cheaper than commercial sealers, it's fairly safe to make and use. Use it to seal wood on decks, fences, outdoor furniture, and the like.

Yield: 1 gallon

INGREDIENTS

1½ cups boiled linseed oil *or* 3 cups exterior varnish (*not* polyurethane)
1 ounce paraffin wax
mineral spirits

SUPPLIES

rubber work gloves
penknife or double boiler
2-gallon bucket
stirrer
paintbrush

☛ **BE SAFE.** *Wear rubber gloves to protect your hands. Ingredients are flammable. Avoid open flames. Do not smoke. Make sure the area is well-ventilated. If you melt paraffin, do it in a double boiler; do not melt over direct heat.*

With a penknife, shave paraffin and set aside. Shaved paraffin works perfectly well and requires no melting. You may melt paraffin in the top of a double boiler and set aside. Pour either oil or varnish, *not both,* into the bucket, and add mineral spirits to make 1 gallon of liquid. Add paraffin and stir until well-mixed. Brush liberally onto wood.

➡ **Notes:** *Buy linseed oil and mineral spirits at paint supply stores and hardware stores. Paraffin is available in the canning section of supermarkets and hardware stores.*

GOOD IDEA!

When applying wood sealers or preservatives with a brush, don't be miserly. Brush the sealer on heavily so it will seep deeply into the wood. Use a natural-bristle brush. Natural bristles hold preservatives better than synthetic bristles do.

Try to save your work for a cloudy day or, if possible, move the wood into the shade. Working in direct sunlight will cause the sealer to dry before it has a chance to penetrate the wood.

GOOD IDEA!

To remove white rings from tabletops, mix together some baking soda and toothpaste (not the gel kind). The proportions aren't important. With a damp cloth, rub this mixture into the stained area, working with the grain of the wood until the ring disappears. Then wash the area with oil soap. If the ring persists, repeat the process. Then, apply a coat of good-quality furniture wax.

If you have some brass polish on hand, you can try rubbing the stain with that instead of the baking soda and toothpaste mixture.

Black Ring Repair

Black rings are tougher than white rings. They're caused by water that has penetrated the wood finish and worked its way into the wood. They're often found under potted plants.

SUPPLIES

#100- and #150-grit sandpaper

rubber work gloves

chlorine bleach (optional)

clean, lint-free cloths

vinegar (optional)

wood stain to match original color

wax filler stick

varnish

#0000 steel wool

furniture wax

☛ **BE SAFE.** Wear rubber gloves to protect your hands. Never mix bleach and vinegar.

To remove the finish over the stained area, sand it as lightly as possible with #100-grit sandpaper, followed by #150-grit sandpaper to feather the edges. Once the finish is removed, try light sanding to remove the stain. If this doesn't work, put on rubber gloves and bleach the wood. After the stain has faded to near the original color of the wood, rinse off the bleach completely; then neutralize the wood with vinegar.

After you've removed as much of the black stain as possible, apply matching wood stain to all bleached areas. Fill dents or scratches with a wax filler stick. Then apply several light coats of varnish to match the original finish. Feather the varnish edges with #0000 steel wool. Finish with furniture wax.

✿ **Variation:** As an alternative to bleaching the stain, you can apply false wood graining (see page 228) over the affected area. This is the method most often used by restoration experts.

➠ **Note:** *Wax filler sticks are sticks of pigment suspended in wax, somewhat like a crayon or colored pencil. Buy these at well-stocked paint supply stores and supply houses that serve the cabinetmaking trade.*

Wood Finish Revivers

If simply cleaning old furniture or woodwork doesn't do the job, and you'd like to avoid totally refinishing the wood, try these wood finish revivers. They will improve the appearance of wood surfaces that are darkened and clouded with age or slightly alligatored. To determine which reviver will do the job, test on an inconspicuous area of the woodwork or piece of furniture. Begin with the first formula, which is the least harsh. If that doesn't give good results, move on to the second, and so on. Stop with the formula that gives you the improvement you're looking for.

Reviver 1: 1 part boiled linseed oil, 1 part turpentine, and 1 part vinegar

Reviver 2: 1 part lacquer thinner and 1 part denatured ethyl alcohol

Reviver 3: denatured ethyl alcohol only

Reviver 4: lacquer thinner only

First, remove old wax from the furniture or woodwork you're reviving by wiping the piece down with mineral spirits. Then, mix each of the formulas in its own glass jar with lid. As you work, keep the jar sealed because the revivers evaporate quickly. Wear rubber work gloves and work outside or in a well-ventilated area. Avoid open flames and do not smoke when using these revivers—they are flammable.

To apply, simply dip a wad of #0000 steel wool into the reviver and squeeze out the excess. Very gently wipe the moistened steel wool over the piece to remove a thin layer of cloudy finish. As you work, discard steel wool that becomes gummy. After you've gone over the entire piece, apply a coat of tung oil or high-quality wax, such as carnauba.

Super Cleaner and Reviver for Wood

This rejuvenates old, dirty varnished woodwork.

Yield: varies by amount of ingredients chosen

INGREDIENTS

1 part boiled linseed oil
1 part turpentine
1 part white vinegar

SUPPLIES

rubber work gloves
container, such as a coffee can
stirrer
#0000 steel wool
clean, lint-free cloths

☛ **BE SAFE.** Wear rubber gloves to protect your hands. Turpentine and linseed oil are flammable. Avoid open flames. Do not smoke. Work in a well-ventilated area.

Wearing rubber gloves, thoroughly mix all ingredients in the container. Dip a wad of steel wool into the formula and lightly scrub the surface. Stir the formula, as needed, to keep the vinegar suspended. Wipe with a clean cloth.

➡ **Note:** Buy linseed oil at paint supply stores.

Wood Bleach

Here's one way to get wood whiter than white pine.

SUPPLIES

rubber work gloves
#0000 steel wool
chlorine bleach
white vinegar
#220-grit sandpaper
tack rag

☛ **BE SAFE.** *Wear rubber gloves to protect your hands. Never mix bleach and vinegar.*

Wearing rubber gloves, dip steel wool into bleach and rub a liberal amount into the wood, working with the grain. Repeat as needed until wood is uniformly lightened. When the bleach dries, apply vinegar to neutralize it. When dry, sand down any raised grain, buff the entire piece with steel wool, wipe the surface with a tack rag, and apply a finish.

High-Quality Furniture Wax

This is suitable for finishing and waxing wood.

Yield: about 2 quarts

INGREDIENTS

1 pound yellow beeswax
1 pint boiled linseed oil
1 pint turpentine

SUPPLIES

double boiler with a 2-quart insert
rubber work gloves
stirrer
resealable container, such as a coffee can

☛ **BE SAFE.** *Wear rubber gloves to protect your hands. Turpentine and linseed oil are flammable. Avoid open flames. Do not smoke. Work in a well-ventilated area. Melt wax in a double boiler; do not melt over direct heat.*

Melt wax in the top of a double boiler. Turn off heat and, wearing rubber gloves, remove double boiler to a heat-proof surface. Add oil and turpentine and mix thoroughly. Pour into the container; cool with lid off. Wax is ready to use when it's cool and solid.

➠ **Notes:** *Buy linseed oil at paint supply stores. Yellow beeswax is simply beeswax that has not been bleached to make candles. Buy it from beekeepers. See page 444 for another source.*

GOOD IDEA!

For a professional-looking, hand-rubbed wax finish for furniture, apply the furniture wax to only a small area at a time with a soft cloth, rubbing vigorously. Allow the wax to sit for a few minutes, then polish with another cloth. Buff to a high gloss.

GOOD IDEA!

If you want to varnish or shellac over wood stain, first seal the stain with a light coating of 2 ounces of shellac flakes mixed into 1 cup of denatured ethyl alcohol. Lightly sand the surface, then apply the normal topcoating of varnish or shellac.

All-Purpose Oil-Based Wood Stain

You can make your own oil-based wood stain in any color you like, including shades of brown, red, green, or blue. Mix this basic formula adding any pigment desired. To ensure consistent color in subsequent batches, record the amount of each ingredient used.

Yield: varies by amount of ingredients chosen

INGREDIENTS

1 part boiled linseed oil
2 ounces Japan drier
2 parts turpentine
up to ½ pound dry artist's pigment

SUPPLIES

rubber work gloves
sealable container
paint stirrer

☛ **BE SAFE.** Wear rubber gloves to protect your hands. Linseed oil and turpentine are flammable. Avoid open flames. Do not smoke. Work in a well-ventilated area.

Wearing rubber gloves, mix linseed oil, Japan drier, and turpentine in the container, then stir in artist's pigment to get the desired color. The pigment does not dissolve. It is suspended in the linseed oil and turpentine. When not using the stain, keep the container sealed to prevent evaporation.

➾ **Notes:** Buy linseed oil at paint supply stores. Buy dry artist's pigments at well-stocked paint supply stores or supply houses that deal with the woodworking and cabinetmaking trade. See page 444 for another source. Japan drier is a clear, colorless liquid that hastens the drying time of normally slow-drying linseed oil. Buy it at art supply stores and well-stocked hardware stores.

All-Purpose Water-Based Wood Stain

You can make your own water-based wood stain in a variety of traditional stain colors. The aniline dyes produce varying shades of brown. To ensure consistent color in subsequent batches, record the amount of each ingredient used.

Yield: 1 pint

INGREDIENTS

water-soluble aniline dye powder, such as Vandyke brown and Bismarck brown

1 pint warm water

1 drop vinegar

SUPPLIES

rubber work gloves

sealable glass container for each dye color

paint stirrer

☛ **BE SAFE.** *Wear rubber gloves to protect your hands. Aniline dyes are highly toxic. Keep dyes and any product made with dyes away from children and pets. Label containers of stain POISON.*

Wearing rubber gloves, stir dye powder into water in the container. Add as much or as little powder as is necessary to get the color you want. Add a drop of vinegar. If you like, combine batches of different colors to get the shade you want.

↦ **Note:** *Buy powdered aniline dyes by the pound at well-stocked paint supply stores. See page 444 for another source.*

G O O D   I D E A !

To **eliminate the fuzzy look and feel of wood caused by water-soluble aniline dyes,** first wipe the wood with a wet cloth or sponge to raise the grain; let it stand overnight. Next, sand it lightly with very fine sandpaper before applying the dye. Various aniline dyes may be soluble in water, alcohol, or hydrocarbon solvents. For wood stains, be sure to buy the water-soluble type. Water-soluble aniline dyes provide the most brilliant colors of all the aniline dyes available.

Fumed Oak Finish

This oak finish is the trademark of the early twentieth century mission-style furniture. Here's a home-brew version of how they did it.

SUPPLIES

ammonia

saucer or bowl

a see-through plastic bag

☛ **BE SAFE.** Work in a well-ventilated area and avoid breathing ammonia fumes.

Pour ammonia into the saucer or bowl and place it in the plastic bag along with a piece of unfinished oak. Seal the bag. The fumes will start changing the color of the wood very quickly. When the color is to your liking, open the bag and take out the piece of wood.

✿ **Variation:** To fume a whole piece of unfinished furniture, dilute ammonia with water (experiment on an inconspicuous area to get the right concentration) and brush the solution onto the piece with an old paintbrush.

Cleaner for Polyurethane-Coated Hardwood Floors

If your hardwood floors are varnished with polyurethane, you can get them clean with a mixture of warm water and vinegar. Mix 4 cups warm water with 1 cup white vinegar in a plastic bucket. Dip in a cloth, sponge, or sponge mop and wring it *nearly dry*. Clean the floor, then immediately wipe the floor dry.

When cleaning floors, many people tend to use too much cleaner and too much water. Use only enough cleaner to do the job and immediately wipe up any remaining moisture.

GENERAL REPAIRS

You'll find things here to help you out with many different common household repairs. To keep your repairs going smoothly, follow two simple steps: (1) Read *all* of the instructions *before* beginning the repair and (2) buy or borrow the right tools and ingredients.

Hole Patch for Drywall

With just a few tools and a scrap of newspaper, patching a hole in drywall is an easy task.

SUPPLIES

goggles, safety glasses, or face shield

newspapers

drywall joint compound

6-inch drywall knife

☛ **BE SAFE.** *Wear goggles when working with joint compound.*

Wad up a sheet of newspaper and fit it into the void in the wall. The wad should be even with the surface of the existing drywall, not project out past it. Let the wad "settle" to make sure it won't push out beyond the plane of the existing drywall.

Apply a coat of joint compound to the newspaper and let it cure. Apply second, third, or fourth coats as necessary to build the patch up flush with the wall plane. Be sure to allow the compound to cure between coats. Feather the edges of the final coat. When the final coat has cured, sand with #100-grit sandpaper, prime, and paint.

↠ **Note:** *Drywall joint compound is a thick, plasterlike material used normally to apply drywall tape. Buy it at hardware stores, home centers, and paint supply stores.*

GOOD IDEA!

When patching drywall, avoid the novice's mistake of overworking the wet joint compound in an attempt to make it smooth. In fact, it's nearly impossible to get wet joint compound perfectly smooth and flat. Simply apply the compound in a single wiping motion, leaving ridges and rough spots as they are. When the compound is dry, knock the ridges off with a knife and achieve a smooth coat through sanding.

GOOD IDEA!

Think SAFETY when-ever doing any kind of roof work. Wear ten-nis shoes or other shoes with rubber soles to de-crease the likelihood of slipping. If you're climb-ing out a window onto a roof, you may want to tie a sturdy rope around your waist and secure the other end around an interior immovable ob-ject—such as a heavy cast-iron radiator—for extra security. Never do roof work when no one else is around. Be sure that when you get ready to go out onto the roof, someone else knows where you're going and stays within shouting dis-tance.

Soldered Patch for Metal Roof or Gutter

For holes in roofs or gutters made of copper or ferrous metal, the only long-term fix is a soldered patch. Tar or "roof coating" patches don't last and may attack the protective coating on the metal. A soldered patch won't adhere to rusted metal. You can patch an isolated area of rust, but if a large area of roof or gutter is rusted, it's probably time to replace it. *This does not work on aluminum roofs.*

SUPPLIES

wire brush

tin snips

ruler

pencil

square metal patch about 2 inches larger than hole

bag of BBs, slightly smaller than the patch

heat-resistant gloves

ruby fluid

acid brush

200-watt or more electric or 3- to 5-pound gas-heated soldering iron

50/50 lead-tin solder

clean rag

mineral spirits

paintbrush

metal primer

☛ **BE SAFE.** Wear heavy gloves when working with the soldering iron, and watch out for any stray drops of hot solder. If you use a gas-fired pot to heat your soldering iron, it could turn over and start a fire. Keep water or a fire extinguisher nearby.

With the wire brush, thoroughly clean the area to be patched down to shiny metal. Cut a square patch about 2 inches larger than the hole, from the *same type of metal as the metal you're patching.* Don't mix materials. Placing two different metals in direct contact may cause corrosion, which can eat up a roof or gutter within weeks.

Starting at a corner, measure ½ inch along the perimeter. Mark a point. Starting at the same corner, measure ½ inch along the perimeter in the other direction and mark a point. Repeat this process for the remaining three corners (there should be eight points altogether). For each corner, draw a line connecting each pair of points and cut off the resulting corner triangle. Then fold the outer edges of metal under ½ inch to form a double thickness along the outer edge. Cut off four more ½-inch triangles at the corners, as before; this eliminates easily damaged sharp points.

Place the patch metal over the hole; then set a bag of BBs over the patch to hold it in place. The patch *must not move* while the solder is being applied. Wearing heavy gloves, apply ruby fluid around the edges of the patch with the acid brush. Use the soldering iron to melt the solder *into and over* the seam. If the patch moves before the solder cools, you have to start over. Finally, wipe the area with mineral spirits and apply a primer suitable for metal.

➺ **Note:** *Lead-tin solder comes in bars. One or two bars should be enough for a patch. Buy soldering supplies at well-stocked sheet metal supply stores. Buy mineral spirits at paint supply stores.*

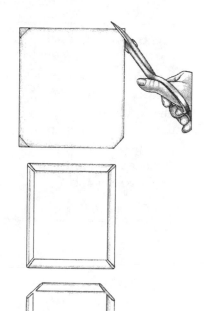

Preparing a metal patch

Rust Remover for Porcelain Tubs

Porcelain-enameled cast-iron tubs sometimes show rust stains where rusty water drips on the tub surface. Here's an easy way to remove minor stains. *This method is for porcelain-enameled tubs only, not modern fiberglass tubs.*

SUPPLIES

old towel or paper towels
white vinegar

Soak an old towel or two or three layers of paper towels in vinegar and drape over the stain. Check the stain after 3 or 4 hours. If it's gone, remove the towels and rinse with clear water. If the stain is stubborn, re-wet the towels with vinegar and leave them in place overnight.

GOOD IDEA!

To **remove rust from bathtubs better,** before using vinegar, make both the bathtub and the room temperature as warm as possible.

GOOD IDEA!

To restore the shine to brass parts, rub them with #0000 steel wool soaked in ammonia. Do this in a well-ventilated area to avoid breathing ammonia fumes.

TSP Paint Stripper for Metal

You can strip paint from metal hardware such as door-knobs, hinges, door bolts, and the like with twenty-dollar-a-gallon paint stripper, or you can do it almost free with TSP.

Yield: 1 gallon

INGREDIENTS

1 gallon water
1 pound trisodium phosphate (TSP)

SUPPLIES

rubber work gloves
goggles, safety glasses, or face shield
8-quart old pot
stirrer
newspapers
#0000 steel wool or kitchen scrubber

☛ **BE SAFE.** Wear rubber gloves to protect your hands. Wear goggles when working with this formula. Avoid skin contact.

Wearing rubber gloves and goggles, place water in the pot and stir in TSP to dissolve. Heat to near boiling. Remove from heat, drop in the metal hardware, and leave it out at room temperature overnight. In the morning, wearing rubber gloves, remove a piece of the hardware. If the paint is loose, place hardware on newspaper and scrub off paint with the steel wool or scrubber. If paint still clings to the metal, heat the water again and let the hardware soak for several more hours.

➻ **Note:** Buy trisodium phosphate at well-stocked hardware stores and paint supply stores.

Wood-Ash Paint Stripper for Metal

You can strip paint from metal parts using only wood ashes as the active ingredient. Don't use this method with wood, though; it'll raise the grain and turn the wood gray.

Yield: 1 gallon

INGREDIENTS

1 gallon water
   about 2 pounds wood ashes

SUPPLIES

rubber work gloves
goggles, safety glasses, or face shield
8-quart old pot (*not* aluminum)
stirrer
newspapers
#0000 steel wool or old kitchen scrubbing pad

☛ **BE SAFE.** *Wear rubber gloves to protect your hands. Wear goggles when working with this formula. Avoid skin contact.*

Wearing rubber gloves and goggles, place water in the pot and stir in wood ash. Heat water to near boiling, stirring occasionally (most of the ash will not dissolve). Remove from heat, drop in metal hardware, and leave it out at room temperature overnight. In the morning, wearing rubber gloves, remove a piece of the hardware. If the paint is loose, place hardware on newspaper and scrub off paint with the steel wool or scrubber. If paint still clings to the metal, heat the water again and let the parts soak for several more hours.

GOOD IDEA!

To remove dirt, lacquer, and paint from solid brass hardware, vinegar and salt are all you need. Place the hardware in a stainless steel pot and add enough vinegar to completely cover it. Then, pour salt directly onto the surface of the submerged hardware, enough to cover it. Place the pot on the stove, and heat on low for about 15 minutes. Remove the hardware from the hot vinegar bath with kitchen tongs. After it is cool, buff the hardware to a shine with very fine steel wool.

This treatment does not work for brass-plated hardware; it works only for solid brass. If in doubt, check the hardware with a magnet. Magnets won't stick to solid brass.

For a near-perfect match, be sure to patch furniture with the same type of varnish as the original. The two main types of varnish, polyurethane and oil-based, come in a range of glosses, from high gloss to satin to low gloss. But if your furniture is older, its varnish finish may have become less glossy because of wear. If this is the case, you don't want your patch to stand out as new and shiny, so choose a patch varnish with a gloss that matches the rest of the piece. If you're unsure of what gloss to use, buy a small quantity of varnish and patch a small, inconspicuous area first.

Cigarette Burn Repair

Repairing a burn is quite similar to repairing a black ring. Both flaws are not only in the finish, but also in the wood itself. The difference is, to remove a burn, you must sand more deeply than for a black ring.

SUPPLIES
#100- or #150-grit sandpaper
pencil
masking tape
wax filler stick
oil-based varnish (*not* polyurethane)
#0000 steel wool
furniture wax

To sand out a burn, wrap sandpaper around the eraser end of a pencil and tape it in place. Roll the sandpaper in the burned area until you reach sound wood. Use a wax filler stick to fill in the depression left from sanding. Then, spot varnish. Rub the area with steel wool to feather the edges of the touch-up. Apply a coat of wax.

✿ **Variation:** If you're good at it, fill in the area and then apply false wood graining (see page 228). It gives good results.

➺ **Note:** Wax filler sticks are sticks of pigment suspended in wax, somewhat like a crayon or colored pencil. Buy these at well-stocked paint supply stores and supply houses that serve the cabinetmaking trade.

Wallpaper Stripper

For best results with interior painting or wallpapering, don't apply paint or new wallpaper over old wallpaper. Frequently, the glue on the old paper will fail within in a few days and ruin your decorating job. If you have strippable modern wallpaper, just loosen a ceiling-level seam and pull it down. If you have unstrippable paper or, worse yet, many layers of old paper, remove them with this easy method.

INGREDIENTS

very hot water
photographer's wetting agent

SUPPLIES

plastic drop cloth
masking tape
spray bottle
wallpaper scraping knife

Protect floors by rolling out a drop cloth and securing it with masking tape to the baseboard. Fill a spray bottle with water and add a few drops of wetting agent—a little goes a long way. Spray the solution on a floor-to-ceiling swath about 4 feet wide. Let it soak in. Repeat spraying this same area until the wallpaper is saturated with water. Then, scrape the wallpaper off, using the wallpaper scraper.

✿ **Variation:** Add vinegar or trisodium phosphate (TSP) to the water in addition to the wetting agent. Vinegar is an acid that attacks the glue. TSP is a strong detergent that does essentially the same thing.

➥ **Note:** The wetting agent helps the water thoroughly penetrate the wallpaper. Buy photographer's wetting agent at well-stocked camera stores. Buy trisodium phosphate at well-stocked hardware stores and paint supply stores.

GOOD IDEA!

To make wallpaper stripping less of a chore, use a real wallpaper scraping knife, which you can buy at paint supply stores and hardware stores. This tool, which looks like a wide putty knife, features a beveled leading edge to aid in paper removal. As you remove the paper, try not to gouge the walls. You'll have to spackle and sand all the gouges before papering or painting.

Chapter Seven

Housekeeping

by Patricia Fisher

As you glance through these pages, you'll find plenty of helpful advice for making numerous household formulas. Making your own formulas means you can save money, plus you will know what's in the product. You can also make just what you need to do the job. But before making your first batch, keep these guidelines in mind.

- Before using a cleaning formula on an entire item, always test it first. Use a bit of the formula on a hidden area—on the seam allowance of a shirt, on a carpet in the closet, on the underside of a chair. Use the cleaning procedure recommended in the instructions and watch for any alteration in color, texture, or finish.

- To prevent accidental poisoning or injury, always label your homemade products clearly and store them in a safe place, preferably in a locked cabinet, away from children and pets. Never put cleaning products or other strong chemicals in recycled food containers unless very clearly labeled.

- Realize that cleaners work differently on various surfaces and under different conditions. The laundry product that does a marvelous job removing baby food stains from white cotton may not perform as well on chocolate stains on polyester. It's impossible to list every use and result for these formulas, so use your own common sense and experience in deciding whether or not a formula will work for you.

- Follow directions and read all of the "Be Safe" information before mixing any formula. Also remember that just because ½ cup ammonia does the job, that doesn't mean that a whole cup of ammonia will do even better. Don't change the amounts of the ingredients, and don't mix in additional ingredients not called for in the directions.

- Above all, exercise the same careful and sensible precautions you'd use with store-bought household products. With ordinary care, you'll find that using homemade household products is as easy and enjoyable as it is to make them.

SPIFFY BRICK, STONE, AND CONCRETE

To tackle the heavy-duty dirt of a well-used fireplace or oil-stained garage floor, you need a heavy-duty formula. These cleaners work on soot, smoke stains, accumulated grime, and even floors stained with motor oil.

Brick or Stone Floor Cleaner

Try this cleaner when sweeping isn't thorough enough.

Yield: 2 gallons

INGREDIENTS

½ cup washing soda

2 gallons warm water

SUPPLIES

rubber work gloves

2½-gallon bucket

mop

☛ **BE SAFE.** *Washing soda is toxic and may irritate skin, eyes, and mucous membranes. Wear rubber gloves when handling this formula.*

Wearing rubber gloves, put soda in the bucket. Pour in water to dissolve. Mop, rinse, and let dry.

➡ **Note:** *Buy washing soda, also called sal soda, in the detergent section of most supermarkets and hardware stores.*

GOOD IDEA!

To clean stubborn soot off glass fireplace doors, lay them inside a heavy-duty garbage bag. Cover each panel with a thick layer of paper towels saturated with undiluted ammonia. Close the bag and let sit for about 10 minutes. Scrub away the softened soot with a plastic mesh scrubber.

GOOD IDEA!

To clean brick or slate surfaces easier, seal them with linseed oil, available at paint supply stores. Rub a very light coating over the surface of the brick or stone with a soft cloth. For easier spreading, thin linseed oil with a little paint thinner. If you use paint thinner, wear rubber work gloves and work in a well-ventilated area.

Fireplace Brick and Stone Cleaner

This mixture removes baked-on soot, dirt, and grease from brick or stone fireplaces.

Yield: about 1½ quarts

INGREDIENTS

- 1 cup laundry soap flakes
- 4 cups hot water
- ½ pound powdered pumice
- ½ cup ammonia

SUPPLIES

1-gallon bucket
stirrer
scrub brush

Dissolve soap flakes in water. Stir in pumice and ammonia and use to scrub the bricks or stones. Rinse by scrubbing with clean water. If necessary, repeat until the bricks or stones are clean.

➡ **Note:** Powdered pumice is ground volcanic rock frequently used as a polishing agent. Buy powdered pumice in hardware stores or from a jeweler who makes settings and mounts stones.

GOOD IDEA!

To clean painted concrete, use a gentle cleaner. Clean painted floors with a solution of ¼ cup mild dishwashing liquid in 2 gallons warm water. Rinse with clear water.

Concrete Floor Cleaner

Use this mixture as a thorough, all-over cleaner of any unpainted concrete floor.

Yield: 2 gallons

INGREDIENTS

- ¼ cup washing soda
- 2 gallons warm water

SUPPLIES

rubber work gloves

2-gallon bucket

mop or scrub brush

☛ **BE SAFE.** *Washing soda is toxic and may irritate skin, eyes, and mucous membranes. Wear rubber gloves when handling this formula.*

Put on rubber gloves. Then, in the bucket, dissolve soda in water. Wash the floor with the mop or scrub brush. Rinse with clean water and allow to dry.

✿ **Variation:** *If your floor is particularly dirty, use ½ to ¾ cup washing soda.*

➺ **Note:** *Buy washing soda, also called sal soda, in the detergent section of most supermarkets and hardware stores.*

Garage Floor Cleaner

Use this cleaner to scrub away old oil stains.

SUPPLIES

rubber work gloves

goggles, safety glasses, or face shield

trisodium phosphate (TSP)

water

scrub brush or push broom

☛ **BE SAFE.** *Wear rubber gloves and goggles when handling this cleaner. Avoid skin contact.*

Wearing rubber gloves and goggles, spread TSP over oil stains. Sprinkle with enough water to thoroughly dampen the powder. Let sit ½ hour, scrub, and rinse well.

➺ **Note:** *Buy trisodium phosphate at well-stocked hardware stores and paint supply stores.*

GOOD IDEA!

To remove stubborn stains on unpainted concrete floors, mix 1 cup chlorine bleach with 2 gallons warm water. Wearing rubber gloves, scrub stains with this solution and rinse thoroughly. Scrub any remaining stains with a solution of washing soda and water.

GOOD IDEA!

To clean fresh oil spills on concrete, sprinkle new cat litter heavily over the spill. Let sit for 15 minutes, then sweep up. Wrap the litter in newspaper and dispose of according to your municipality's regulations. Scrub remaining stains with a mild detergent or trisodium phosphate solution.

CLEANING CARPETS, CLOTHING, AND CHAIRS

Here's a handy reference with stain-removal and cleaning formulas for almost every fabric in your home.

OUT, OUT DARNED SPOT! Stain Removal Formulas for Washable Fabrics		
Stain	**Remove With**	**Instructions**
Alcohol	Mild dishwashing liquid	Rinse immediately in warm water; sponge with dishwashing liquid.
	Hydrogen peroxide	For bleach-safe fabrics, sponge lightly with hydrogen peroxide.
Baby formula	Enzyme detergent	Launder in enzyme detergent; or use enzyme presoak.
	Meat tenderizer	Cover stains with a paste of meat tenderizer and water; let sit 15 minutes, then wash as usual.
Ballpoint pen ink	Hair spray	Saturate stains with hair spray and wash out with warm water.
	Rubbing alcohol	Sponge stains with rubbing alcohol, then rinse in clear water.
Blood	Ammonia	First wash stains with plain cold water, then with mild dishwashing detergent in cold water. If stains remain, sponge with a solution of 3 Tbs. ammonia in a gallon of cold water.
	Hydrogen peroxide	For set stains on bleach-safe fabrics, sponge with hydrogen peroxide.
	Enzyme detergent	Launder in cold water with enzyme detergent.
Candle wax	Rubbing alcohol	Sandwich the fabric between two layers of paper towels and apply a hot iron. Paper towels will absorb the wax. Remove remaining stains with a solution of rubbing alcohol and water.
Chewing gum	White vegetable shortening	Rub gum with an ice cube to harden. Scrape off as much as possible. Work shortening into remaining gum and wash out with warm water. Repeat shortening and warm water until gum is removed.
Chocolate	Mild dishwashing liquid	Treat fresh stains with dishwashing liquid and warm water. Treat remaining stains with commercial spot remover.
	Enzyme detergent	Rub enzyme detergent into stains before laundering.

Stain	Remove With	Instructions
Coffee	Boiling water	Stretch fabric over a bowl, hold in place with a rubber band, and pour boiling water through stains.
	Hydrogen peroxide	For bleach-safe fabrics, sponge with hydrogen peroxide.
	Borax	Sponge with a solution of 1 Tbs. borax in 1 cup water.
Crayon	White vegetable shortening	Work shortening into stains; then wash out shortening and crayon with mild dishwashing liquid and water. Treat remaining stains with commercial spot remover.
Cream or butter	Mild dishwashing liquid	Wash with dishwashing liquid and warm water; treat remaining stains with commercial spot remover.
	Enzyme detergent	Rub enzyme detergent into stains before laundering.
Egg	Salt	Soak stains in solution of 1 Tbs. salt in a cup of cold water. Then pretreat stains with enzyme detergent before washing.
Fruit juice	Hydrogen peroxide	Stretch bleach-safe fabric over a bowl, hold in place with a rubber band, and pour boiling water through stains. Sponge remaining stains with hydrogen peroxide.
	Glycerine	If stains have set, work in glycerine; let sit 30 minutes. Then rinse with white vinegar. Launder as usual.
	Chlorine bleach	On white or color-fast cotton or cotton blends, soak 2 to 4 minutes in 1 part bleach to 4 parts water. Rinse with white vinegar and launder as usual.
Grass or pollen	Rubbing alcohol	Sponge with rubbing alcohol to remove most plant stains.
	Hydrogen peroxide	For bleach-safe fabrics, sponge stubborn stains with hydrogen peroxide.
Grease	Talcum powder	Sprinkle stains with powder, let sit for 15 minutes, brush off, then wash in mild dishwashing liquid and warm water.
	Enzyme detergent	Pretreat stains with enzyme detergent, then wash as usual.
	Petroleum jelly	Rub dry grease stains with petroleum jelly, then wash with mild dishwashing liquid.
Greasy cuffs and collars	Shampoo	Lather shampoo into stains, then launder as usual.

(continued)

	OUT, OUT DARNED SPOT!—*Continued*	
Stain	**Remove With**	**Instructions**
Latex paint	Rubbing alcohol	Wash fresh paint as soon as possible with soap and warm water. Soak dried latex in rubbing alcohol before laundering.
Lipstick	Glycerin	Soften stains with glycerin before laundering as usual.
Makeup foundation or powder	Baking soda	Dip toothbrush into baking soda and water. Brush until stains disappear.
Mud	Mild dishwashing liquid	Let mud dry completely. Brush to remove surface dirt. Pour cool water through stains to remove more dirt. Wash with mild dishwashing liquid.
Oil paint	Turpentine	Provide adequate ventilation and wear rubber work gloves, then sponge on turpentine until paint softens. Scrape off excess paint. Launder as usual.
Rust stains	Lemon juice and salt	Rub stains with lemon and salt. Leave white fabrics in sun for a few hours to bleach; leave colored fabrics indoors for a few hours. Rinse and launder as usual.
Tar	Glycerin	Scrape off surface tar. Work glycerin into remaining stains. Launder. Treat remaining stains with commercial spot remover.
Urine	White vinegar	Wash first with mild dishwashing liquid and cool water. Then saturate stains with vinegar to remove odor. Wash as usual.

First-Aid for Carpet Stains

For carpet-cleaning emergencies, keep on hand paper towels or some absorbent cloths, a bottle of plain club soda, and a box of cornstarch. Here's the procedure.

For nongreasy spills: Blot up as much of the liquid as possible with paper towels or absorbent cloths. Don't rub. Rubbing forces the stain deeper into the carpet fibers. Blot! Absorb! Lift! Pour a little plain club soda over the stain and blot that up. Repeat until no more seems to be coming up. If any stain remains, you can treat it later with the proper spot remover, but many spills, especially food and beverage stains, come up nicely with club soda.

For greasy stains, such as salad dressing or butter: Blot up as much as possible with paper towels or cloths, then sprinkle the spot liberally with cornstarch to absorb the oil. Let the cornstarch do its work for 10 minutes or so, then vacuum up. Any remaining stain may be treated later with the appropriate spot remover.

Rug and Carpet Shampoo

This is an easy-to-make foam carpet shampoo that does a good job of removing light soil. It can also be used for spot cleaning of heavy traffic areas.

Yield: 1 pint

INGREDIENTS

½ cup mild dishwashing liquid
2 cups boiling water

SUPPLIES

4- to 5-quart bowl
hand eggbeater or electric mixer

☛ **BE SAFE.** *Use this shampoo on synthetic fiber carpets and rugs only. The dyes in wool carpets may not be colorfast; have wool carpets professionally cleaned. Before using on any carpet, test for colorfastness. First treat a small hidden portion of the carpet, then check for any color change before cleaning the rest of the carpet.*

Pour dishwashing liquid into the bowl. Pour water over dishwashing liquid and allow to cool. When the mixture has cooled and turned to a thick, jellylike substance, whip the mixture with the eggbeater or electric mixer into a thick foam.

To use, working with a small area of carpet at a time, spread the foam over a portion of carpet with a clean cloth or sponge. Rub gently over any heavily soiled areas. Rinse by sponging with clean water until no traces of suds remain. Do not soak any area of the carpet. Let dry thoroughly. Vacuum to restore nap and remove any remaining detergent residue.

GOOD IDEA!

To remove spots from carpets, use a gentle cleaning solution. Stir 1 teaspoon mild dishwashing liquid and 1 teaspoon white vinegar into 2 cups warm water. After absorbing as much liquid from the stain as possible with paper towels or absorbent cloths (or after scraping up as much solid matter as possible), gently sponge stains with this solution. Don't rub or scrub. Just sponge the cleaner into the fibers with an easy press-and-lift motion. Rinse by sponging with a cloth or sponge rinsed out in clean water. Don't get the carpet too wet when rinsing; be sure the cloth or sponge is well wrung out. Repeat, if necessary, until the spot disappears.

Upholstery Cleaner

Use this on any colorfast, washable upholstery fabric.

Yield: about 3 quarts

INGREDIENTS

3 quarts hot water
2 ounces castile soap, grated or chipped
1 tablespoon borax (1/2 ounce)
1/4 cup glycerin (2 ounces)

SUPPLIES

1-gallon jug or bottle with lid

BE SAFE. Even though borax is a commonly used laundry product, it is poison and can cause death when ingested. Keep it out of the reach of children.

Place water and soap in the jug or bottle, replace lid, and shake to dissolve. Add borax and glycerin, shaking to dissolve. Allow to cool. To use, sponge onto fabric. Do not soak furniture. Do a small area at a time. Rinse by sponging with water.

Notes: Castile soap is a fine, hard soap made from olive oil and is available at health food stores and specialty gift shops. Buy borax (99.5 percent pure sodium borate) at paint supply stores, hardware stores, and in the detergent section of supermarkets. Glycerin is nontoxic and safe to handle. Buy it at pharmacies or craft supply stores.

Upholstery First-Aid

Try these techniques to remove spots from upholstery. If the upholstery is washable, refer to "Out, Out Darned Spot!" on page 266. Before using any of these treatments, test a hidden spot to make sure the fabric is colorfast.

For greasy stains: Sprinkle the spot with a generous layer of cornstarch. Let dry 20 to 30 minutes; then vacuum up the powder and the grease.

For wine and colored juices: Sponge the stain with club soda or seltzer water.

For smelly spots: Treat odorous spots, such as pet accidents, by sponging the area with white vinegar then rinsing with clear water.

Vinyl Cleaner

Use this cleaner to remove dirt and stains from any kind of vinyl object.

Yield: varies by amount of ingredients chosen

INGREDIENTS

1 part calcium carbonate (whiting)

3 parts baking soda

1 teaspoon mild dishwashing liquid

2 quarts warm water

SUPPLIES

mixing bowl or bucket

stirrer

sponge

3-quart bowl

Combine whiting and baking soda in the bowl or bucket. Stir well. Rub powder onto the vinyl with a damp sponge. Mix dishwashing liquid and water in the 3-quart bowl to make a sudsy solution and wash off the baking soda mixture. Rinse and wipe dry.

➡ **Note:** *Buy calcium carbonate at hardware stores.*

GOOD IDEA!

It's easy to restore softness to vinyl products, such as furniture, car tops, or toys, that often become dried out and stiff with age. To restore softness, rub petroleum jelly into the vinyl. Allow the petroleum jelly to soften the vinyl for a few minutes, then buff vigorously with a soft, dry cloth to leave a soft shine. Vinyl that has become gummy with age can be restored by rubbing in a little cornstarch with a cloth.

Laundry Presoak for Delicate Fabrics

When you need brightening and stain removal for fabrics that cannot be subjected to harsh bleaches and strong detergents, try this gentle but effective presoak.

Dissolve 2 tablespoons cream of tartar in 1 gallon hot water. Then let the mixture cool. Soak delicate fabrics, synthetic knits, baby clothes, and clean diapers to remove minor stains and restore whiteness.

How to Handle Lye Safely While Making Laundry Soap

Lye is a highly caustic, crystalline substance that dissolves easily in water. Lye crystals alone react with skin moisture to cause burns; a water solution of lye can also cause serious burns. Lye is also highly toxic if swallowed. When adding crystalline lye to water, wear rubber gloves, a face mask, and goggles. Keep 1 cup of white vinegar on hand at all times while handling lye. If lye solution splashes on your skin, flood the area first with vinegar and then with cool water to stop the burning. Adding lye to water causes a chemical reaction that generates heat and gives off harsh fumes. Be sure your work area is well-ventilated before you begin making soap. *Be sure to add the lye crystals to the water. Do not add the water to the lye.*

To dissolve the lye crystals, use an 8-quart pan made of stainless steel, stoneware, or enameled cast iron. Use the same type of pan to hold the rendered fat for the final soap-making step. You may also use a glass pan, but it must be especially manufactured to withstand high temperatures, like Pyrex. Use a long-handled stainless steel or wooden spoon or an old broomstick for stirring. When working with lye, never use aluminum, tin, iron, or nonstick-coated pans, such as Teflon or Silverstone.

If you must store a partially used can of lye crystals, keep the leftovers tightly sealed. You can also store lye crystals in a jar: *Label the jar* and seal tightly. Lye crystals exposed to moisture will sometimes form a solid mass and become unusable. If you have children in your household, avoid the possibility of accidental poisoning by disposing of leftover lye crystals. Simply pour small amounts (less than ½ cup) of the crystals down a kitchen drain and immediately flood the drain with a heavy stream of cold water for 2 to 3 minutes.

Laundry Soap

This soap is easy and economical to make. If you don't have a supply available, your local butcher or supermarket may be able to supply you with fat at low cost. Because this is a true soap rather than a synthetic detergent, fabrics come out of the wash soft and fluffy without the use of fabric softeners. It's especially nice for towels.

Yield: about 5 pounds

INGREDIENTS

11 cups cold water

1 can 100 percent pure lye crystals (13 ounces)

9 cups rendered and strained fat (see "How to Render Fat for Making Soap" on page 274)

2 cups borax

SUPPLIES

two 8-quart, lye-proof cooking pots (stainless steel, stoneware, or enameled cast iron)

rubber work gloves

goggles, safety glasses, or face shield

face mask

1 cup white vinegar (used as safety precaution only)

stainless steel or wooden spoon

dairy, meat, or candy thermometer

stainless steel potato masher or wooden meat mallet

2 shoe boxes or similar size wooden boxes lined with plastic wrap

blender, food processor, or hand grater

☛ **BE SAFE.** *Lye is very caustic; it can destroy skin by chemical action. Handle it very carefully. Read "How to Handle Lye Safely While Making Laundry Soap" on the opposite page before making this soap. Even though borax is a commonly used laundry product, it is poison and can cause death when ingested. Keep it out of the reach of children.*

Place water in a lye-proof pot. Put on the rubber gloves and other safety gear. Have the vinegar handy. Very slowly add lye crystals to water, constantly stirring until lye is dissolved. As lye is added to water, the water temperature will rise to around 150°F. Place the thermometer in the water and allow it to cool to 95° to 98°F.

As the water is cooling, slowly heat rendered fat in an 8-quart lye-proof pot until it reaches 95° to 98°F. When both lye and fat are in the same 95° to 98°F temperature range, slowly pour lye into fat, stirring constantly until well-mixed.

Set the entire mixture aside, well away from children and pets, stirring slowly and evenly every half hour, for several hours. The mixture will begin to look like cottage cheese. As chunks form, break them up with a potato masher or meat mallet. Allow the mixture to stand for two to three days, stirring occasionally and breaking up large chunks of soap.

After three to four days, the soap should be a nearly dry, solid, but crumbly mass. Place the soap in a plastic-

(continued)

lined box and allow it to dry further for another one to two days. When completely dry, grate the soap in batches in a blender or food processor or on a hand grater until very fine. Mix the entire batch of grated soap with borax. Store in boxes, plastic bags, or jars. Use as you would commercial soap flakes in your washer or for hand laundry.

➺ **Notes:** Lye is crystalline sodium hydroxide or potassium hydroxide. It is usually sold in the drain cleaner section of supermarkets and hardware stores. Buy pure lye crystals or flakes, not lye sold as a liquid drain cleaner. Buy borax (99.5 percent pure sodium borate) in paint supply stores, hardware stores, and in the detergent section of supermarkets.

How to Render Fat for Making Soap

To render fat, begin with clean, fresh animal fat, such as beef tallow or pork lard. First cut away all traces of sinew, muscle, or cartilage. Place the chunks of fat in a heavy casserole or cooking pot and heat over low heat until completely melted. Strain the melted fat through a double layer of cheesecloth into an empty soapmaking pot or into a clean glass jar, warmed first with hot water, then dried thoroughly. This prevents cracking when pouring the hot fat into the jar. Cover tightly and store in the refrigerator if you are not making soap immediately.

GOOD IDEA!

Before using a laundry presoak, test the product on a hidden area first. Presoaks containing bleach may damage or remove color from some fabrics.

Heavy-Duty Laundry Presoak

Use this presoak for removing stains and for brightening dull, grayed whites and colorfast colors.

Yield: about 2 gallons

INGREDIENTS

2 gallons hot water
½ cup chlorine bleach
½ cup automatic dishwasher detergent

SUPPLIES

2-gallon clean plastic bucket
stirrer

Mix all ingredients in the bucket. Soak white cottons and washable synthetics for 2 hours (longer if heavily stained). For bleachable, colorfast colors, allow the mixture to cool first, then soak for 30 minutes. Pour off liquid and launder as usual.

Detergent Booster

Sand, the surprising ingredient in this formula, improves the cleaning power of your detergent.

Yield: 2 quarts

INGREDIENTS

5 cups masonry sand

3 cups washing soda

SUPPLIES

1-gallon sealable container

☛ **BE SAFE.** Washing soda is toxic and may irritate skin, eyes, and mucous membranes. Do not use this formula to handwash clothes.

Add sand and soda to the container, cover, and shake to mix. Add 1 to 2 tablespoons detergent booster per washer load.

➺ **Notes:** Buy masonry sand at well-stocked building supply stores. Buy washing soda, also called sal soda, in the detergent section of supermarkets and hardware stores.

GOOD IDEA!

If you use soap instead of detergent In your washer, use vinegar as a fabric softener. It helps remove fabric-stiffening soap scum from clothing, even from delicate washables, such as wool and silk. Add 1 cup white vinegar to the rinse cycle of your washer.

GOOD IDEA!

Borax freshens laundry and removes a variety of laundry odors without adding a heavy perfume scent. To freshen one average washer load, add ½ cup borax to the washer along with your regular laundry soap or detergent. Borax is toxic. Keep it out of the reach of children.

Laundry Starch

You can easily make your own laundry starch to stiffen collars and cuffs, table linens, and other fabrics.

Yield: 1½ cups

INGREDIENTS

1 cup cornstarch
½ cup wheat starch

SUPPLIES

stirrer
1-pint container with lid

Stir cornstarch and wheat starch together and cover tightly to store. To use, dissolve 2 teaspoons in 1 cup water. Apply to damp fabric with a spray bottle or dilute with more water and moisten fabrics in a starch bath.

➥ **Note:** Buy wheat starch at supermarkets, health food stores, and flour mills.

GOOD IDEA!

To keep your wool clothing in excellent shape, hang dry woven wool garments on padded or shaped hangers. Before hanging, empty pockets, remove belts, and zip or button all closures. Store knitted woolens gently folded in drawers. Always dry-clean woolens before storing them.

Wool Wash for Hand Washables

You don't need to buy special products for handwashing wools. Just use this simple formula.

Yield: 3 gallons

INGREDIENTS

2 tablespoons mild dishwashing liquid
3 gallons lukewarm water (80° to 90°F)

In the sink, dissolve dishwashing liquid in water. Turn the garment inside out and submerge it. Let soak for 3 to 5 minutes, then squeeze suds through the fabric to remove soil without twisting or wringing. Rinse two or three times in clean water, squeezing gently to remove all suds. Compress the garment against the side of the basin to remove water. Don't wring or twist the garment.

To help speed drying, roll the item between two large, absorbent bath towels and press to absorb as much moisture as possible before air-drying. Shape the garment to its original size and shape. Let it dry flat at room temperature. Never hang knits to dry because they will stretch out of shape.

FLOORS, WALLS, AND WINDOWS

Here you'll find formulas for coping with everything from crayon on wallpaper to black heel marks on vinyl flooring. The floor-care formulas cover the best ways to care for wood, marble, linoleum, and vinyl flooring.

Floor Mop Oil

For oil-finished, painted, and other unwaxed wood floors, use this mixture to attract dust to your dust mop.

Yield: 2 cups

INGREDIENTS

1¾ cups mineral oil
¼ cup turpentine

SUPPLIES

rubber work gloves
mixing container, such as a coffee can
22-ounce plastic spray bottle

☛ **BE SAFE.** *Turpentine is flammable. Avoid open flames. Do not smoke. Wear rubber gloves to protect your hands. Work in a well-ventilated area. Don't use this for dusting waxed floors; it will ruin the wax coating.*

Wearing rubber gloves, mix oil and turpentine in the container. Pour into the spray bottle. Lightly spray on your dust mop before dusting floors.

GOOD IDEA!

To protect the shine on both waxed and no-wax floor coverings, dust mop daily. Dust mops pick up more dirt than brooms and are especially gentle on the glassy surface of no-wax floors. To speed dust mopping, buy a wide dust mop from janitorial supply stores.

Liquid Floor Polish

Use this formula to polish oiled floors that should not be waxed.

Yield: about 2 quarts

INGREDIENTS

¼ cup shredded paraffin wax
2 quarts mineral oil

SUPPLIES

double boiler with 3-quart insert
spoon or paddle
2-quart bottle with lid

☛ **BE SAFE.** Ingredients are flammable. Always use a double boiler to melt wax; never place over direct heat. Never leave hot wax unattended.

Boil water in a double boiler with the insert empty. Turn off heat and remove double boiler to a heat-proof surface. *Then* place paraffin and mineral oil in the insert. Stir until paraffin melts into the oil. Store tightly sealed.

To use, apply a small amount of polish to a small section of floor, rubbing it in well. Then buff the floor with a clean cloth to remove excess oil.

➡ **Note:** Buy paraffin in the canning section of supermarkets and hardware stores.

Floor Cleaner
for Polyurethane-Finished Floors

If your polyurethane-covered floor shows grease and dirt accumulation, try this mild detergent solution.

Yield: 1 gallon

INGREDIENTS

1 tablespoon mild dishwashing liquid
2 tablespoons ammonia
1 gallon warm water

SUPPLIES

stirrer
2-gallon bucket
soft cloth or sponge
terrycloth towel

Mix all ingredients in the bucket to make a sudsy solution. Wash the floor using this solution and a soft cloth or sponge, working on a small area at a time. After washing, dry the floor thoroughly with a towel to eliminate water spots and restore a high gloss to the floor.

Shiny Vinyl Basics

To keep your vinyl floor in top condition, dust mop it daily and then damp mop with a vinegar-and-water solution. Just mix ½ cup vinegar with 2 quarts warm water and mop as usual. Rinsing is unnecessary. Once a week, mop with a mild detergent solution and rinse with clear water. If you can't remove spots with mild detergent, try the following techniques.

To remove black heel marks and similar dark smudges: Sprinkle a little baking soda on a damp sponge or cloth and rub the spots until they disappear. Rinse with a little water. A dab of toothpaste on a paper towel also removes many dark smudges. You can sometimes erase black heel marks with an ordinary pencil eraser.

To remove food stains: Dab the stains lightly with a little rubbing alcohol, then rinse. No-wax floors should need no follow-up; polished floors may need a fresh coat of polish.

To remove paint spots: Soften the spots with full-strength vinegar; then rub spot with nylon netting.

To remove asphalt, tar, or glue: Lift the spot with a cloth dipped in lighter fluid (wear rubber gloves and work in a well-ventilated area); then wash with a mild detergent solution.

GOOD IDEA!

It is rarely necessary to remove old wax before applying fresh wax, unless the old wax finish is extremely dirty or discolored. Wax is self-cleaning in that the new wax dissolves the previous wax finish. The most crucial step in waxing is buffing. Vigorous buffing removes all but a very thin film of wax, leaving just enough for protection and a hard, glossy finish.

Floor Wax Stripper

In most cases, you do not need to strip old wax from well-buffed waxed floors before rewaxing. Heavily soiled floors, floors with buildup of improperly buffed wax, or floors covered with clear, water-based, acrylic polish may require a more thorough cleaning. Use this to remove grime, old wax, or old acrylic polish before rewaxing.

Yield: 2¼ quarts

INGREDIENTS

1   cup ammonia
¼   cup washing soda
2   quarts water

SUPPLIES

rubber work gloves
stirrer
1-gallon bucket
sponge or sponge mop
plastic mesh scrubber

☞ **BE SAFE.** Washing soda is toxic and may irritate skin, eyes, and mucous membranes. Wear rubber gloves when handling this formula.

Wearing rubber gloves, mix all ingredients in the bucket. Sponge or mop the cleaner onto a small area of floor, getting the floor quite wet. Let sit for 5 minutes to soften the wax. Loosen the wax by scrubbing with the scrubber. Then sponge up the cleaner and loosened wax. Rinse with clear water. Repeat for the rest of the floor. If any wax residue remains, repeat the stripping treatment over the entire floor.

➡ **Note:** Buy washing soda, also called sal soda, in the detergent section of supermarkets and hardware stores.

Parquet Floor Cleaner

Normally, parquet floors need only frequent vacuuming and, if they have a wax finish, waxing once or twice a year. But if your parquet floor is really dirty and needs a more heavy-duty cleaning, this cleaner should do the job.

Yield: about 3½ cups of concentrate, enough for about 2 gallons of cleaner

INGREDIENTS

2¼ cups mineral oil
¾ cup oleic acid
2 tablespoons ammonia
5 tablespoons turpentine

SUPPLIES

rubber work gloves
1-quart bucket or other mixing container
stirrer
1-quart jar with lid

☛ **BE SAFE.** *Wear rubber gloves to protect your hands. Turpentine is flammable. Avoid open flames. Do not smoke. Work in a well-ventilated area.*

Wearing rubber gloves, mix together mineral oil and oleic acid in the bucket or other container, then stir in ammonia and turpentine. Mix vigorously to distribute ammonia throughout the formula. Store in a sealed jar or use immediately. To use, dilute 1 cup cleaner with ½ gallon water. Wash the floor with a mop or sponge well wrung out in the cleaning solution. If the floor has a wax finish, apply a fresh coat of wax after the floor has dried.

➡ **Note:** *Oleic acid, a yellow to red viscous liquid, is a fatty acid derived from animal tallow. Most pharmacists can order it for you.*

> **GOOD IDEA!**
>
> **T**o keep frequently **moved furniture from scratching a wood floor,** glue circles of felt or moleskin to the feet of tables and chairs. Moleskin is usually available in 3 × 5-inch sheets. Buy it in the foot-care section of pharmacies.

GOOD IDEA!

Polished marble in good condition only needs to be dusted and wiped occasionally with a damp cloth. If heavily soiled, wash with 1 tablespoon powdered laundry soap (not detergent) mixed with 1 quart hot water. Rinse; wipe dry.

GOOD IDEA!

To remove chewing gum, caulk, or blobs of glue from concrete floors, apply dry ice. The gooey mess will become brittle and easy to break up and remove with a spatula.

Marble Cleaner Poultice

A poultice made with hydrogen peroxide will remove a variety of stains from marble.

Yield: 1 tablespoon

INGREDIENTS

1 tablespoon cornstarch
1 teaspoon 3-percent hydrogen peroxide

Mix cornstarch and hydrogen peroxide into a paste right in the tablespoon. Spread on the stain and let dry for an hour or two. Wash with clear water.

Floor Sweeping Compound

This sweeping compound is wonderful for garage and basement floors, workshops, porches, patios, or anywhere dust flies when you sweep.

Yield: 9½ cups

INGREDIENTS

6 cups sifted sawdust
2 cups rock salt
1½ cups mineral oil

SUPPLIES

2-quart container with lid or plastic garbage bag
stirrer

Mix all ingredients in the container. Or, put all ingredients in the plastic garbage bag and shake and knead until well-combined. To use, sprinkle the compound on the floor and sweep it up.

➽ **Notes:** Buy sawdust from sawmills and woodshops. Buy rock salt at hardware stores and supermarkets, especially in the winter. Be sure to buy real rock salt, not a chemical de-icer.

Linoleum Polish

This liquid polish spreads easily and requires little buffing. Use it on old-fashioned linoleum that needs waxing.

Yield: 2½ pints

INGREDIENTS

½ cup shredded carnauba wax
2 tablespoons shredded paraffin wax
¼ cup yellow beeswax
4 cups turpentine

SUPPLIES

rubber work gloves
double boiler with 2-quart insert
stirrer
2-quart glass or plastic bottle with lid

☛ **BE SAFE.** *Ingredients are flammable. Avoid open flames, Do not smoke. Always use a double boiler to melt wax. Never place over direct heat. Never leave hot wax unattended. Work in a well-ventilated area. Wear rubber gloves to protect your hands.*

Boil water in the double boiler with the insert empty. Turn off heat and remove double boiler to a heat-proof surface. Place carnauba, paraffin, and beeswax in the insert. Let the wax melt, stirring to blend and hasten melting. When the wax is fully melted, stir in turpentine. Let the mixture cool before pouring it into a tightly capped bottle for storage. To use, apply a very thin layer of wax to the floor with a cloth or sponge mop, let dry, then buff vigorously with a clean cloth to a shine.

Notes: Buy carnauba wax at stores that specialize in custom paints and wood finishes. Buy paraffin in the canning section of supermarkets. Yellow beeswax is simply beeswax that has not been bleached to make candles. Buy it from beekeepers. See page 444 for other wax sources.

GOOD IDEA!

To prevent wax buildup around room edges and under furniture, apply wax to these areas every other waxing session.

GOOD IDEA!

To move heavy furniture without scratching waxed floors, place each leg of the furniture piece in the bottom half of a clean cardboard milk carton.

General-Purpose Wall Cleaner

This mild cleaner is good for all washable painted walls as well as walls covered with washable vinyl wallpaper.

Yield: 1 gallon

INGREDIENTS

2 tablespoons mild dishwashing liquid
1 cup borax
warm water

SUPPLIES

2-gallon bucket
sponge or cloth

☛ **BE SAFE.** Even though borax is a commonly used laundry product, it is poison and can cause death when ingested. Keep it out of reach of children.

Put dishwashing liquid and ½ cup borax in the bucket and add warm water from the tap to produce a gallon of sudsy mixture and to dissolve the borax. Wash walls with a sponge or cloth wrung out in the cleaner. To rinse, dissolve the remaining ½ cup borax in clean warm water. Using a clean sponge, rinse with this mixture.

☞ **Note:** Buy borax (99.5 percent pure sodium borate) at paint supply stores, hardware stores, and in the detergent section of supermarkets.

Painted Wall Cleaner

This cleaner is safe for all washable painted walls.

Yield: about 1 quart

INGREDIENTS

¾ cup cornstarch

½ ounce copper sulfate

⅛ teaspoon alum

1 quart hot water

SUPPLIES

rubber work gloves

stirrer

½-gallon bucket or mixing container

☞ **BE SAFE.**   Copper sulfate is poisonous. Alum is toxic if ingested in large amounts. Keep this formula out of the reach of children. Wear rubber gloves and protective clothing when using this formula.

Mix cornstarch, copper sulfate, and alum in the bucket or other container. Slowly add water, stirring constantly, until the mixture is well-blended. To use, sponge walls with the cleaner, then rinse by sponging with clear water.

➺ **Notes:**   Buy copper sulfate crystals through your pharmacist. In some areas, crystalline copper sulfate, also known as blue vitriol or blue stone, is available at livestock supply stores, where it is sold as an antifungal agent to control hoof diseases in sheep or goats. Buy alum (ammonium aluminum sulfate) in the pickling and canning section of supermarkets.

GOOD IDEA!

To remove grease and dirt on wood wall paneling without harming the finish, clean with a solution of 1 tablespoon white vinegar plus 1 tablespoon olive oil in a quart of warm water. Dip a cloth in the solution, wring it out well, then rub down wood paneling, cabinets, or furniture. Wipe dry and finish with a coat of paste wax, if desired.

Wallpaper Spot Remover

Clean regular, nonvinyl wallpaper with care. This formula uses a combination of absorbent powders to blot up grease, dirt, and many types of stains. But first test the cleaner on a hidden area to make sure the paper won't be damaged by this treatment. Work gently. Don't scrub. Simply blot the cleaner on.

Yield: about 3½ pints

INGREDIENTS

6 cups calcium carbonate (whiting)

1 cup diatomaceous earth

3 tablespoons powdered rottenstone

2 teaspoons lemon oil

SUPPLIES

dust mask

stirrer

½-gallon storage container with lid

☛ **BE SAFE.** Do not inhale powdered ingredients. Wear a dust mask when mixing this formula. Lemon oil is flammable. Avoid open flames. Do not smoke.

Put on a dust mask. Stir together whiting, diatomaceous earth, and rottenstone in the container. Sprinkle lemon oil on the mixture and stir to combine.

To use the cleaner, mix some of the cleaning compound with enough warm water to make a thick, spreadable paste. Working on a small area of wall at a time, spread a thin layer of the paste on the wallpaper, gently dabbing it on rather than scrubbing it on. Let the paste dry, then vacuum off using a soft dusting brush attachment on your vacuum cleaner.

⊷ **Notes:** Buy calcium carbonate at hardware stores. Diatomaceous earth is available at well-stocked garden supply stores and through mail-order garden suppliers. Buy powdered rottenstone at hardware stores and well-stocked paint supply stores. Buy lemon oil from herb shops and craft shops.

Heavy-Duty Wood Wash

Use this wash on heavily soiled, greasy, or sticky wood surfaces. It shouldn't damage the finish, although the wood may need polishing after cleaning to restore a rich luster.

Yield: about 1 quart

INGREDIENTS

3 tablespoons linseed oil
2 tablespoons turpentine
1 quart hot water

SUPPLIES

rubber work gloves
stirrer
½-gallon bucket

☛ **BE SAFE.** *Linseed oil and turpentine are flammable. Avoid open flames. Do not smoke. Wear rubber gloves to protect your hands.*

Wearing rubber gloves, mix all ingredients in the bucket. To use, rub the cleaner over the wood surface with a clean cloth. Wipe dry. Repeat, if necessary, until the finish is clean. Polish, if needed, to restore gloss.

➥ **Note:** *Buy linseed oil at paint supply stores and hardware stores.*

The Wall Clean Journal

If you just have a few spots to remove from a wall and don't want to wash or clean the entire surface, try one of these quick spot removers.

For washable walls and vinyl wallpaper: Use toothpaste or baking soda to remove crayon marks, pen and pencil marks, fingerprints, and other spots and smudges. To remove mildew, dab with a cloth moistened in rubbing alcohol (70 percent isopropyl). To remove smoke stains or grease, mix 1 ounce borax and ½ teaspoon ammonia in 1 quart water. Use to wash off areas blackened by smoke or grease and rinse.

For wallpaper: Dab a paste of cornstarch and water onto grease spots and crayon marks. Let the paste dry, then brush or vacuum off. For pencil marks and other miscellaneous spots, gently dab or rub with an art gum eraser, a slice of bread (Italian or French bread works best), or wheat bran sewn into a double cheesecloth bag or light muslin bag.

BATH AND KITCHEN CARE

The next time you're in line at the supermarket, calculate how much of your weekly grocery budget goes for cleaning products. Whether it's 5 percent or 25 percent, you can easily cut that figure in half by cutting back on the number of specialty cleaners you buy. The formulas here help you make your own bath and kitchen cleaners with ordinary ingredients you already have on hand.

All-Purpose Cleaner

Use this cleaner anywhere you would use a commercial all-purpose cleaner.

Yield: 2½ quarts

INGREDIENTS

2 cups rubbing alcohol (70 percent isopropyl)
1 tablespoon mild dishwashing liquid
1 tablespoon ammonia
2 quarts water

SUPPLIES

stirrer
3-quart mixing bowl
22-ounce spray bottle and 64-ounce storage bottle
with lid

☛ **BE SAFE.** Use dishwashing liquid made for hand-washing dishes. Automatic dishwasher detergents often contain chlorine bleach, which must never be mixed with ammonia. Don't use a recycled bleach bottle for storing this formula.

Stir all ingredients together in the bowl. Fill the spray bottle with cleaner and store the rest, tightly sealed, in the large bottle. Use with a cloth or sponge to clean bathroom fixtures, kitchen fixtures, appliances, chrome, plastic countertops, and painted surfaces. Rinse using a clean cloth or sponge after cleaning.

GOOD IDEA!

Store homemade cleaners in recycled containers. Use 22-ounce recycled spray window cleaner bottles for spraying homemade cleaners. Use recycled liquid detergent bottles for storing leftover cleaners. Be sure to completely rinse each bottle before filling it with a new homemade cleaning solution.

All-Purpose Quick Shiner

This shiner is mild and safe for all surfaces.

Yield: 2½ cups

INGREDIENTS

1¼ cups white vinegar
1¼ cups water

SUPPLIES

22-ounce plastic spray bottle

Pour vinegar and water into the spray bottle. Shake gently to combine. To use, spray on and wipe off.

Ceramic Tile Floor Cleaner

This formula works and is less expensive than commercial tile sprays.

Yield: 1 gallon

INGREDIENTS

2 tablespoons trisodium phosphate (TSP)
1 gallon warm water

SUPPLIES

rubber work gloves
2-gallon bucket
stirrer

☛ **BE SAFE.** *Wear rubber gloves to protect your hands. Avoid skin contact.*

Wearing rubber gloves, dissolve TSP in water in the bucket. To use, wash tile with cleaner and a sponge mop or cloth. If grout is heavily stained, apply and let sit 15 minutes. Then rinse with clear water and a clean sponge.

➴ **Note:** *Buy trisodium phosphate at well-stocked paint supply stores and hardware stores.*

> **GOOD IDEA!**
>
> **F**or extra cleaning power and a nice shine, use vinegar and water when wiping countertops, appliances, sinks, bathroom fixtures, and tile. Keep vinegar and water in a spray bottle on your counter to use for quick cleanups.

GOOD IDEA!

To prevent glass fogging from moisture or temperature changes, dip a damp soft cloth into a little dishwashing liquid. Wring it out so it is just lightly moistened with detergent. Wipe the window, leaving a thin film of detergent on the glass. Let dry.

GOOD IDEA!

To remove shallow surface scratches from glass, try a polishing paste made with 1 ounce water, 1 ounce glycerin, and 1 ounce iron oxide jewelers' rouge. Glycerin is available at pharmacies, and jewelers' rouge is available from jewelers who make settings and mount stones. Rub the polishing paste gently on scratched glass with a soft cloth and rinse with clear water.

Window and Glass Polish

This polish is useful for adding extra shine to dull, scratched, especially dirty windows.

Yield: 1½ cups

INGREDIENTS

1¼ cups calcium carbonate (whiting)
2 tablespoons ground quassia
2 tablespoons ammonium carbonate

SUPPLIES

stirrer
glass jar with lid

☛ **BE SAFE.** Ammonium carbonate is a traditional component of smelling salts. It exudes irritating fumes, especially if heated.

Mix all ingredients in the jar. Store tightly sealed. To use, apply the compound to windows with a damp cloth or sponge, then polish off with a clean damp cloth or sponge.

➺ **Notes:** Buy calcium carbonate at hardware stores. Ground quassia is the powdered bark of a tropical tree. Buy it at health food stores and herb shops. Your pharmacist can order ammonium carbonate for you.

All-Purpose
Window and Glass Cleaner

Vinegar cuts grease and leaves windows sparkling clean. Best of all, this simple mixture is absolutely safe. It's your best choice if you have young children in the house.

Yield: about 1 quart

INGREDIENTS

¼ cup white vinegar
1 quart water

SUPPLIES

2-quart bowl or container or plastic spray bottle

Pour vinegar and water in the bowl or container. Or, mix the ingredients in the spray bottle. Clean windows directly with a sponge dipped in the bowl or spray on windows and wipe clean.

Outdoor Window and Glass Cleaner
for Cold Weather

The alcohol in this mixture keeps it from freezing on the glass when you use it in cold weather.

Yield: about 1 quart

INGREDIENTS

3 cups rubbing alcohol (70 percent isopropyl)
1½ tablespoons mild dishwashing liquid
¾ cup water

SUPPLIES

1-quart plastic spray bottle

Mix all ingredients in the spray bottle. Use on outdoor windows in below-freezing weather.

GOOD IDEA!

Many people swear **by newspaper** as an inexpensive cleaning "rag" to shine and polish windows. Paper towels work just as well, and they leave your hands cleaner.

GOOD IDEA!

If you don't have an **empty 1-quart spray bottle,** look in garden supply centers for spray bottles sold for mixing plant sprays. Quart-size spray bottles are the most convenient size for big jobs, such as washing windows.

GOOD IDEA!

For mixing cleaners, save and reuse plastic food containers, such as margarine tubs or ice cream cartons. Be sure to permanently mark all containers used for nonfood purposes and to store them in your shop or garage well away from containers for food.

Grout Cleaner

When that nice, white grout on the bathroom tile floor starts turning a little gray, first try a commercial cleaner. But if the grout has been neglected, and no cleaner will touch the dirt, try this.

Yield: about 1 quart

INGREDIENTS

4½ cups water
½ cup muriatic acid

SUPPLIES

masking tape
2-quart container
goggles, safety glasses, or face shield
rubber work gloves
paint stirrer
old paintbrush

☛ **BE SAFE.** Muriatic acid will burn skin and eyes. Wear skin and eye protection. Wear protective clothing. Be sure to add the acid to the water. Do not add the water to the acid. Do not try to make a stronger solution by adding more acid; a stronger acid solution may damage some household surfaces.

To prevent pitting of woodwork and porcelain bathroom fixtures, cover them with masking tape before you start this project. Place water in the container. Wearing the proper clothing and saftey gear, stir acid into the water. Stir for a minute or so to mix thoroughly. Apply a coat of the solution to the stained grout and let stand for up to an hour or until the color of the grout improves. Rinse the surface with clean water.

➻ **Note:** Buy muriatic acid at hardware stores, home centers, and masonry supply houses.

Tile Cleaner

Use on tile and grout to remove and retard mildew.

Yield: 1 quart

INGREDIENTS

2 cups chlorine bleach

2 cups water

SUPPLIES

rubber work gloves

1-quart plastic spray bottle

☛ **BE SAFE.** *Chlorine bleach irritates skin. Wear rubber gloves when using this formula.*

Wearing rubber gloves, pour bleach and water into the spray bottle. Spray on tile and scrub off with a sponge or brush. Rinse thoroughly with clear water.

> ### GOOD IDEA!
>
> **T**o remove very heavy mildew, apply tile cleaner with a sponge, let sit for a few minutes, and scrub with a stiff brush. Use an old toothbrush for getting into tiny cracks and crevices.

Tile Grout Cleaner

This mixture removes dirt and mildew stains and kills mold spores to retard the regrowth of mildew.

Yield: about 1 quart

INGREDIENTS

¾ cup chlorine bleach

3 cups water

SUPPLIES

rubber work gloves

1-quart spray bottle

☛ **BE SAFE.** *Chlorine bleach irritates skin. Wear rubber gloves when using this solution.*

Wearing rubber gloves, pour bleach and water into the spray bottle. Spray solution on grout. For heavily soiled grout, use a scrub brush. Rinse with clear water.

WASH YOUR TROUBLES DOWN THE DRAIN
Drain and Garbage Disposer Cleaners and Fresheners

Name	Ingredients	Instructions	Comments
Drain opener	½ cup borax; 2 cups boiling water. Yields 1 treatment.	Pour borax into the drain, then slowly pour in water. Let sit 15 minutes, then flush with additional water.	This drain opener is a good alternative to lye-based drain cleaners. It's safer to use and has less hazardous effects on the environment. Buy borax (powdered sodium borate) in the cleaning supplies section of supermarkets.
Noncaustic drain cleaner	1 cup baking soda; 1 cup salt; ¼ cup cream of tartar. Yields 2¼ cups.	Mix all ingredients and store in a 1-qt. covered container. To use, pour ¼ cup cleaner into the drain. Add 1 cup boiling water. Let sit 10 minutes, then flush with cold water. Use weekly to keep drains clear.	This drain cleaner is safe for all types of plumbing, including polyvinyl chloride (PVC) pipes. Keep this cleaner dry or it will lose its effectiveness.
Heavy-duty drain cleaner	2 Tbs. washing soda; 1 qt. hot water. Yields 1 quart.	Dissolve washing soda in water. Pour the entire qt. of solution slowly down the drain. Let sit 10 minutes, then flush with hot water.	This cleaner is stronger than noncaustic drain cleaner, but safer than commercial lye-based cleaners. Washing soda irritates mucous membranes and skin. Wear rubber gloves.
Drain freshener	¼ cup automatic dishwashing detergent; 1 qt. hot water. Yields 1 quart.	Dissolve dishwashing detergent in water. Slowly pour entire solution down the drain. Flush with hot water.	This mixture freshens musty, sour-smelling drains. Automatic dishwashing detergent irritates skin. Wear rubber gloves.
Garbage disposer cleaner	1 cup vinegar; 1 cup water. Yields 2 cups.	Mix vinegar and water and use to fill one or more ice-cube trays. Freeze. Remove the cubes and grind them through the garbage disposer. Flush the disposer with cold water for 1 minute.	This unique method of cleaning your garbage disposer scours food particles from the walls and blades and removes odors.

Shower Head Cleaner

Mineral deposits and corrosion soak away in this simple cleaner to unclog and shine your shower head.

Yield: 1 quart

INGREDIENTS

2 cups white vinegar

2 cups warm water

SUPPLIES

2-quart bowl

cloth or plastic mesh scrubber (optional)

Pour vinegar and warm water into the bowl. Remove shower head and let soak in the solution several hours or overnight. After soaking, rinse the shower head to remove any clinging deposits, scrubbing lightly with a cloth or scrubber, if necessary. Replace the shower head.

Mildew Inhibitor

After cleaning mildew stains, use this inhibitor to retard renewed growth.

Yield: about 1 gallon

INGREDIENTS

2 cups table salt

1 gallon hot water

SUPPLIES

2-gallon bucket

sponge

In the bucket, dissolve salt in water. Wipe tile walls generously with the solution, then let dry. To retard mildew growth on vinyl shower curtains, soak them in this formula and rehang without rinsing.

GOOD IDEA!

To clean a **nonremovable shower head,** wrap it in a small towel or washcloth soaked in a solution of half vinegar and half water. Tie a plastic bag around the wrapped shower head to keep it moist. After several hours, remove the bag and wrapping and wipe away the softened mineral deposits and dirt.

GOOD IDEA!

A perfect polish for **all chrome bathroom fixtures** is plain vinegar. Simply moisten a cloth or sponge with vinegar and use it to polish chrome. No rinsing is necessary.

GOOD IDEA!

To remove white calcium deposits from sinks, tubs, and faucets, mix 1 cup white vinegar with 1 cup water. Use this to wash areas coated with calcium deposits. Or soak a cloth in the solution and lay it over crusty faucets and faucet handles for 10 minutes, then wash with clear water.

Faucet Cleaner

This removes soap scum, mineral deposits, and stains from chrome or plastic fixtures and leaves them shining.

Yield: ½ cup

INGREDIENTS

4 teaspoons table salt
½ cup white vinegar

SUPPLIES

sponge or clean, soft cloth

Dissolve salt in vinegar right in the measuring cup. With a sponge or soft cloth, wash faucets and handles. Rinse thoroughly and polish dry with a clean cloth.

Plastic Shower Curtain Cleaner

The grubbiest plastic shower curtain or liner will be clean after this wash.

INGREDIENTS

1½ cups chlorine bleach
¼ cup laundry detergent

SUPPLIES

2 old, bleach-safe towels

Fill the washer with warm water and add bleach and laundry detergent. Do *not* use cold water; it may cause the shower curtain to crack or shed. Put the shower curtain and two towels in the washer and run it through the entire cycle—wash, rinse, and spin. Remove curtain and rehang immediately.

Tub and Sink Stain Remover

This gentle paste removes stains from chrome, stainless steel, porcelain, plastic laminate, acrylic, and marble fixtures.

INGREDIENTS

cream of tartar

3-percent hydrogen peroxide

SUPPLIES

small cup

stirrer

soft brush, such as old toothbrush

In the cup, mix cream of tartar with hydrogen peroxide to make a medium-thick paste. With the brush, scrub the paste onto the stains, then rinse thoroughly. If stains remain, apply again, let dry for an hour, then gently scrub off.

Removing Stains from Acrylic and Fiberglass Bath Fixtures

Do not use abrasives on nonporcelain fixtures. Try these treatments for stains that won't wash away with mild soap and water.

To remove mold and mildew: Make a paste of baking soda and cool water and spread it over the entire surface of the unit. Allow the paste to sit for a few minutes, then rinse with warm water.

To remove heavy soap deposits: Apply a nonabrasive, ammonia-based household cleaner with a sponge and scrub.

To remove deep, dark stains: Soak clean, white cotton rags with 3-percent hydrogen peroxide. Apply the rags to the stain and let sit overnight. Rinse thoroughly with cold water.

To remove hard-water scale deposits: Sponge with white vinegar until deposits disappear. Rinse with cold water.

To restore dull or scratched units: Apply an automotive white polishing compound with a clean cotton rag. Rub scratches and dull areas vigorously. Wipe off residue. Follow with a coat of white automotive paste wax. Do not wax areas where you walk or stand.

To remove adhesive, such as from labels or decals: Saturate a small, white cotton rag with nail polish remover and rub vigorously until the adhesive dissolves and disappears. Nail polish remover is flammable, so use caution.

GOOD IDEA!

To make cleaning an acrylic or fiberglass shower enclosure easier, try changing your shower habits just a little bit. After every shower, wipe down the walls of your shower stall with a small towel. This simple routine takes less than a minute, and it eliminates hard-water deposits and soap scum accumulation from the shower walls. If you keep your shower stall polished, you'll only need to clean the shower floor regularly.

Nonporcelain Tub and Shower Cleaner

Many newer bathtubs and shower enclosures are made of acrylic or fiberglass finished with a clear coating. Use this as a regular cleaner instead of harsh abrasives or scouring powders that can damage the finish. The wax will make daily cleaning easy and will protect the shine and finish of the unit.

Yield: 1 treatment

INGREDIENTS

1 tablespoon mild dishwashing liquid

2 quarts warm water

SUPPLIES

1-gallon bucket

white automotive paste wax

soft cloth or towel

☛ **BE SAFE.** Do not wax areas where you stand or walk; it will be slippery.

Make a sudsy solution with dishwashing liquid and water in the bucket. Clean as usual. Every six months or so, after cleaning, apply a thin coat of paste wax and buff to a high shine with the cloth or towel.

Stain Remover for Porcelain

This formula removes rust and mineral stains. It's safe for tubs and sinks that may not be acid resistant.

Yield: 1 gallon

INGREDIENTS

1 bar naptha soap, chipped or grated

1 gallon hot water

½ cup mineral spirits

SUPPLIES

rubber work gloves
2-gallon bucket
stirrer
scrub brush

☛ **BE SAFE.** *Wear rubber gloves to protect your hands. Mineral spirits is highly flammable. Avoid open flames. Do not smoke. Make sure the area is well-ventilated.*

Wearing rubber gloves, add soap and water to the bucket, stirring to dissolve the soap. Stir in mineral spirits. Scrub stains and rinse with clear water.

➡ **Notes:** *Buy naptha soap at supermarkets, drug stores, and hardware stores. Buy mineral spirits at hardware stores and paint supply stores.*

GOOD IDEA!

To make your toilet bowl sparkle, use chlorine bleach, which cleans and disinfects a toilet bowl quickly and easily. Pour 1/2 cup bleach into the bowl. Brush the inside of the bowl thoroughly, let sit for 10 minutes, and flush to rinse. Don't use this method if your water contains iron.

Heavy-Duty Help for Porcelain Tubs, Sinks, and Toilets

To clean tough stains in tubs and sinks, try a mineral oil/kerosene mixture. Stir 1 cup mineral oil and 1 cup deodorized kerosene together in a 1-pint plastic or glass jar with a lid. If, desired, add a few drops of an essential oil or oil-soluble scent, such as lemon oil. Apply to stained porcelain using a clean rag.

Do not use this cleaner on acrylic or fiberglass fixtures. Kerosene may damage the finish on nonporcelain fixtures. Kerosene is flammable, so avoid open flames and do not smoke. Be sure your working area is well-ventilated. This heavy-duty cleaner should not be used daily.

Wear rubber gloves to protect your hands.

Buy deodorized kerosene at hardware stores and paint supply stores. Buy essential oils at drug stores, cosmetic counters, and craft shops.

To remove stubborn stains from a toilet bowl, try a pumice stone. Pour a bucket of water into the toilet bowl to flush it without refilling. Wet the stone and use it to gently scrub out stains. Keep the pumice stone wet at all times to prevent scratching. When the stains are gone, flush the toilet to rinse. Buy pumice stones at hardware stores.

Cleaners for Cast-Iron and Enameled Stove Burners

To remove heavy, burned-on grease from cast-iron stove burners, dissolve ¼ cup washing soda in 1 gallon water in a 6- to 8-quart, nonaluminum pot. Submerge the burners in the solution and bring to a boil. Boil gently for 10 minutes. Remove burners with tongs and rinse, scrubbing stubborn spots with a plastic mesh scrubber. To prevent rust, dry by placing in a hot oven for 10 minutes.

Buy washing soda in the detergent section of most supermarkets and hardware stores. Washing soda is toxic and may irritate skin, eyes, and mucous membranes. Wear rubber work gloves to protect your hands.

To clean enameled stove burners and drip pans, place the stove parts in a sealable container large enough to hold them. Working in a well-ventilated area, pour a cup of ammonia over them, seal, and leave overnight. The next day, rinse in clear water, removing loosened soil with a plastic mesh scrubber. Wash the parts in hot, sudsy water, rinse, and dry.

GOOD IDEA!

To clean a greasy, crusty barbecue grill, sandwich the grill between layers of paper towels and place it inside a large plastic garbage bag. Pour 1½ cups ammonia into the bag, saturating the paper towels. Tie the bag shut and let the grill soak outdoors overnight. The next day, wash in hot, soapy water, using a plastic mesh scrubber to remove any stubborn deposits. Rinse with clear water. This treatment also works well for heavily soiled oven racks.

Oven-Cleaning Powder

This formula makes a dry powder. At oven-cleaning time, mix the powder with water to make a spray.

Yield: 2 cups of powder, enough for 2 quarts of spray

INGREDIENTS

½ cup trisodium phosphate (TSP)
½ cup washing soda
1 cup sodium perborate
2 tablespoons laundry soap flakes

SUPPLIES

1-pint sealable container
rubber work gloves
22-ounce plastic spray bottle
goggles, safety glasses, or face shield
clean cloth or sponge

☛ **BE SAFE.** TSP, washing soda, and especially sodium perborate are all skin irritants. Wear rubber gloves when mixing the powder and gloves and goggles when using the spray. Store each ingredient and this formula well away from children.

For the powder, combine all ingredients in the container and store tightly sealed. To clean your oven, mix only the amount of spray cleaner you need for one cleaning. Don rubber gloves and dissolve ½ cup cleaning powder in 1 pint water. Pour into the spray bottle and, wearing goggles, spray the oven interior, thoroughly coating all surfaces. Avoid spraying light bulbs and heating elements. Let sit 1 hour. Wipe away the cleaner and oven soil with a damp cloth or sponge. To rinse, wipe with a clean damp cloth.

➦ **Notes:** Buy trisodium phosphate at well-stocked paint supply stores and hardware stores. Buy washing soda, also called sal soda, in the detergent section of supermarkets and hardware stores. Order sodium perborate, a white powder, from your pharmacist.

Overnight Oven Cleaner

Replace expensive, caustic commercial oven cleaners with this simple cleaning routine.

Yield: about 2 quarts

INGREDIENTS
½   cup ammonia
2   tablespoons mild dishwashing liquid
2   quarts hot water

SUPPLIES
measuring cup
2-quart pot
plastic mesh scrubber

☛ **BE SAFE.** Keep children away from ovens being treated with ammonia.

Pour ammonia into the measuring cup and place in the oven. Close the oven door and leave overnight. The next day, remove the ammonia. Mix dishwashing liquid and water in the pot. Use the scrubber to wash out loosened grease and grime. Rinse with clear water.

> **GOOD IDEA!**
>
> **T**o remove oven cleaner residue left after cleaning your oven, spray the surfaces with a solution of equal parts vinegar and water, then wipe down with a damp sponge. This simple trick eliminates smoking the first time you use your oven after cleaning.

GOOD IDEA!

To quickly eliminate food odors in your microwave and generally freshen it up, fill a microwave-safe cup with a cup of water and 2 tablespoons lemon juice. Place the cup in the microwave and heat to boiling. Turn off the microwave and leave the solution in the oven for 5 minutes.

Microwave Cleaner

Use this two-step treatment to remove dried-on spatters and spills from the interior of your microwave.

Yield: 1 quart

INGREDIENTS

1 cup water
¼ cup baking soda
1 quart warm water

SUPPLIES

microwave-safe cup
sponge or cloth

Put 1 cup water in the microwavable cup and heat in the microwave until it boils; turn off the microwave and let the water sit for 1 minute. Steam softens dried-on food.

Dissolve baking soda in 1 quart warm water and, using a sponge or cloth, wash the interior of the microwave with this solution to clean and deodorize it.

How to Freshen a Refrigerator That's Been in Storage

One of the worst refrigerator or freezer odors is the odor left when the turned-off unit has been closed for a while. Usually mold grows in the closed box. This multistep treatment kills mold spores and destroys bad odors.

Mix equal parts chlorine bleach and water. With a sponge or cloth, thoroughly wash out the interior of the refrigerator or freezer, including shelves and bins. Also remove and wash out the condensation pan that rests beneath or behind many frost-free units. Rinse with clear water and dry thoroughly. This treatment will remove mold and kill any remaining mold spores. Then spread 8 ounces activated charcoal in a shallow pan, place it in the refrigerator or freezer, close the door, and turn on the unit. Leave the charcoal in the unit for one week, then check to see if any odor persists. If odor is still present, replace the charcoal with fresh activated charcoal and leave it for another week to ten days.

Buy activated charcoal at pet shops that sell aquarium supplies.

Refrigerator Refreshers

To keep your refrigerator sweet-smelling during daily use, keep an open 1-pound box of baking soda in the back of a middle shelf. Replace the box once a month.

To remove strong odors, pour baking soda into a shallow pan. The more baking soda exposed to air, the more odors absorbed.

To eliminate the odor of spoiled food, wash out the interior of the refrigerator or freezer with a solution made of 1 part vinegar and 1 part water. After this treatment, let the interior of the refrigerator air-dry.

To impart a pleasant scent to your newly cleaned refrigerator, saturate a small sponge with vanilla extract. Wipe out the interior of the refrigerator, but don't rinse. Allow to air-dry.

Cleaner for Dishwasher Interiors

If you have a heavy calcium content in your water, it could cause chalky white mineral deposits to build up in your dishwasher. This can clog up the filtering mechanism and inhibit the efficient operation of the machine, leaving you with less-than-sparkling dishes. Use this treatment to dissolve mineral deposits.

SUPPLIES

citric acid

Put 1 tablespoon citric acid in each section of the detergent dispenser of the machine. Run the machine (empty) through the entire wash and rinse cycle.

Note: Citric acid is a crystalline white powder often used to preserve food color in home canning. Buy it in the spice section or canning section of supermarkets.

GOOD IDEA!

To remove food stains on the interior of your dishwasher, start the regular wash cycle with an empty machine. Just before the first wash cycle, open the door and pour in ½ cup chlorine bleach. Run the machine through the entire wash and rinse cycle. Do not use this method to remove iron stains. Use a commercial iron stain cleaner, such as Iron-Out or Rover.

Small Appliance Cleanup

Blenders: To quickly clean a blender, put a drop of mild dishwashing liquid into the blender jar and add 1 cup water. Cover and turn on the blender to low speed. Blend for 1 minute, then empty and rinse. Frequently remove the blade and bottom assembly from the jar to wash out hidden food particles.

Can Openers: Spray the cutter assembly with rubbing alcohol (70 percent isopropyl) and wipe dry.

Automatic Drip Coffee Makers: To remove mineral deposits and prevent clogging, pour a quart of white vinegar into the water chamber. Put a paper filter into the coffee basket and run the machine through the brewing cycle. Pour the vinegar back into the water chamber and let sit 30 minutes, then run through the brewing cycle again. Finally, run a fresh pot of water through the brewing cycle twice.

Percolators: To remove mineral deposits, fill with vinegar and perk for 10 minutes. Rinse thoroughly with clear water. To clean tubes without a brush, saturate a small piece of cotton with sudsy water and poke through with a knitting needle.

Toasters, Toaster Ovens, and Irons: To remove melted plastic, heat the appliance just enough to soften the plastic, then scrape off as much as possible with a hard plastic cooking spatula. Let cool. Remove any residue by polishing with a cloth dipped in rubbing alcohol.

Steam Irons: To clean out mineral deposits, fill the water chamber half with white vinegar and half with water. Heat to highest "steam" setting and leave on for 5 minutes. Unplug and let cool. Empty vinegar mixture, along with loosened mineral deposits. If the iron is still clogged, repeat the treatment with full-strength vinegar. To remove starch buildup, rub the faceplate with a cake of beeswax, then wash with a damp sponge and a little baking soda. Rinse and dry.

Wood Cabinet Polish

This polish removes grease and grime from kitchen cabinets and leaves them with a warm, rich glow.

Yield: 1 cup

INGREDIENTS

⅔ cup white vinegar
⅓ cup safflower oil

SUPPLIES

blender
soft cloth

Pour vinegar into the blender. With the blender running, add oil in a thin stream. Blend until the mixture is emulsified. Apply with a soft cloth and buff to a shine.

Woodwork/Wood Cabinet Cleaner

This cleaner removes grease, dirt, and yellowing.

Yield: about 1 quart

INGREDIENTS

2 tablespoons olive oil
4 tablespoons white vinegar
1 quart warm water

SUPPLIES

2-quart bottle with lid
soft cloths

Combine all ingredients in the bottle and shake to mix. Dampen a cloth with the solution and wipe cabinets. Dry with a clean cloth. Shake the bottle frequently to keep the oil dispersed in the water.

> ### GOOD IDEA!
>
> **To remove grease and soil from painted cabinets,** try using 1 cup ammonia and 1/4 cup washing soda mixed with 1 gallon warm water. Wearing rubber gloves, sponge onto the cabinets, then rinse with clear water. Buy washing soda, also called sal soda, in the detergent section of supermarkets and hardware stores.

Seasoned Skillets

To season and condition new or freshly cleaned cast-iron pans, spread a thin layer of unsalted vegetable oil or white vegetable shortening all over the inside of the pan. Coat the entire cooking surface thoroughly. Place in a 350-degree oven for 2 hours, rubbing a little oil or shortening around the inside every 1/2 hour or so. (Wear thick hot mitts; the pan will be extremely hot.) After 2 hours, turn off heat and leave the pan in the oven until it is cool enough to handle. Wash the pan with hot water; but *do not* use soap. Dry thoroughly by placing the pan in a warm oven for 10 minutes. Always dry cast iron pans thoroughly to prevent rust.

The next few times you use the pan, spread a thin film of oil or shortening around the inside before cooking and after washing and drying it. This continues the seasoning process and protects the pan from rust. After four or five uses, discontinue additional greasing. Simply wash and dry the pan carefully after each use.

For unseasoned cast-iron pans that have burned-on grease, scour with scouring powder and steel wool before reseasoning. Or clean the pan in a self-cleaning oven during the cleaning cycle. After heavy cleaning, or after washing a cast-iron pan in an automatic dishwasher, reseason the pan before using.

LITTLE THINGS MAKE A DIFFERENCE

In the following pages, you'll find a collection of formulas for cleaning and preserving ordinary household articles as well as personal valuables.

Metal Polishing Cloth

This easy-to-use polishing cloth is gentle and safe for shining any metal surface.

Yield: four 12 × 12-inch polishing cloths

INGREDIENTS

1 quart paraffin oil
½ cup mineral oil

SUPPLIES

stirrer
mixing container, such as a coffee can
four 12 × 12-inch squares lightweight cotton flannel
sealable glass or metal container

☛ **BE SAFE.** Oils are flammable. Avoid open flames. Do not smoke. As with any oily rag, these polishing cloths may spontaneously ignite if stored in a hot place near other flammable materials. Store the polishing cloths in a sealed glass or metal container in a cool place away from other combustibles.

Stir oils together in the container. Saturate the flannel squares with the oil mixture, squeezing out any excess. Store the cloths tightly sealed.

⮞ **Note:** Paraffin oil is a derivative of paraffin wax. Buy it at stores that specialize in custom paints and wood finishes. See page 444 for another source.

GOOD IDEA!

For a super-quick copper cleaner, simply pour plain ketchup on the copper surface and rub vigorously with a damp cloth. Rinse and buff to a glow with a soft cloth.

GOOD IDEA!

To brighten discolored aluminum pans, dissolve 1 tablespoon cream of tartar in 1 quart water. Boil this solution in the pan for 5 minutes. Then wash in hot, soapy water and rinse. To remove stains from aluminum objects, dissolve cream of tartar in hot water and soak the stained aluminum in it.

METAL MAGIC
Quick-and-Easy Metal Polishes

Name	Ingredients	Instructions	Comments
Aluminum polish	1 cup alum; 1 cup talc; 1½ cups calcium carbonate (whiting). Yields 3½ cups.	Wearing a dust mask, combine all ingredients and mix thoroughly. Store in a sealed 1-qt. jar. Apply with a soft damp cloth or sponge, rubbing briskly. Rinse and polish dry with a soft clean cloth.	Store formula out of the reach of children. Alum is poisonous if ingested in large enough quantities. Talc is hazardous if inhaled. Buy alum in supermarkets where pickling supplies are sold. Buy talc through your pharmacist. Buy whiting at hardware stores.
Brass polish	1 tsp. salt; 1 cup white vinegar; 1 cup flour. Yields about 1½ cups.	Dissolve salt in vinegar. Stir in flour to form a paste. Apply to brass and let sit 15 minutes; rinse with water and polish with a soft cloth.	This polish also revives old, dull pewter.
Copper polish	2 Tbs. flour; 2 Tbs. salt; 2 Tbs. white vinegar. Yields 6 tablespoons.	Mix all ingredients to make a smooth paste. Scrub tarnished copper with the paste on a soft cloth. Rinse and polish with a clean cloth.	To keep polished copper shining after each use, spray with white vinegar and rub the vinegar-coated surface with salt. Rinse and dry.
Gold polish	1 cup fuller's earth; 1 cup calcium carbonate (whiting); 2 tsp. ammonium sulfate. Yields about 2¼ cups.	Stir all ingredients together and store in a sealed 1-qt. container. Apply with a damp cloth. Buff with a clean cloth.	Store this formula out of the reach of children. Ammonium sulfate is toxic if ingested. Order both fuller's earth and ammonium sulfate through your pharmacist. Buy whiting at hardware stores.
Metal polish	½ cup ammonia; ½ cup denatured ethyl alcohol; 1 cup diatomaceous earth; ¼ cup water. Yields about 1½ cups.	Mix ammonia and denatured ethanol. Don a dust mask and gradually stir in diatomaceous earth. Stir in water to bring the mixture to the consistency of a thick cream. Store in a sealed 1-pt. jar. Before using, shake thoroughly.	Use to polish any metal, except silver or gold. Store this formula out of the reach of children. Denatured ethyl alcohol is toxic and flammable. Diatomaceous earth is hazardous to breathe. Wear a dust mask when handling it. Buy denatured ethyl alcohol at hardware stores and paint supply stores. Buy diatomaceous earth at aquarium supply stores and garden centers.

GOOD IDEA!

To remove grease, such as shortening or automotive oil, from gold jewelry, simply dip the gold briefly into rubbing alcohol (70 percent isopropyl), then wipe away grease with a soft cloth. Rinse briefly in cool water and wipe dry with a soft cloth. Do not dip gemstones, pearls, or other nongold elements into alcohol.

Gold Jewelry Cleaner

Remove grease and dirt from gold necklaces, chains, and rings with this gold jewelry cleaner. However, use with caution on jewelry set with inexpensive stones that may be glued into their settings. Soaking in the detergent and ammonia solution could soften the glue and loosen the stone. This wouldn't normally happen with more expensive pieces containing precious stones, such as diamonds set with prongs rather than glue.

Yield: 1 quart

INGREDIENTS

1 teaspoon mild dishwashing liquid
1 teaspoon ammonia
1 quart warm water

SUPPLIES

small bowl
soft toothbrush
chamois cloth

In the bowl, mix dishwashing liquid and ammonia in water to make a sudsy solution. Immerse the gold to be cleaned in the solution for a few minutes, then brush gently with the toothbrush to get into crevices and cracks and other hard-to-reach places. Rinse in lukewarm water and allow to dry. After drying, rub gold lightly with the chamois cloth to restore a lustrous shine.

Pearly White

Pearls are quite delicate and should be treated as such. Don't subject them to harsh cleaners or abrasives. To remove body oils, perspiration, cosmetics, or perfume that can discolor or damage pearls, simply swish the pearls in a mild, soapy solution. In a bowl, combine 1 teaspoon mild dishwashing liquid with 1 quart lukewarm water. Lightly agitate the solution until warm suds form. Swish the pearls through the soapy bath and rinse briefly with cool water. Pat dry with a very soft cloth.

Silver Cleaner

This polish easily removes tarnish and aids in buffing silver to a bright shine.

Yield: about 1 pint

INGREDIENTS

2 tablespoons stearic acid

1½ cups water

½ teaspoon washing soda

½ teaspoon trisodium phosphate (TSP)

1 cup diatomaceous earth

SUPPLIES

double boiler with 1-pint insert

rubber work gloves

stirrer

dust mask

1-pint jar with lid

☛ **BE SAFE.** *Stearic acid is flammable. Melt in a double boiler, not over direct heat. Washing soda and TSP are skin irritants. Wear rubber gloves when handling this polish. Avoid skin contact. Wear a dust mask when handling diatomaceous earth.*

With the insert empty, boil water in the double boiler. Turn off heat and remove double boiler to a heat-proof surface. Wearing rubber gloves, place stearic acid and 1½ cups water in the insert. Stir until stearic acid is melted. Wearing a dust mask, stir in remaining ingredients to make a smooth, creamy paste. Pour into the jar; cool before using.

➡ **Notes:** *Buy stearic acid at craft shops that sell candlemaking supplies or through your pharmacist. See page 444 for other sources. Washing soda, also called sal soda, is available in the detergent section of supermarkets and hardware stores. Trisodium phosphate is available at well-stocked paint supply stores and hardware stores. Diatomaceous earth is available at well-stocked garden supply stores and through mail-order garden suppliers.*

GOOD IDEA!

Prevent silver tarnish by limiting air contact with silver pieces or by storing silver in flannel bags especially treated to prevent tarnish. If you don't have treated flannel bags, wrap each piece in plastic wrap, eliminating as much air as possible.

Store plastic-wrapped silver in a cool, dry drawer. Rubber may corrode or permanently etch the silver. Never leave silver—even plastic-wrapped pieces—in contact with rubber bands or any other rubber item.

Also, don't leave silver in prolonged contact with these common corrosive substances: salt, eggs, olives, salad dressings, sulfur, vinegar, fruit juices, and alcohol, including perfume or cologne.

Electrolytic Silver Cleaner

This process depends on a chemical reaction to remove heavy accumulations of tarnish quickly without rubbing. It is not recommended for frequent use as this treatment may dull the surface shine of silver.

Yield: 2 quarts

INGREDIENTS

2 quarts boiling water

4 teaspoons baking soda

SUPPLIES

3-quart or larger enameled pan large enough to hold the silver to be cleaned

aluminum foil

soapy water

soft cloth

Line the bottom of the pan with aluminum foil. Place silver on the foil. Pour water over silver, covering it completely. Sprinkle in baking soda. Let silver sit in the solution for 5 minutes, then remove it. Wash the silver in hot, sudsy water, rinse, and dry. Buff to a shine with a soft cloth.

Save That Stone

Besides diamonds, there are many other precious and semiprecious gemstones found in jewelry: agates, emeralds, rubies, opals, moonstones, turquoise, and jade, to name just a few. Because each has such different properties and because exact identification is sometimes not known, especially with less-expensive jewelry, it is wisest to have such pieces cleaned professionally by the jeweler. While most such stones will not be harmed by a simple detergent solution, washing with anything stronger may soften glues. Brushing may scratch soft surfaces, and other unforeseen damage may result.

Diamond Cleaner

Clean diamonds in a mild detergent solution. This cleaner may be used on rings, necklaces, bracelets, or other jewelry. It is an excellent cleaner for routine maintenance.

Yield: 1 quart

INGREDIENTS

1 teaspoon mild dishwashing liquid
1 quart warm water

SUPPLIES

2-quart bowl
soft toothbrush
lint-free cloth

To make a warm, sudsy bath, mix the dishwashing liquid and water in the bowl. Brush the diamonds to be cleaned with the sudsy water. Rinse and pat dry with a soft lint-free cloth.

> **GOOD IDEA!**
>
> **To clean diamond jewelry that is truly grimy,** combine 1 cup ammonia and 1 cup cold water in a small bowl. Soak the jewelry in the solution for 30 minutes. Wearing rubber gloves, lift out and dislodge loosened dirt by gently using a soft toothbrush around the back and front of the mounting. Swish the jewelry in the solution once more, rinse, and drain on paper towels.

Lemon Oil Furniture Polish

This polish is easy to make and use.

Yield: 1 quart

INGREDIENTS

1 bottle mineral oil (1 quart)
1 tablespoon lemon oil

☛ **BE SAFE.** Oils are flammable. Avoid open flames. Do not smoke.

Add lemon oil into the bottle of mineral oil. Shake to mix. To use, wipe it on and wipe it off with a clean cloth.

➺ **Note:** Buy lemon oil in herb shops and craft shops.

Furniture Polish

This polish provides a good protective finish.

Yield: 1 quart

INGREDIENTS

1 quart mineral oil
2 tablespoons chipped or shredded carnauba wax

SUPPLIES

double boiler with 2-quart insert
stirrer
1-quart bottle with lid

☛ **BE SAFE.** *Ingredients are flammable. Avoid open flames. Do not smoke. Always use a double boiler to melt wax; never place over direct heat.*

With the insert empty, bring water to a boil in the double boiler. Turn off heat and remove double boiler to a heat-proof surface. Put oil and wax in the insert and stir until wax is melted. Let cool and store in the bottle.

➥ **Note:** Buy carnauba wax at stores that specialize in custom paints and wood finishes. See page 444 for another source.

Cleaning Plastic

Plastics are all over the house these days. Here are some spot removers for common stains on various plastic surfaces.

For food stains: For stains from tomato products, fruit juice, coffee, tea, and miscellaneous stains, rub the surface vigorously with a damp cloth dipped in baking soda. Rinse with plain water.

For ballpoint pen ink: Spray the stain with hair spray, then wipe with a damp cloth.

For all types of stains in containers, plastic bottles, cups, vases, and the like: Fill the container with water, then drop in one or two foaming denture cleaning tablets. Let articles soak for 15 to 20 minutes, then rinse.

For adhesives, tar, and similar sticky substances: Wearing rubber gloves, rub the stain with a little lighter fluid until it's gone, then wash with mild detergent and water. Rub adhesives from stickers and labels with cooking oil until glue is dissolved and rubbed away. Wash in mild detergent and water to remove oil.

Lacquered Wood Cleaner

This contains no solvents; it won't remove lacquer.

Yield: about ½ cup

INGREDIENTS

1 cup flour
½ cup olive oil

SUPPLIES

stirrer
1-pint measuring cup or bowl
soft clean cloth

Stir flour and oil into a paste in the cup or bowl. Smooth on wood with a soft cloth, then wipe off with a clean cloth. Buff to a gloss with a dry, clean cloth.

Leather Oil

This oil keeps leather smooth, supple, and crack-free.

Yield: 3 cups

INGREDIENTS

1½ cups neat's-foot oil
1½ cups mineral oil

SUPPLIES

1-quart bottle with lid

☛ **BE SAFE.** *Oils are flammable. Avoid open flames. Do not smoke.*

Combine oils in the bottle. Shake to mix. Store tightly sealed. To use, wipe onto leather with a cloth, let sit 10 to 15 minutes, then buff vigorously with a clean cloth.

➡ **Note:** *Buy neat's-foot oil at hardware stores, saddlery and tack shops, and backpacking supply stores.*

GOOD IDEA!

To make furniture scratches less noticeable, mix 1 tablespoon finely ground pecans with 1 teaspoon mineral oil in a small cup. Rub the nut and oil paste into the scratches with a soft cloth. Polish away excess with a clean soft cloth. Small scratches often disappear.

GOOD IDEA!

One way to preserve leather is to rub it with an oil mixture that's 1 part neat's-foot oil and 1 part castor oil. Heat the oil mixture over very low heat until it's just warm. Rub the warm oil into the leather with a soft cloth. Let sit 15 minutes; then buff with a clean soft cloth.

GOOD IDEA!

To remove dirt and grease from leather, mix 1½ cups water and ¾ cup denatured ethyl alcohol in a 1-quart bowl. Stir in ½ cup white vinegar. Dampen a soft cloth or sponge with this solution and wipe leather clean.

Denatured ethyl alcohol is toxic and flammable. Store this and all cleaning fluids away from children. Do not use near open flames. Buy denatured ethyl alcohol at paint supply stores and hardware stores.

Saddle Soap Leather Cleaner

Saddle soap is the traditional cleaner and conditioner for leather. Make your own with this formula.

Yield: about 4½ cups

INGREDIENTS

3½ cups water
¾ cup soap powder
¼ cup neat's-foot oil
½ cup chipped or shredded beeswax

SUPPLIES

2-quart saucepan
spoon or paddle
double boiler with 2-quart insert
margarine tubs or other sealable containers

☛ **BE SAFE.** Neat's-foot oil and beeswax are flammable. Avoid open flames. Do not smoke. Always heat in a double boiler; never place over direct heat.

In the saucepan, bring water to a simmer over low heat. Add soap powder and stir until dissolved. Remove from heat and set aside. With the insert empty, boil water in a double boiler. Turn off heat and remove double boiler to a heat-proof surface. Blend oil and wax in the insert until the wax is melted. Add the oil and wax mixture to the soap solution, stirring until thickened. Pour the soap mixture into the tubs or other containers and let cool completely.

➡ **Notes:** Be sure to use soap powder, such as Ivory Snow; don't use detergent. Buy neat's-foot oil at hardware stores, saddlery and tack shops, and backpacking supply stores. Buy beeswax at hardware stores, beekeepers, and craft supply stores. See page 444 for other sources.

Paper Preservative

Save newspaper clippings, magazine articles, and other papers almost indefinitely with this treatment.

Yield: about 1 quart

INGREDIENTS

2 tablespoons milk of magnesia

1 quart club soda

SUPPLIES

1½-quart bowl

stirrer

shallow pan, large enough to hold papers in a single layer

paper towels

In the bowl, blend milk of magnesia into club soda. Refrigerate overnight. The next day, pour the mixture into the pan. Lay the papers in the solution. Let soak for 1 hour. Remove soaked clippings and blot between paper towels to absorb as much moisture as possible. Spread clippings on a flat surface to dry thoroughly.

Bottle/Vase Cleaner

This is a great way to clean narrow-necked containers.

Yield: about ⅓ cup

SUPPLIES

¼ cup white vinegar

2 tablespoons uncooked rice

Pour vinegar into the bottle or vase, then add rice. Cover with one hand and shake vigorously. The vinegar cleans while the rice loosens dirt without scratching.

GOOD IDEA!

Here's a simple method for preserving newspaper clippings and other special papers. Spread a thin layer of white craft glue over the entire piece. Let dry. The glue stiffens and strengthens the paper and prevents yellowing. You can coat just the side you want to preserve, or you can coat both sides. Just let the first side dry before coating the reverse side. Be sure to choose white craft glue or paper glue that dries to a clear coat.

GOOD IDEA!

Clean combs and brushes in 1 teaspoon dishwashing liquid plus 1 tablespoon borax dissolved in 2 quarts warm water. Soak items for 30 minutes; then rinse in hot running water. Borax is toxic. Keep it out of the reach of children.

GOOD-BYE TO HOUSEHOLD PESTS

Here are simple but effective remedies for our most unwelcome guests—flour weevils, ants, mice, and cockroaches. We all wish them gone instantly, and we all hate dousing our homes with poison to hasten their departure. The remedies that follow provide some interesting alternatives to commercial fumigants and poisons.

Cockroach Powder

Make this formula with either borax or boric acid. Boric acid is somewhat stronger than borax, however, borax is less expensive.

Yield: about 3 tablespoons

INGREDIENTS

2 tablespoons borax or boric acid
2 teaspoons sugar

SUPPLIES

small cup
stirrer

☛ **BE SAFE.** Borax and boric acid, while safer to use than insecticides, are still poisons and can cause death when ingested. Do not store or sprinkle this formula where children or pets can get into it.

In the cup, mix together borax or boric acid and sugar. To control roaches, sprinkle behind cabinets and appliances, under and behind sinks, and other places where cockroaches run and congregate. If heavily infested, repeat applications every two weeks until cockroaches are gone. Then repeat once a month or so to prevent reinfestation.

➼ **Notes:** Buy borax (99.5 pure sodium borate) at paint supply stores, hardware stores, and the detergent section of supermarkets. Buy boric acid through your local pharmacist.

GOOD IDEA!

To rid your home of **silverfish,** insects that feed on paper and even drapery linings, discard old papers and books and sprinkle boric acid in cracks and hiding places. Repeat weekly until bugs are gone. Boric acid is toxic. Do not use it around children or pets.

GOOD IDEA!

To kill cockroaches, use a "gourmet" chocolate formula. Mix ¼ cup borax, 2 tablespoons flour, and 1 tablespoon cocoa powder. Apply where cockroaches congregate. Borax is toxic. Keep it away from children and pets.

Clothing Storage Formula

This mixture helps to repel moths and give stored clothing, linens, and other fabrics a sweet aroma. Proportions of the herbs may be mixed to your preference.

Yield: varies by amount of ingredients chosen

INGREDIENTS

powdered sandalwood
whole or ground cloves
dried lavender
dried sweet woodruff

SUPPLIES

bowl
small squares of double-layer cheesecloth or muslin

Mix all ingredients in the bowl and tie or sew a little into each square of cloth. Spread sachets among layers of packed clothing or hang them in garment bags or closets to keep the fabrics fresh and sweet-smelling.

➦ **Note:** *Grow these herbs in your garden or buy them at herb shops. See page 444 for other sources.*

GOOD IDEA!

For a quick and inexpensive way to keep stored clothing smelling fresh, spread packets of activated charcoal throughout the layers of clothing. Simply wrap ordinary activated charcoal (available from aquarium supply dealers and hardware stores) in tissue paper. Be sure to keep the charcoal from touching fabric. It can stain.

Along Came a Spider

Most spiders are harmless yet helpful since they keep other insect pests under control. But if you wish to reduce the number of spiders in your home, try these tips.

- To keep out both spiders and the insects they hunt, make sure all door and window screens are in perfect order.
- Check firewood, plants, and cut flowers before bringing them into the house. Be sure to check for egg cases as well as live spiders.
- Regularly sweep or vacuum behind appliances, furniture, and other dark hiding places where spiders like to congregate.
- Vacuum webs and egg cases found in the home and empty the bag immediately into a tightly sealed plastic garbage bag. Or remove the egg cases to your garden where they will be beneficial.
- To prevent venomous spider bites—a pretty unlikely occurrence—check and shake out shoes or clothing that have been stored. Don't poke your hand or foot in a dark hole, such as a chimney, before checking for spiders. If a spider does crawl on your arm, brush it off rather than swatting it. A spider is unlikely to bite when quickly brushed off.

GOOD IDEA!

To moth-proof cloth-
ing in drawers, scatter
loose herbal moth repel-
lent between layers of tissue paper. Be sure to protect fabric from direct
contact with the herbal
mixture. The oils in some
spices can stain fabrics.

Herbal Moth Repellent

This mixture is a great replacement for moth balls.

Yield: about 1¼ cups

INGREDIENTS

½ cup whole cloves
½ cups whole black peppercorns
3 or 4 sticks of cinnamon bark, broken into small
    pieces

SUPPLIES

1-pint bowl
small squares of double-layer cheesecloth or muslin

Mix all ingredients in the bowl. Tie or sew a little into each square of cloth. Hang in closets or scatter in drawers and boxes to keep moths away.

GOOD IDEA!

A fairly effective
ant stopper is ordinary
white vinegar. Simply
track down the ants to
where they are entering
your home. Liberally
wash down all entry
areas and areas where
ants congregate with full-
strength white vinegar.
Let the area air-dry.

Ant Traps

These are safe, nonpoisonous traps.

Yield: 4 to 6 traps

INGREDIENTS

¼ cup sugar
¼ cup baking yeast
½ cup molasses

SUPPLIES

2-cup measure
spatula
six 3 × 5-inch index cards

Mix all ingredients in the measure. Smear a thin layer of the mixture on the index cards. Place the cards, syrup side up, in areas where ants travel.

Herbal Flea Treatment

This natural combination of herbs is a safe alternative to chemical flea treatments for your pet's bedding.

Yield: about 1 cup

INGREDIENTS

½ cup dried pennyroyal

3 tablespoons dried thyme

3 tablespoons dried wormwood

3 tablespoons dried rosemary

SUPPLIES

1-pint bowl

Stir all ingredients together in the bowl. Open a seam of your pet's bedding item and insert the herbs. Resew the seam. The herbs should help repel fleas.

➠ **Note:** Grow these herbs in your garden or buy them at herb shops. See page 444 for other sources.

GOOD IDEA!

To treat a flea-infested carpet, sprinkle flea-repellent herbs liberally over the affected area and let sit a few days. Then vacuum up thoroughly. Be sure to discard your vacuum bag after cleaning up fleas. Herbs that repel fleas include pennyroyal, yellow dock, fennel, and eucalyptus.

No More Flour Bugs

Smart use of your freezer will put an end to those nasty worms and bugs that show up in flours, grains, and other dry staples. Simply wrap packages of newly purchased flours, meals, and grains in plastic freezer bags or plastic wrap. Place the wrapped goods in the freezer for 24 hours. Freezing destroys any eggs that may hatch into worms or bugs. After 24 hours, remove the products from the freezer and store them at room temperature.

When storing treated staples at room temperature, the best course is to store them in airtight containers or tightly closed plastic bags to prevent new infestation from outside. To minimize infesting your existing supplies, be sure to freeze all new supplies as soon as you get them home and before putting them into the pantry.

If you have room in the freezer, store flours, meals, and grains there permanently. They'll stay fresh as well as bug-free. Whole-grain flours and meals grow rancid quickly at room temperature, and freezer storage will keep them fresh and flavorful. Don't store wheat germ in the freezer, however, as freezing destroys the vitamin E content.

Bedbug Exterminator

Bedbugs hide and lay eggs behind loose wallpaper, in wall and floor cracks, in nail holes, in lightswitch boxes, and on door and window frames. They can also hide in wooden bed frames. If you have a problem with bedbugs, send out your mattress and pillows to be fumigated. Thoroughly vacuum the entire room and everything in it. Wash bed linens and blankets in the hottest water possible. Apply this exterminating powder in all cracks and crevices where bedbugs might be hiding.

Yield: 1 cup

INGREDIENTS

¾ cup powdered alum
2 tablespoons boric acid
2 tablespoons salicylic acid

SUPPLIES

stirrer
1-pint bowl
new garden dusting equipment (optional)

☛ **BE SAFE.** Ingredients are toxic, especially if ingested. Keep children and pets away from areas where this powder is spread.

Stir all ingredients together in the bowl. Sprinkle all infested areas. Or buy a garden duster to blow the powder into crevices. Do not use a garden duster that has previously held garden insecticides or fungicides.

➡ **Notes:** Buy alum sold as an astringent (potassium aluminum sulfate) not alum sold as a pickling agent. Alum, boric acid, and salicylic acid can be ordered through your pharmacist.

HOME COMFORTS

These formulas are for those extra touches—scented soaps and potpourris—that make home a special place to be. Some of these formulas make inexpensive and unique gifts requiring little cash to make. Before you set out to make any of the soaps though, do read "Using Lye Safely" on page 322. To make soap, all you need is familiarity with lye precautions and several hours of unhurried time to enjoy the whole process.

Liquid Pump Soap

If you like the convenience of liquid pump soaps, but not the exorbitant prices, make your own. This formula makes a thick, creamy liquid soap.

Yield: about 2½ cups

INGREDIENTS

2 cups mild laundry soap flakes

10 ounces hot water

2 tablespoons baby oil or mineral oil

SUPPLIES

1-quart bowl

spoon or paddle

24-ounce recycled soap pump bottle

Place soap in the bowl, stir in water, and mix. Add oil and blend well. Pour into the pump bottle. Since the soap does tend to separate, shake it occasionally before using. Adding oil helps keep the mixture from drying up.

✿ **Variation:** To make a scented soap, add a few drops of an essential oil, such as rose oil.

➥ **Note:** Buy essential oils at drug stores, cosmetic counters, and craft shops.

> **GOOD IDEA!**
>
> **To make your own premoistened towelettes,** mix a few tablespoons of baby oil with a cup of soapy water. Soak paper towels in this solution and tuck them into plastic bags to use in the nursery. Or carry them in a diaper bag or purse for quick cleanups anywhere.

Using Lye Safely

Lye is a highly caustic, crystalline substance that dissolves easily in water. Lye crystals alone react with skin moisture to cause burns; a water solution of lye can also cause serious burns. Lye is also highly toxic if swallowed. When adding crystalline lye to water, wear rubber gloves, a face mask, and goggles. Keep 1 cup white vinegar on hand at all times while handling lye. If lye solution splashes on your skin, flood the area first with vinegar and then with cold water to stop the burning. Adding lye to water causes a chemical reaction that generates heat and gives off harsh fumes. Be sure your work area is well-ventilated before you begin making soap. *Be sure to add the lye crystals to the water. Do not add the water to the lye.*

To dissolve the lye crystals, use a large-enough pot to hold all the lye and water called for in the recipe with extra room to allow for stirring without splashing. Use a pot made of stainless steel, stoneware, enameled cast iron, or heat-proof glass, such as Pyrex or Corning Ware. Use a long-handled stainless steel or wooden spoon or an old broomstick for stirring. Use the same type of pan and stirring implement to hold and stir the fat and lye mixture in the final soap-making step. When working with lye, never use aluminum, tin, iron, or nonstick-coated pans, such as Teflon or Silverstone.

Store leftover lye crystals tightly sealed in the original can. You can also store lye crystals in a jar. *Label the jar* and seal it tightly. Lye crystals exposed to moisture will sometimes form a solid mass and become unusable. If you have children in your household, avoid the possibility of accidental poisoning by disposing of leftover lye. Pour small amounts (less than ½ cup) of the crystals down the kitchen drain and immediately flood the drain with a heavy stream of cold water for 2 to 3 minutes.

GOOD IDEA!

To make scented soap, add any of the following oils before pouring soap in molds: cinnamon, citronella, cloves, lavender, lemon, lemongrass, rose, rose geranium, rosemary, and sassafras.

Basic White Hand Bar

This is a basic, pure bar of soap. Adding oils, coloring, or scents makes it richer, prettier, or more fragrant.

Yield: about ½ pound

INGREDIENTS

1 cup cold water

2 tablespoons pure lye crystals

1 cup rendered and strained fat (see "How to Render Fat for Making Soap" on page 274)

SUPPLIES

two 1-quart lye-proof cooking pots (stainless steel, stoneware, or enameled cast iron)

rubber work gloves

goggles, safety glasses, or face shield

face mask

1 cup white vinegar (used as safety precaution only)

stainless steel or wooden spoon

dairy, meat, or candy thermometer

hand eggbeater

flexible plastic soap molds, such as margarine tubs or cardboard or wooden boxes lined with plastic wrap

☛ **BE SAFE.** *Lye is very caustic; it can destroy skin by chemical action. Handle it very carefully. Read "Using Lye Safely" on the opposite page before making this soap.*

Place water in a lye-proof pot. Put on rubber gloves and other safety gear. Have the vinegar handy. Very slowly add lye crystals to water, constantly stirring until lye is dissolved. As lye is added to water, the water temperature will rise to around 150°F. Place the thermometer in the water and allow it to cool to 95° to 98°F.

As the water is cooling, slowly heat rendered fat in a lye-proof pot until it reaches 95° to 98°F. When both lye and fat are in the same 95° to 98°F temperature range, slowly pour lye into fat, stirring constantly until well-mixed. Beat mixture very gently with the eggbeater to the consistency of thick honey. Avoid splashing.

Pour the mixture into molds. Cover with a blanket and set aside to dry for 24 hours, well away from children or pets. After 24 hours, carefully turn the soap out of the molds and leave in a dry, airy place for at least two weeks. A fine white powder may appear on the surface when the soap is a few days old. This is sodium carbonate. Wash it away when the soap is mature; it tends to make the skin dry.

➡ **Note:** *Lye is crystalline sodium hydroxide or potassium hydroxide. It is usually sold in the drain cleaner section of supermarkets and hardware stores. Buy pure lye crystals or flakes, not lye sold as a liquid drain cleaner.*

Vegetable-Oil Soap

If you have trouble getting animal fat, or don't want to render it down, this soap is for you. This formula makes a mild soap rich with coconut oil and olive oil.

Yield: about 5½ pounds

INGREDIENTS

1	quart cold water
10¼	ounces pure lye crystals
23	ounces white vegetable shortening
42	ounces olive oil
16	ounces coconut oil

SUPPLIES

2-quart lye-proof cooking pot *plus* 8-quart lye-proof cooking pot (stainless steel, stoneware, or enameled cast iron)

rubber work gloves

goggles, safety glasses, or face shield

face mask

1 cup white vinegar (used as safety precaution only)

stainless steel or wooden spoon

dairy, meat, or candy thermometer

hand eggbeater

flexible plastic soap molds, such as margarine tubs or cardboard or wooden boxes lined with plastic wrap

☛ **BE SAFE.** Lye is very caustic; it can destroy skin by chemical action. Handle it very carefully. Read "Using Lye Safely" on page 322 before making this soap.

Place water in the 2-quart lye-proof pot. Put on rubber gloves and other safety gear. Have the vinegar handy. Very slowly add lye crystals to water, constantly stirring until lye is dissolved. As lye is added to water, the water temperature will rise to around 150°F. Place the thermometer in the water and allow it to cool to 95° to 98°F.

As the water is cooling, slowly heat the vegetable short-ening and oils in the 8-quart lye-proof pot until it reaches 95° to 98°F. When both lye and fats are in the same 95° to 98°F temperature range, slowly pour lye into fat, stirring constantly until well-mixed. Beat mixture very gently with the eggbeater to the consistentcy of thick honey. Avoid splashing.

Pour the mixture into molds, cover with a blanket, and set aside to dry for 24 hours, well away from children or pets. After 24 hours, carefully turn the soap out of the molds and leave it in a dry, airy place for at least two weeks. A fine white powder may appear on the surface when the soap is a few days old. This is sodium carbonate. Wash it away when the soap is mature; it tends to make the skin dry.

•➔ **Notes:** Lye is crystalline sodium hydroxide or potassium hy-droxide. It is usually sold in the drain cleaner section of supermar-kets and hardware stores. Buy pure lye crystals or flakes, not lye sold as a liquid drain cleaner. Buy coconut oil from drug stores and health food stores.

Lavender and Spice Luxury Bar

This hand and face soap is scented with lavender and cinnamon and enriched with coconut oil and olive oil.

Yield: about 6 pounds

INGREDIENTS

- 1 quart cold water
- 13 ounces pure lye crystals
- 38 ounces rendered and strained fat (see "How To Render Fat for Making Soap" on page 274)
- 3 cups coconut oil
- 1½ cups olive oil
- ½ ounce finely ground lavender
- 1 tablespoon ground cinnamon

> ### GOOD IDEA!
>
> **T**o **make decorative soaps for gifts,** pur-chase decorative candy molds from candymaking supply stores. Make soaps in a variety of small, pretty shapes and decorate with dried flow-ers as described in "Good Idea!" on page 329.

(continued)

GOOD IDEA!

To dry your own lavender for soap, cut the stems just as the flowers open. Hang them in bunches or spread them on screens in a shaded, well-ventilated, dry, and warm place. You can also tie them in bunches and suspend them from rafters in an attic or shed. Keep out of direct sunlight.

After the flowers have dried, strip the tiny blossoms from the stem and store in a sealed jar until ready to use.

For the strongest fragrance, grind the blossoms just before using.

SUPPLIES

2-quart lye-proof pot *plus* 8-quart lye-proof pot (stainless steel, stoneware, or enameled cast iron)

rubber work gloves

goggles, safety glasses, or face shield

face mask

1 cup white vinegar (used as safety precaution only)

stainless steel or wooden spoon

dairy, meat, or candy thermometer

hand eggbeater

flexible plastic soap molds, such as margarine tubs or cardboard or wooden boxes lined with plastic wrap

☛ **BE SAFE.** Lye is very caustic; it can destroy skin by chemical action. Handle it very carefully. Read "Using Lye Safely" on page 322 before making this soap.

Place water in the 2-quart lye-proof pot. Put on the rubber gloves and other safety gear. Have the vinegar handy. Very slowly add lye crystals to water, constantly stirring until lye is dissolved. As lye is added to water, the water temperature will rise to around 150°F. Place the thermometer in the water and allow it to cool to 95° to 98°F.

As the water is cooling, stir rendered fat and oils in the 8-quart lye-proof pot. Slowly heat until fats reach 95° to 98°F. When both lye and fat are in the same 95° to 98°F temperature range, slowly pour lye into fat, stirring constantly until well-mixed. Beat very gently with the eggbeater to the consistency of thick honey. Avoid splashing. Stir in lavender and cinnamon.

Pour the mixture into molds, cover with a blanket, and set aside to dry for 36 hours, well away from children or pets. After 36 hours, carefully turn the soap out of the molds and leave in a dry, airy place for at least two weeks. A fine white powder may appear on the surface when the soap is a few days old. This is sodium carbonate. Wash it away when the soap is mature; it tends to make the skin dry.

➻ **Notes:** Lye is crystalline sodium hydroxide or potassium hydroxide. It is usually sold in the drain cleaner section of supermarkets and hardware stores. Buy pure lye crystals or flakes, not lye sold as a liquid drain cleaner. Buy coconut oil from drug stores and health food stores. Buy dried lavender at herb shops and craft shops.

Olive-Almond Soap

The almond meal in this soap makes it an especially good cleanser for your skin. For a beautiful, sweet-smelling soap, add food coloring and your favorite essential oils.

Yield: about 3 pounds

INGREDIENTS

- 2¼ cups cold water
- 6½ ounces pure lye crystals
- 18 ounces rendered and strained fat (see "How To Render Fat for Making Soap" on page 274)
- 12 ounces olive oil
- 12 ounces coconut oil
- 2 ounces fine almond meal
- 10 drops yellow food coloring (optional)
- 4 to 8 drops essential oil (optional)

SUPPLIES

2-quart lye-proof cooking pot *plus* 6- to 8-quart lye-proof cooking pot (stainless steel, stoneware, or enameled cast iron)

rubber work gloves

goggles, safety glasses, or face shield

face mask

1 cup white vinegar (used as safety precaution only)

stainless steel or wooden spoon

dairy, meat, or candy thermometer

hand eggbeater

flexible plastic soap molds, such as margarine tubs or cardboard or wooden boxes lined with plastic wrap

(continued)

GOOD IDEA!

Buy essential oils instead of trying to make them. Essential oils, fragrant substances extracted from flowers and leaves, make wonderful additions to soaps. But making them is no easy task. Essential oils are extracted by steam distillation. With the proper equipment, a huge amount of herbs or flowers, and lots of steadfastness, you can distill your own pure essential oils. But in the long run, it is a better bet to buy them from a reputable company.

GOOD IDEA!

Here's a great way to use those soap pieces that are too small to keep but too big to throw out. Place ½ cup soap bits and pieces with 2 tablespoons water in a small saucepan. Bring to a gentle boil over medium heat, stirring continuously until the pieces are completely melted. Continue to boil for a minute or two to remove excess water. Pour soap into a mold and let stand for a few days until the bar is dry and hard. A plastic margarine tub or a small box lined with plastic wrap makes a nice mold.

☛ **BE SAFE.** Lye is very caustic; it can destroy skin by chemical action. Handle it very carefully. Read "Using Lye Safely" on page 322 before making this soap.

Place water in the 2-quart lye-proof pot. Put on rubber gloves and other safety gear. Have the vinegar handy. Very slowly add lye crystals to water, stirring constantly until lye is dissolved. As lye is added to water, the water temperature will rise to around 150°F. Place the thermometer in the water and allow it to cool to 95° to 98°F.

As the water is cooling, slowly heat the rendered fat and oils in the 6- to 8-quart lye-proof pot. Heat until fat reaches 95° to 98°F. When both lye and fat are in the same 95° to 98°F temperature range, slowly pour lye into fat, stirring constantly until well-mixed. Beat very gently with the eggbeater to the consistency of thick honey. Avoid splashing. Stir in the almond meal and, if you are using them, food coloring and essential oil.

Pour mixture into molds, cover with a blanket, and set aside to dry for 24 hours, well away from children or pets. After 24 hours, carefully turn the soap out of the molds and leave in a dry, airy place for at least two weeks. A fine white powder may appear on the surface when the soap is a few days old. This is sodium carbonate. Wash it away when the soap is mature; it tends to make the skin dry.

➠ **Notes:** Lye is crystalline sodium hydroxide or potassium hydroxide. It is usually sold in the drain cleaner section of supermarkets and hardware stores. Buy pure lye crystals or flakes, not lye sold as a liquid drain cleaner. Buy coconut oil at drug stores and health food stores. Buy almond meal at health food stores, or make your own by grinding fresh almonds in a food processor. Buy essential oils at drug stores, cosmetic counters, and herb shops.

Decorated Soaps

Perfect as gifts, these decorated soaps can be made in any size with a variety of decorations.

Yield: 1 decorated bar soap

SUPPLIES

new bar of soap with at least one plain side

water

small decorative picture on thin paper, such as a
flower picture from a greeting card

2 tablespoons chipped or shredded paraffin wax

small, heat-proof custard cup

small pot of hot water

small, shallow pan, such as a single section of a frozen
dinner tray

old towel or foil-covered baking sheet

clear plastic wrap

☛ **BE SAFE.** Paraffin is flammable. Heat it over hot water;
never place over direct heat.

Moisten a plain side of the soap with water, then place
the picture on it, pressing down so it adheres to the wet
soap.

Place paraffin in the cup. To melt, set the custard cup
in the hot water. Pour the melted wax into the shallow pan,
then dip the picture side of the soap into the wax. Set the
wax-coated soap on the towel or baking sheet and allow to
harden. Wrap the finished soap in plastic wrap to protect it
until ready to use. For more bars, simply multiply the ingredients as needed.

↦ **Note:** Buy paraffin in the canning section of supermarkets
and hardware stores.

GOOD IDEA!

Use a variety of ma-
**terials to decorate
soaps,** such as tiny, flat
dried flowers or bits of
lace or ribbon. Any small,
flat, lightweight item that
will adhere to the soap
and can be completely
covered with paraffin is
suitable.

GOOD IDEA!

If you have a **woodstove,** fill a covered cast-iron casserole with water, herbs, and spices and simmer on the hot stove with the lid slightly ajar. For a Christmas evergreen fragrance, add a few sprigs of fresh pine or spruce, a few whole cinnamon sticks, and some whole cloves or allspice. Be sure to check the water level in the casserole frequently and to remove the casserole from the woodstove when you retire at night.

Aromatic Simmer

A lovely way to add fragrance to your home is to set a pot of spices and herbs simmering on the stove. Guests will think you've been baking all day.

Yield: 3 cups

INGREDIENTS

2 three-inch pieces of stick cinnamon

5 whole cloves

5 whole allspice berries

3 strips orange peel

1 teaspoon almond extract

3 cups water

SUPPLIES

skillet or shallow pan

Place all ingredients in the skillet or pan. Place it on the stove and gently heat to a simmer. Turn the heat down as low as possible and let the mixture barely simmer for at least 20 minutes or as long as desired. Add water as necessary to prevent the pan from boiling dry.

Quick-and-Easy Sachets

Think of how refreshing it is to open a lingerie drawer and smell the fragrance of a sachet. There is nothing better than the "aroma therapy" of herbs and flowers to perk up the spirits.

The ingredients for sachets are the same as for potpourris (see Potpourri Mix on page 366), but they are ground and crumbled rather than used whole. Then, they are stuffed into festive pillows or bags.

A really quick method of making the decorative pouches for sachets is to use discarded panty hose. First wash the panty hose and cut off the feet. Then think of making sausages. Tie one end of a leg with pretty ribbon, stuff some sachet mixture inside, tie the other end, and cut it from the rest of the leg. Continue tying, stuffing, and cutting until you've used up a leg. You can make as many sachets as the leg is long without any sewing. It's easy to make a dozen or so sachets in just 15 minutes.

Use the recipes in Potpourri Mix to create rose-lilac, herbal bouquet, or spicy sachets. Put them in dresser drawers, lingerie boxes, or suitcases in storage.

Basement Freshener

Clean up stale, musty basement odors with this odor- and moisture-absorbing mixture.

Yield: 15 pounds

INGREDIENTS

10 pounds new cat litter (clay or cedarized)

5 pounds baking soda

SUPPLIES

5 or 6 shallow pans, such as cat litter pans or large baking pans

plastic garbage bags

Mix together cat litter and baking soda. Place an inch or two of the mixture in shallow pans and distribute around the room. If the basement is very large, you will want to use more pans and more freshener. Replace the mixture with new freshener once a week. Store any leftovers in plastic garbage bags.

GOOD IDEA!

To help damp and musty-smelling basement floors, sprinkle a mixture of new cat litter and baking soda liberally over the floor. Let it sit for a few days, then vacuum.

Homemade Odor-Eaters

Tired of strong cooking odors lingering for hours—sometimes days—after a meal? What smelled taste-tempting in the evening seems stale and unpleasant by morning. Here are some fresh ideas for fresh-smelling homes.

- Stir 2 teaspoons ground cinnamon into 2 cups water and bring to a simmer on the stove. The sweet scent of cinnamon will quickly replace less pleasant odors.
- While cooking strong-smelling vegetables, such as cabbage, sauerkraut, or cauliflower, lay a layer of celery leaves on top of the vegetables to prevent odors. Or, add a table- spoon of vinegar to the water to help cut the odor.
- Smother smoking food drips in the oven with a generous layer of salt. Salt stops the smok- ing, eliminates odors, and makes cleanup much easier once the oven is cool.
- Minimize the odor left by smoking guests by hiding small bowls of ammonia, vinegar, or activated charcoal around the room.
- To get smoke odor out of carpeting, sprinkle generously with baking soda, let sit 20 to 30 minutes, then vacuum up thoroughly.

GOOD IDEA!

Make your rose jar special by thinking of shades of meaning. That means selecting roses by their colors. Red means passion and desire. Pink stands for simplicity and happy love. White signifies purity and innocence. Yellow means jealousy and perfect achievement. Thinking color is an ideal way to make a rose jar a special gift for a friend or to celebrate a happy occasion.

Rose Jar: Love That Rose

Keep a jar of rose-based potpourri to scent your home for special occasions or for adding a relaxing atmosphere to a late-night supper. In this rose-based potpourri, a salt treatment preserves and dries the flower petals.

Yield: about 1 cup

INGREDIENTS

2 cups petals from freshly picked roses
½ cup table salt
1 teaspoon dried, grated lemon peel
6 drops rose oil

SUPPLIES

old window screen or shallow pan
1-pint jar or tin with lid

Pick fresh roses early in the morning and shake off any moisture. Remove the petals carefully and spread a thin layer of petals on a screen or in a shallow pan. Sprinkle the petals with salt. Place another thin layer of petals on top of the first and sprinkle with additional salt. Continue loosely layering petals and salt to a thickness of no more than an inch.

Place the petal-covered screen or pan in a dry, dark place away from sunlight. Check daily to make sure the petals are drying and not mildewing. If necessary, stir gently to speed even drying.

When thoroughly dry, shake off salt. Place petals and lemon peel in the jar or tin and shake gently. Sprinkle rose oil over the mixture and shake gently until well-combined. Keep the jar or tin covered to preserve fragrance. Open it to release fragrance, when desired.

Notes: Roses from a florist usually are not suitable; they don't have enough scent. Buy rose oil at some pharmacies, cosmetic counters, and herb shops.

Rose Jar: Rose Mint

Mint and spice perk up the essential rose aroma of this fragrant mixture. Make this potpourri in the summer from your own roses and mint plants. In mid-winter, release the fragrance to chase away the stuffy, musty odors that creep into every long-closed home.

Yield: about 1 cup

INGREDIENTS

 1 cup dried rose petals (follow directions for "Rose Jar: Love That Rose" on the opposite page)

10 mint leaves, dried and crushed

½ teaspoon orrisroot powder

¼ teaspoon ground cinnamon

¼ teaspoon ground allspice

¼ teaspoon ground nutmeg

SUPPLIES

1-pint jar or tin with lid

Add all ingredients to the jar or tin and gently shake until well-combined. Keep the jar or tin covered to preserve the fragrance. Open it to release fragrance, when desired.

➤ Notes: *Roses from a florist usually are not suitable for drying; they don't have enough scent. Orrisroot powder is a fixative, a substance that slows down the release of fragrant oils into the air. When used in a potpourri, it makes the fragrance last longer. Buy orrisroot at craft shops,, floral supply stores, and pharmacies.*

GOOD IDEA!

Growing mint in a pot on a windowsill is easy. Give your potted mint good air circulation and high humidity. Water when the surface soil feels dry. Remember, mint likes to be moist. When the plants get crowded, repot in a container that is wider than it is deep. Mint plants remain productive for six months or more. Harvest by trimming or cutting individual stems.

Mints vary in the quality of their fragrance. Buy plants that smell good to you. It's best to buy mint plants rather than start them from seed because there is no guarantee that all of the seeds in a packet will have a nice fragrance. Plus, mint is difficult to start from seed.

Chapter Eight

Crafts

by Diane K. Gilroy

On the following pages, you'll find a wide assortment of crafts formulas, some simple enough to entertain a child and many sophisticated enough to challenge an experienced adult. Many of these formulas require only commonplace ingredients from your kitchen cupboard or basement workshop. Some of these crafts may bring back happy childhood memories of rainy days spent cutting paper dolls or carving boats from soap bars. That's intentional. All of the easy formulas here, whether for finger paint or egg dye, are intended to provide plain old-fashioned pleasure for children as well as the young-at-heart.

Candlemaking, for example, may be complex enough to interest serious hobbiests or simple enough to offer gratifying results for children. My own personal interest in candlemaking began with a childhood experience in recycling candle wax. One year, my brothers and sisters and I, supervised by our mother, made new candles from old stubs and paraffin, using vegetable cans and milk cartons as molds. The results were pretty ordinary, but we were proud of our efforts and gladly presented them as gifts to doting relatives. Of course, we had also created something far more precious and permanent than candles—the memory of our family having fun together. As a side benefit, we learned about an age-old craft because we had actually been part of the process.

Through the years, I've worked with other crafts, such as baker's clay, finger paint, pomanders, egg dyes, and bubble mixes. These crafts are so inexpensive and easy to do that they lend themselves beautifully to group activities. Whether you use a craft formula once or many times, you'll find that the greatest joy of these crafts is that they lend themselves to sharing and learning experiences—the stuff that memories are made of.

So look over the offerings here. No matter which craft you try, you'll find all the basics needed to succeed. For each craft formula, always read through the directions first to find out how much time is required as well as what ingredients and supplies you'll need. Then turn your imagination loose and let the fun begin!

OLD AND NEW CRAFTS

Many old-time crafts are perfect for our homes and lifestyles. From batik, which was first done in Indonesia, to candlewicking, a part of our colonial heritage, the items to make in this section include decorative objects, items to wear, or gifts for special occasions—fun to make and enjoyable to use.

Batik Decorating

Batik is a method of decorating and dyeing natural-fiber cloth, traditionally cotton. To work in batik, you simply apply a wax design to fabric and then dye the fabric in a cold-water dye bath. The wax design resists the dye. After the wax is removed, the undyed area stands out. You may create a multi-faceted, many-colored design using multiple wax applications and dye baths. If you'd like to make more than one wax-and-dye application, begin with the lightest dye color and finish with the darkest. The most recently applied color will be preserved under the next layer of wax.

Traditional batik artists apply the design with a special wax dispensing device called a tjanting tool. But the materials and equipment suggested here work perfectly for an introduction to the craft. A scarf or placemat is a good first project.

Yield: 15 ounces of wax, enough for several small projects

INGREDIENTS
powdered cold-water dye or liquid household dye, assorted colors

6 ounces paraffin wax

9 ounces beeswax

water

GOOD IDEA!

To remove wax from heat-proof items, set them in a low-heat oven for a few minutes. Wipe clean with paper towels. Chlorine bleach will help remove dyes from enamel pans.

GOOD IDEA!

Try an all-cotton T-shirt for your first batik project. Just be sure to place layers of newspaper between the front and back to absorb excess when you're adding or removing the wax.

(continued)

GOOD IDEA!

For a child's batik project, heat paraffin and crayons in a muffin tin. Place the muffin tin in a baking pan filled with ½ inch of water and heat the baking pan over a stove or hot plate. Use old craft brushes to apply wax designs.

SUPPLIES

scissors

prewashed, 100-percent cotton fabric

stiff, heavy cardboard or old picture frame

snap clothespins

plastic apron

rubber work gloves

2 or more plastic basins or large enamel pans

pint jar (if using liquid dye)

double boiler with 1½- to 2-quart insert

wooden spoon

candy thermometer

stiff-bristle art brushes in various sizes

old towel

newspaper

paper towels

electric iron with ironing board

☛ **BE SAFE.** Wax is flammable. Always use a double boiler to melt wax; never place it over direct heat. Never leave hot wax unattended. Also, to avoid unwanted dye stains, wear rubber gloves and a plastic apron.

Cut fabric to a size several inches larger than the finished size of your project. Cut cardboard to the same measurement as the fabric. With clothespins, fasten the fabric edges to the cardboard edges. Or mount fabric on an old picture frame instead of cardboard. Set aside.

Don apron and gloves and mix cold-water dye in a basin or pan following the manufacturer's instructions and set aside.

Or follow these instructions for liquid dye. Combine ½ cup liquid dye with ½ cup hot water in a pint jar. Mix well. In a basin, mix this dye solution with 3½ quarts of room-temperature water. Set aside. Do *not* use a hot-water dye bath as recommended on most commercial household dye containers; the heat might melt the wax.

In the top part of a double boiler, melt paraffin and beeswax together and stir. Insert the thermometer and heat to between 160° and 200°F. Turn off heat and remove the double boiler to a heat-proof surface. Leave the hot wax in the top insert, and as you work, reheat the water as needed to maintain the proper wax temperature.

Dip a brush in hot wax and brush your design on the fabric. Use a small brush for fine lines. For a spatter design, load a brush with wax and shake it over the fabric.

When the wax design is completed, fill a basin with clear, cool water. Remove the fabric from the frame and place it in the clear-water bath. Then completely immerse it in the dye bath. Soak it until it is slightly darker than the desired color, at least an hour. It dries to a lighter color. Rinse the fabric in clear, cold water until no color runs from it.

Using the clothespins, stretch a piece of old towel over the cardboard frame and then stretch the fabric to dry on that. Or simply lay the dyed fabric flat on an old towel. When the fabric is dry, repeat the waxing and dyeing steps as many times as desired. After the final waxing and dyeing, stretch and dry the fabric completely and prepare to remove the wax.

On an ironing board, layer as follows: ½-inch layer of newspaper, layer of several paper towels, batiked fabric (waxed side down), layer of several paper towels. Set a *steam-free* electric iron on slightly lower heat than is recommended for the fabric. Slide the warm iron over the top layer of towels. As you iron, the paper towels will absorb the wax. Each time a few newspapers and paper towels become coated with wax, replace them. Stop ironing when the papers no longer absorb any wax. Wax does not harm the surface of the iron. Remove wax from the iron by ironing over clean paper towels until no more wax comes off.

✿ **Variation:** For a crackled effect in the wax design, use more paraffin and less beeswax. Before placing the fabric in the dye bath, "bend" the fabric to crack the dried wax.

➦ **Notes:** Buy paraffin in the canning section of supermarkets and hardware stores. Cold-water dyes purchased through art supply stores and craft shops work best. Beeswax is available from hardware stores, beekeepers, and craft supply stores. See page 444 for other sources.

GOOD IDEA!

To ensure successful batik projects, select the right fabric. Muslin or old cotton bedsheets are ideal batik fabrics. If you're using new fabric, wash it several times to remove sizing before beginning batik.

To keep colors bright, dry-clean batiked fabrics. But if you don't mind slight color fading, wash them in cold water.

GOOD IDEA!

It's easy to store **bread-glue dough for future use.** Wrapped tightly in plastic wrap and placed in a plastic bag, bread dough keeps in a refrigerator for several weeks. To ease dough handling, moisten your hands with a little glycerin or hand lotion.

GOOD IDEA!

Bread-glue dough **pins, barrettes, and earrings are simple to make.** Buy pin backs, barrette forms, or earring posts at craft supply stores and decorate them with your bread-glue creations. Then just glue each completed figure in place with epoxy. These make great craft fair items as well as inexpensive gifts.

Bread-Glue Dough

Handcraft your own jewelry, doll house decorations, and more from this clay.

Yield: about ¼ cup

INGREDIENTS

 3 slices day-old white bread
 2 tablespoons white household glue, such as Elmer's
 ½ teaspoon glycerin or hand lotion
    food coloring
    water (optional)

SUPPLIES

shallow cereal bowl

plastic wrap

waxed paper

toothpicks or floral wire

block of floral foam or Styrofoam

artist's brush (optional)

tempera paint (optional)

Remove crust from bread and discard. Break bread into pea-size pieces in the bowl. Drizzle with glue and glycerin or hand lotion. Knead until it has the consistency of dough, 8 to 10 minutes. Separate into portions.

To color dough, add food coloring one drop at a time, mixing after each drop until the desired shade appears. Wrap each colored portion separately in plastic wrap. For best results, work with only one batch of dough at a time. If dough dries out as you work, add a few drops of water.

Cover the work surface with waxed paper. Use toothpicks or floral wire stuck in a foam block to hold shapes as you work or to hold completed pieces while they dry. Simply mold the dough into delicate shapes with your fingers. Roll it into balls, cylinders, and teardrop shapes. Flatten or elongate them as you experiment.

After molding the piece, if desired, apply details and finishing touches with tempera paint. Then set the piece on waxed paper or on toothpicks as described above and allow it to air-dry for at least a week. When drying on waxed paper, turn the piece every few hours the first day to dry it evenly. Air-dried pieces will have a bisquelike finish.

✿ **Variation:** For a smooth, porcelain-like finish, mix equal parts of white household glue and water and brush on several coats. Let each coat dry completely before applying another.

➡ **Notes:** Use white household glue, not white school glue. Glycerin is nontoxic and safe to handle. Buy it at pharmacies and craft supply stores.

GOOD IDEA!

For more vivid colors on bread-glue dough pieces, omit the food coloring and paint finished bread-glue dough pieces with acrylic paints. You may also seal pieces with clear acrylic spray instead of glue and water.

Making a Bread-Glue Rose

A rose makes a classic earring or barrette decoration. To make a bread-glue rose, first make a small teardrop shape as the flower center. (If you want the rose on a stem, place a drop of white glue on the tip of a floral wire and glue the teardrop in place.) Roll eight to ten small dough balls, about ⅛ inch in diameter. Flatten each ball into a concave shape. Rub the outer edge of the concave shape between your thumb and fingers until the edge is very thin. This makes a single rose petal. Add the first petal by wrapping one edge tightly around the larger end of the teardrop. Make sure to place the petal with the concave center on the inside and the thin edge curling slightly outward. Moisten the petal edge where the pieces join.

Continue adding one petal at a time, moistening the lower edge and slightly overlapping the petal that was most recently added. When you're pleased with the petal configuration, add a leaf or two at the base, if you wish. If the rose will be glued to a flat jewelry base, flatten the bottom somewhat before setting the piece out to dry. If the rose is on a stem, wrap the floral wire with green floral tape, adding artificial or glycerinized leaves as you wrap.

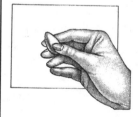 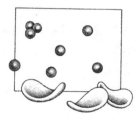 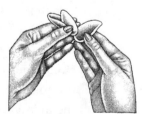 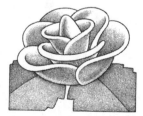

GOOD IDEA!

To remove wax from heat-proof utensils, place them on a foil-covered tray in an oven set at WARM. When wax softens, wipe it off with paper towels.

GOOD IDEA!

To make easy candle molds, use milk cartons, metal cans, juice cans, paper cups, and cardboard cans. Because the finished candle must be removed through the top of the mold, make sure the top is at least as large as the bottom.

Hand-Crafted Candles

With some basic kitchen equipment and a few purchased materials, you're on your way to basking in the glow of your own wax creations. Set aside plenty of time, this activity will probably take an entire day.

Yield: about 2¼ pounds of wax, enough for 2 pillar candles, 2½ inches in diameter and 3¾ inches high

INGREDIENTS

1½   pounds paraffin wax

¼   pound beeswax

½   pound stearic acid

5   teaspoons powdered household hot-water dye (optional)

⅛   teaspoon scented oil (optional)

SUPPLIES

two 10½-ounce soup cans for candle molds or commercial molds of similar size

vegetable oil

awl or ice pick

scissors

30-ply flat-braided candlewicking (see "Notes")

pencil

electrical or floral putty

metal cookie sheets or trays

waxed paper

double boiler with 2- to 3-quart insert

wooden spoon

candy thermometer

hot mitts

metal ladle

heat-proof 2-cup glass measure

knitting needle

sharp knife

aluminum foil (optional)

☞ **BE SAFE.** *Wax and stearic acid are flammable. Always melt them wax in a double boiler; never place over direct heat. Do not leave hot wax unattended. Use hot mitts to protect your hands. Supervise children closely if they are participating.*

To prepare the molds, first lightly coat the inside of each mold with vegetable oil. Next, with the awl or ice pick, punch a small hole in the center of the mold bottom. Cut a length of wicking at least 4 inches longer than the height of the mold. Thread the wick up through the hole. Fasten the top end of the wick by knotting it tightly around a pencil placed across the top of the mold. Knot the wick tightly at the bottom of the mold; seal the bottom hole on the outside with putty. To ease clean-up of spilled wax, place prepared molds on cookie sheets or trays lined with waxed paper. Set aside.

To prepare the wax, place paraffin, beeswax, and stearic acid in the top part of a double boiler. Place over medium heat and stir well as the mixture melts. Insert the thermometer in the wax.

If you're making colored candles, add dye when stearic acid has completely dissolved. As wax continues to melt thoroughly, mix in dye. Molten wax will be a brighter color than the finished candle. Note whether the amount of dye added gives a satisfactory color so that you can change the color or duplicate it in later projects.

As wax continues to heat, watch the thermometer for the proper pouring temperature. For glass or cardboard molds, pour wax when it reaches 150° to 165°F. For acrylic plastic molds, pour at around 185°F. For metal molds, pour when it reaches 190° to 200°F.

When wax has reached the desired temperature, turn off heat. Wearing hot mitts, remove double boiler to a heat-proof surface. Thoroughly mix in scented oil, if desired. Pour or ladle wax into the measure. Some dye residue will remain in the pan. Simply discard the residue when it cools.

To pour wax without air bubbles, first tilt the mold toward you. Slowly add just enough wax to coat the bottom of the mold. Check for leaks and add more putty if necessary. Now tilt the mold toward you again and pour wax slowly until you must set the mold upright to finish. Fill to

(continued)

GOOD IDEA!

As **candle diameter increases,** wick size and the melting point should be increased. To make larger candles, increase the proportion of beeswax and stearic acid and increase the wick size.

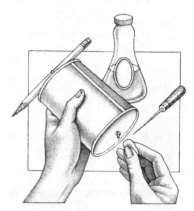

Use a pencil to hold a wick in place.

the top of the mold. During the pour, check the wax temperature. If necessary, reheat wax to keep it near the desired temperature. Set aside leftover wax for filling the center of the candle.

Because wax shrinks as it cools, a hollow area will form near the wick as the candle cools. After the candle has cooled for an hour, push a knitting needle through the top wax crust and into the hollow area. Push the needle along the center of the candle from the top to the bottom of the mold. Reheat leftover wax to the correct pouring temperature and slowly refill this hollow center to within ½ inch below the line of the first pour.

Probe and refill the hollow center one or two more times, at 1-hour intervals, until the well has been completely eliminated. Before the final fill, cut off the knot at the top of the mold. Let the filled mold set at least 5 more hours in a cool, dry place.

To remove the candle from the mold, discard the putty and cut off the knot at the bottom of the mold. Pull firmly on the wick at the top of the mold. If the candle does not slide out, refrigerate the mold for an hour and try again.

To flatten the base of a finished candle, cut cleanly across the bottom with the knife. To make the bottom even smoother, warm a foil-covered cookie sheet in the oven. Set the candle on the warm cookie sheet and turn it in circles to soften the bottom and set it up evenly.

To achieve a lustrous finish and eliminate the seam mark from the soup can molds, roll the candle on a glass or marble surface. Or, using a circular motion, polish it lightly with a nylon stocking. The lighter your touch, the more lustrous the candle will become.

✿ **Variations:** For candlewicking, you may substitute twisted cotton cording, such as twine, but it must be treated following the directions in "Good Idea!" on the opposite page. This formula can be multiplied or divided. If doubling the recipe, be certain the double boiler is large enough to accommodate the wax.

➥ **Notes:** Do not add extra scented oil to this formula. Instead of producing a stronger scent, it may cause the candle to smoke. Buy paraffin in the canning section of supermarkets and hardware stores. Beeswax is available from hardware stores, bee-keepers, and craft supply stores. Stearic acid, a pure white granular substance derived from beef tallow, has a high melting point. It hardens paraffin and beeswax and slows the burning and dripping of candles. Buy it at craft shops that sell candlemaking supplies and from some pharmacists, who may carry stearic acid. For coloring candles, add about 2 teaspoons of powdered household dye to 1 pound wax. Lighter dye shades work best. Crayons also work. But for best color results, purchase special candle color buttons at hobby shops or candlemaking supply houses. Buy scented oils at pharmacies, gift shops, candlemaking supply houses, and some department stores. Scents to try include pine, spearmint, wintergreen, lemon, and bayberry. Candlewicking, available at hobby shops and candlemaking supply houses, is plaited cotton pretreated to burn slowly and evenly. It is sized by ply—the higher the ply number, the thicker the wick. Actually measure the cording at the store to be sure you're buying the right size because thicknesses are not standardized. For soup-can-size candles, buy cording 2 millimeters in diameter. See page 444 for additional sources of candlemaking supplies.

GOOD IDEA!

If you use twisted cotton cording as a candlewicking, pretreat it several days before candlemaking. To treat 3 yards of cording, combine 1 tablespoon salt, 2 tablespoons borax, and 1 cup water. Soak the cording in the mixture overnight. Hang the cord to dry thoroughly, about 24 hours.

Borax is powdered sodium borate. Even though it is a commonly used laundry product, it is poison and can cause death when ingested. Keep it out of the reach of children. Buy borax in paint supply stores, hardware stores, and in the detergent sections of supermarkets.

GOOD IDEA!

For stronger craft plaster, add ¼ cup white household glue for each cup of water used. Be sure that all equipment is free of old plaster residue. Bits of old plaster will keep the new batch from curing correctly.

Craft Plaster

Use craft plaster for dozens of different projects. Carve it into a decorative wall plaque or a three-dimensional figure. Use it as a medium to hold other decorative elements, such as seashells or colored glass. Or pour it into plastic molds to create figures that can be painted and decorated. See page 346 for other plaster craft ideas. Craft plaster hardens very quickly, so mix no more than the exact amount of plaster needed to fill one mold.

Yield: enough plaster to fill a single mold

INGREDIENTS

1   part water
2   parts plaster of paris

SUPPLIES

warm, soapy water
basin or bucket
plaster mold
2-cup or larger measure
set of measuring cups
mixing container, such as a coffee can or milk carton
dust mask
goggles, safety glasses, or face shield
stirrer, such as an old spatula
mold release spray (optional)
acrylic paint or sanding sealer *plus* stain or tempera paint
clear acrylic spray

☞ **BE SAFE.** Wear a dust mask and goggles when working with plaster of paris. When applying finish sprays, work in a well-ventilated area. Avoid open flames. Do not smoke.

Before beginning, place warm, soapy water in the basin or bucket and set aside to clean equipment. To determine how much plaster of paris you need, fill the mold with water; pour water into the measure. The amount of plaster of paris needed will be exactly double the water measure. For example, if the water equals ½ cup, you need 1 cup plaster of paris. Measure the correct amount of plaster of paris and set aside.

To mix the plaster, pour the water into a clean mixing container. Wearing a dust mask and goggles, slowly sift the plaster of paris through your fingers into the water. Let the mixture stand for 3 to 4 minutes. Stir it *very slowly*, to avoid creating air bubbles. Stir until smooth.

To pour the plaster, first make sure the mold is thoroughly dry. If the mold is rigid, apply mold release spray to the inside surfaces. Pour the plaster into the mold until it is half full. Gently tap or jiggle the mold (not the plaster) to release air bubbles. Pour the remaining plaster and jiggle the mold again. (Pour larger molds a third at a time.) Immediately place mixing equipment in the warm, soapy water to prevent plaster residue from hardening in it.

To cure the plaster, place the mold in a warm, dry place. Direct sunlight is perfect. Curing takes 25 minutes to an hour, depending on the size of the mold. The plaster will heat up as it cures. Let it cool completely before removing it from the mold. After removing the figure, let it stand in the air for another hour or so. Wash reusable molds in soapy water.

Decorate with acrylic paint or sanding sealer and stain or tempera paint. Then apply the acrylic spray. Plaster attracts moisture and eventually crumbles if not sealed.

✿ **Variation:** Substitute petroleum jelly for the mold release spray. Just be sure to gently sand off petroleum jelly residue from the finished cast before applying paint and acrylic spray.

➹ **Notes:** Almost anything—heavy paper plates, plastic bowls, aluminum pans, or cardboard containers—can serve as a mold. Hardened plaster residue may clog a sink drain. Strain plaster residue out of clean-up water and dispose of it. Buy plaster of paris at hardware stores. Buy ready-made decorative molds and most of the craft plaster supplies at craft supply stores and art supply stores. See page 444 for other sources.

Paste in a Pinch

Even children can make this paper paste.

Yield: about 1 tablespoon

INGREDIENTS

1 tablespoon flour
2 teaspoons cold water

SUPPLIES

saucer

spoon

Mix flour and water into a smooth paste in the saucer. Use immediately. Multiply recipe for more paste.

Craft Plaster Projects

Plaster crafts can be simple or complex. Here are suggestions for your next project.

Carve a character. Cast plaster in a small milk container or vegetable can. Draw lines on the cast to serve as carving guides. Carve it with a pocket knife, paring knife, or other sharp tool.

Make a mosaic sand casting. Place sand in a box, wet it slightly, and form a design in the sand surface. The sand design will be reversed in the cast plaster. On the surface of the sand design, place stones, small tiles, seashells, or other decorative objects. Be sure to place the objects with their best sides down. Pour plaster over the sand design. When it has hardened, lift it out. The sand design and decorative objects will be embedded in the plaster. The piece will also have a unique sand-textured finish.

Make a child's handprint plaque. Fill an aluminum pie plate with craft plaster. To make a hole for hanging the plaque, push a drinking straw through the plaster to the bottom of the pie plate. Let a child place his hand in the plaster just far enough to make a complete impression. Although the warm plaster may feel a little uncomfortable, no harm is done by this brief skin contact. When the plaster begins to harden, the child may lift his hand out and remove the straw. To release the hardened plaque, simply turn the pie plate over on your hand. Decorate the plaque with acrylic paint, spray with acrylic sealer, and lace a ribbon through the hole for hanging.

Make castings from nature. Wet the smooth side of leaves and place them in an aluminum pie plate. The rough, veined side of the leaves should face up. Add other interesting woody plant material, such as pieces of bark or seed pods with the most interesting side facing up. Fill the pie plate with plaster and make a hole as for the handprint plaque. Remove the hardened plaque from the pie plate, but leave the plant parts in it. Spray acrylic paint around the plant parts and remove them when the paint is dry. The leaf impressions will be silhouetted in the plaster. Finish as described for the hand-print plaque.

Papercraft Glue

Paper projects don't require store-bought paste. In a few minutes, you can produce this excellent glue.

Yield: 1 cup

INGREDIENTS

¼ cup flour
¼ cup sugar
¼ cup cold water
¾ cup hot water
½ teaspoon powdered alum
5 drops clove oil (optional)

SUPPLIES

stirrer
medium saucepan
whisk
plastic or glass container with lid

☛ **BE SAFE.** Store clove oil and alum out of the reach of children. Clove oil is highly toxic. Ingesting less than 1 teaspoon may result in fatal poisoning.

Mix flour and sugar in the saucepan. Add cold water and whisk until mixture is smooth. Using a whisk prevents lumps in the glue. Then add hot water. Place mixture over medium heat and stir constantly until it comes to a boil and thickens. Remove from heat. Stir in alum. Add clove oil for a pleasant scent, if desired. Allow paste to cool before using. Store tightly sealed.

✿ **Variation:** This formula may be halved or multiplied, as desired. Make sure the saucepan is large enough if multiplying.

➼ **Notes:** Buy alum (ammonium aluminum sulfate) in the pickling and canning sections of supermarkets. Clove oil is available at health food stores and herb shops. Or order it through your pharmacist.

GOOD IDEA!

To make paste quickly, use your microwave. Combine the flour and sugar in a microwave-safe bowl. Stir in cold water and combine until smooth. Add hot water and stir. Place the bowl in the microwave and heat on high for 1 minute. Stir mixture. Repeat heating and stirring once or twice at 1-minute intervals. Mixture should be thick. Stir in alum, and add clove oil, if desired.

HOLIDAY CRAFTS

Holidays are times to work with crafts. Celebrate the holidays by making decorations and gifts.

Cinnamon-Applesauce Ornaments

Add a spicy scent to the air with these decorations, which are perfect for adorning packages, trees, or wreaths.

Yield: about 2 dozen 2 × 2-inch ornaments

INGREDIENTS

about 1 cup cinnamon or cinnamon blended with cloves, ginger, or nutmeg
1 cup applesauce, room temperature

SUPPLIES

spoon
1-quart bowl
waxed paper
rolling pin
assortment of cookie cutters
toothpick or drinking straw
cookie sheets
spatula
4 yards ¼-inch ribbon
sealable container, such as a cookie tin

Mix cinnamon or spice blend and applesauce in the bowl until smooth and doughy. Spread waxed paper on a flat surface, sprinkle with cinnamon, and roll dough ¼ inch thick. Dip cookie cutters in cinnamon and cut out shapes. With a toothpick or drinking straw, punch a hole near the top of each ornament. Do not make the hole too close to the edge; the ornament will shrink as it dries.

Carefully place ornaments on cookie sheets lined with waxed paper. Air-dry the ornaments for 3 to 4 days, gently turning them with a spatula several times each day. When

GOOD IDEA!

To add a nice finishing touch to home-made ornaments, match the hanging loop to the ornament. For example, if the shape is a Scottie dog, use a Scotch plaid ribbon. If it's a horse, use a thin leather string. Use red and white ribbons for a candy cane and green for a shamrock.

completely dry, thread ribbon through the holes and tie into loops. Store in a cool, dry place, tightly sealed.

Dyed Eggs

Dyeing eggs is as easy as 1-2-3 if you have food coloring in your kitchen cupboard. This is for dyeing eggs in one color. For each new color, make the recipe again.

Yield: 4 same-color dyed eggs

INGREDIENTS

½ cup boiling water
1 teaspoon vinegar
20 drops food coloring
4 hard-boiled white eggs

SUPPLIES

cup
spoon or wire egg dipper
egg carton
paper towels

Place boiling water in the cup. Mix in vinegar and food coloring. To mix special colors, see "Colorful Combinations" on page 350.

With the spoon or egg dipper, set an egg into the dye. When the desired shade is obtained, lift out and place in an egg carton lined with paper towels. As dye cools and more eggs are colored, it becomes less effective. Color won't rub off.

✿ **Variations:** Draw designs on eggs with crayons before dyeing. The areas that are covered with crayon wax will resist the dye. This formula also works for blown-out eggs. To keep blown-out eggs immersed in the dye, lightly press on them with the spoon or dipper.

GOOD IDEA!

Add salt to the cooking water, when you hard-boil eggs. This little trick makes eggshells absorb dye better. To remove coloring from cups, wipe them with chlorinated bleach before washing in soapy water.

GOOD IDEA!

Dye eggs as you hard-boil them. Add 1½ tablespoons vinegar and 2 cups grape juice (for lavender), beet juice (for pink), carrot tops (for yellow), or purple cabbage (for blue) to the eggs and water in a saucepan. When the eggs are cooked, allow them to stand in the liquid for an hour before rinsing.

COLORFUL COMBINATIONS How to Make Special Colors with Food Coloring		
Color	**Number of Drops of Food Coloring**	
	For Eggs	**For Other Uses**
Orange	6 red, 14 yellow	1 red, 2 yellow
Chartreuse	24 yellow, 2 green	12 yellow, 1 green
Turquoise	15 blue, 5 green	5 blue, 1 green
Purple	10 red, 4 blue	1 red, 1 blue
Rose	15 red, 5 blue	5 red, 1 blue
Peach	—	1 red, 3 yellow
Pale brown*	—	1 green, 4 yellow, 3 red

NOTE: Courtesy of McCormick/Schilling
*Some sources recommend strong coffee to produce a medium brown.

GOOD IDEA!

Pay attention to dryness and moisture for success when working with baker's clay. If the clay is too dry, add a little water by wetting your hands as you knead. If the mix is too sticky, add a little flour during kneading. Dampness may spoil even finished sealed figures. Apply an acrylic or polyurethane sealer to keep moisture out. Keep finished pieces in a cool, dry place.

Baker's Clay

Between your kitchen cupboard and the corner drug store, you'll find all the ingredients you need to make this traditional molding clay.

Yield: 2½ cups

INGREDIENTS

2 cups white flour (*not* self-rising)

½ cup table salt

¾ cup water

2 tablespoons glycerin (optional)

food coloring (optional)

SUPPLIES

1-quart bowl

stirrer

waxed paper

acrylic paint (optional)

sealable container

In the bowl, mix flour and salt. Add water a little at a time. Knead dough on a waxed-paper-covered surface until thoroughly combined, then several minutes longer. If desired, knead in glycerin. It makes the clay stretchy, which helps when making narrow strips like rolled coils. Mold pieces into desired shapes. Air-dry or bake them following the suggestions given in "Success with Baker's Clay" below.

To bake the finished figures, make them with uncolored clay and color with acrylic paint after baking. To air-dry your creations, make them with colored clay.

For colored clay, separate into desired portions and knead food coloring into each (see "Colorful Combinations" on the opposite page). Work with one dough portion at a time; wrap remaining portions in plastic. Store leftover clay in an airtight container for up to two weeks.

➻ **Note:** *Glycerin is nontoxic and safe to handle. Buy it at pharmacies and craft supply stores.*

Success with Baker's Clay

It's a simple, traditional craft, but you'll get the best results with baker's clay if you follow the tips here.

Although baker's clay ornaments can be air-dried, baking figures in a low-temperature oven makes them more break-resistant.

To bake figures, place them on a lightly floured or waxed-paper-covered cookie sheet. Use a low oven temperature to prevent browning and puffing. Baking times and temperatures vary according to the project. In general, bake cookie cutter figures at 150° to 325°F for several hours. Bake thick, three-dimensional figures at 325°F for a slightly longer time.

Check figures every 20 to 30 minutes to see if the clay has fully hardened. To test for proper hardness, remove a sample figure from the oven. When it's barely cool, gently press the top with your fingertips. If the clay "gives," it's not hard enough. Bake for 20 more minutes before testing again. If the top of a sample figure seems hard, check the underside as well. If tops are hard but not undersides, return figures to the oven, top side down. Retest in 20 minutes.

For a shiny finish, brush on a natural glaze before baking. Mayonnaise will produce a shiny finish. On uncolored clay, brush on a mixture made from one egg white and 1 teaspoon water for a light brown finish. One egg yolk with 1 teaspoon water will produce a yellow-brown glaze. For a colored glaze, add tempera or food coloring to the egg-yolk mixture before brushing it on. Maximum temperature for baking glazed items is 250°F.

For best results, decorate baked unglazed clay figures with acrylic paints. After painting, seal figures against moisture by applying two coats of polyurethane varnish.

If a figure breaks after baking, but before painting, epoxy the pieces together. Allow the glue to dry thoroughly. Cover the flaw with an extra coat of paint.

Pomanders

Stud a piece of fruit with cloves, roll it in some spices, let it dry, and what do you have?

A pomander to perfume the air and gladden the hearts of all traditionalists. Although a pomander is a time-honored Christmas present, it's also a thoughtful gift for a housewarming or nice to enclose with new linens at a bridal shower.

Choose an unblemished, firm lemon, lime, orange, apple, or pear. Thin-skinned varieties of citrus work best. Round, green apples and Seckel, Bosc, or Anjou pears work well also.

Yield: 1 pomander

SUPPLIES

1 piece firm, unblemished fruit

½-inch-wide adhesive tape

straight pins

about 2 ounces whole cloves

piercing tool, such as an ice pick, awl, or knitting needle

spoon

⅜ cup half pumpkin pie spice and half powdered orrisroot

shallow bowl

⅜-inch-wide ribbon

To prepare the fruit, run a strip of tape around it from top to bottom. Run tape around the middle of the taped halves, dividing them into quarters. Pin the tape in place wherever needed.

Push the pointed end of several cloves into a small section of the untaped area. Place the cloves as close together as possible; then remove them. Use the resulting holes as a pattern or guide for piercing like-sized holes all over the un-taped areas of the fruit with a piercing tool. Then put cloves in all the holes.

Place spices in the shallow bowl. Roll fruit in the mixture several times a day for 2 to 3 days. The spices will stick to the juices that seep from the fruit.

Set the pomander in the bowl in a dry area. Let it air-dry for 2 to 5 weeks, turning every 4 to 5 days. When the fruit has dried, remove the tape and replace it with ribbon. Make a hanging loop and fasten the ribbon with straight pins.

➡ **Note:** Orrisroot powder is a fixative, a substance that slows down the release of fragrant oils into the air. When used in a pomander, it makes the fragrance last longer. Buy orrisroot at craft shops, floral supply stores, and pharmacies.

Pysanky Eggs

The Ukrainian word "pysanka" means "writing on an egg," and each Ukrainian village has its own traditional pysanky style. Pysanky artisans use a craft technique called wax-resist dyeing. Artisans decorate hollow eggs with minute strokes of melted beeswax and then dye them. The dye colors the eggshell only in areas not covered with beeswax. Successive coats of wax and dye produce an egg design that glows like a jewel.

If you've never tried pysanky before, try a simple two-color design first. With experience you'll be able to create more complex patterns later.

Yield: 12 decorated eggs

INGREDIENTS

12 white eggs, unwashed
    vinegar (optional)
    baking soda (optional)
    water
1 cup prepared dye for each color desired (cold-water dyes preferred)

> **GOOD IDEA!**
>
> **U**se a beeswax candle to apply wax to pysanky eggs. Light the candle and load your decorating pin by dipping it in the soft wax near the flame.

(continued)

GOOD IDEA!

Unwashed eggs
work best for making
pysanky eggs. Supermar-
ket eggs, which have al-
ways been washed, must
be treated with vinegar
or baking soda solution
to remove soap residue.
Try local farms, farmers'
markets, or health food
stores as a source of un-
washed eggs.

SUPPLIES

needle

egg carton

paper and colored markers or crayons

newspaper

1 ounce pure beeswax

double boiler with ½-quart or larger insert

stirrer

candy thermometer

straight pins with heads, various sizes

pencils with erasers

spoon or wire egg dipper

tissues

muffin tin

soft cloth

☛ **BE SAFE.** Wax is flammable. Always melt wax in a double
boiler; never melt over direct heat. Never leave hot wax unattended.

To prepare the eggs, rinse farm-fresh eggs with tap
water. Rinse store-bought eggs with vinegar or a small
amount of baking soda dissolved in a cup of water. *Do not
use soapy water;* it will hinder the wax-and-dye process. To
hollow an egg, push a needle through the pointed end of
the shell. Insert the needle far enough to break the membrane just inside the shell. Puncture a similar hole in the
opposite end and enlarge this hole slightly by picking at it
with the needle. Blow through the small hole until the contents of the egg have all been forced out the larger hole.
Rinse the hollow eggshell inside and out and place in an
egg carton to dry thoroughly, at least a week.

To create a pattern, draw geometric shapes on paper.
Play with the geometric shapes by arranging and rearrang-
ing them. Create different color combinations with markers
or crayons. Plan each consecutive step for creating your
final design and write the steps down for later reference.
For example, note the first pattern to be waxed on the egg,
the first dye color to be applied, the second pattern, the sec-

ond dye, and so on. Traditionally, dyes are applied in this order from first to last: yellow, orange, red, purple, or black.

Cover the work surface with newspaper. Melt beeswax in the top part of the double boiler. Occasionally stir the wax to keep the temperature even throughout. Check wax temperature with a candy thermometer. *Do not let the wax temperature exceed 300°F.*

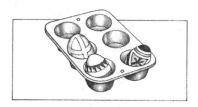

Use various sizes of straight pins to apply wax designs.

Push the point of a straight pin into the eraser end of a pencil. You will use the pinhead to apply wax to the egg. Various pinhead sizes give different wax effects. Practice applying wax to paper with the various pinheads to get an idea of how much wax each pinhead applies at one time. It is usually best to begin at the wider portion of a line because, as the wax is used up, the line will become thinner. Dip a pinhead in the warm wax and draw pattern lines on the egg. If the wax seems to skip, warm it up.

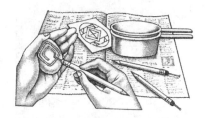

Place eggs in a muffin tin and warm in an oven to remove wax.

When the wax has cooled on the first set of pattern lines, use the spoon or egg dipper to dip the egg in prepared dye. *Do not use hot-water dye;* it will melt the wax. Apply the lightest color first. Remove the egg when it appears slightly darker than the desired shade. Dry carefully and completely with tissues.

Now apply the next set of design lines in wax. Then color the egg with another dye. Continue the wax-and-dye process until you've achieved the desired result.

When you've completed several eggs, set them in the wells of a muffin tin. Place the pan in a preheated oven set at WARM, about 150°F. The wax will soften in only a few minutes. Wipe each egg gently with a soft cloth to remove the wax.

➥ **Notes:** Purchase cold-water dye powders at art supply stores and craft shops. See page 444 for other sources. You can also use ordinary Easter egg dyes or use the formula for Easter egg dye on page 349. Artist's pens for pen-and-ink drawing work well for applying wax to eggs. Purchase a pen with various sizes of nibs at art supply stores.

CRAFTS FOR CHILDREN

The formulas here will brighten up a rainy afternoon or add to birthday party fun.

Finger Paint

With a few items from your pantry, you can make finger paint and save money over the usual variety store cost.

Yield: 3 cups

INGREDIENTS

1 envelope unflavored gelatin (¼ ounce)
1 cup cold water
¾ cup cornstarch
2 cups hot water
½ cup mild laundry soap flakes, such as Ivory Snow
   liquid tempera paint, assorted colors

SUPPLIES

spoon
bowl
medium saucepan
small, sealable containers, such as baby food jars

To make a clear base for paint, stir gelatin into ¼ cup cold water in the bowl. Set aside. In the saucepan, stir cornstarch into remaining cold water until mixture is smooth. Add hot water. Cook over medium heat, stirring constantly, until mixture comes to a boil and is smooth and clear. Remove from heat. Add gelatin mixture and stir well. Add soap flakes and stir until dissolved.

Separate mixture into containers. For each color desired, add ½ tablespoon tempera paint to ½ cup of finger paint. Use immediately or store tightly sealed in a cool, dark place.

GOOD IDEA!

Finger paint can be cooked in a microwave. Cook until it comes to a boil and is smooth and clear. If toddlers will be fingerpainting, use food coloring instead of tempera paint.

Giant Bubbles

This formula makes big bubbles—sometimes even bigger than 2 feet wide. It's spectacular for entertaining kids as well as kids at heart.

Yield: about 5½ cups bubblemaking liquid

INGREDIENTS

½ cup Dawn or Joy liquid dishwashing detergent
4½ cups water
3 to 4 tablespoons glycerin

SUPPLIES

2-quart unbreakable basin
stirrer
yarn, string, twine, or bubble wands
sealable plastic container

☛ **BE SAFE.** *Avoid contact with eyes. Enjoy the bubbles on a paved or gravel surface. The mixture may cause temporary dieback of grass.*

In the basin, mix all ingredients—gently, so that foam doesn't form on top of the water. Skim off any foam that appears; it interferes with bubble making. Knot string into loops of different sizes, up to 30 inches in circumference. (The larger the loop, the larger the bubble.) Let string loops soak for a minute in bubble mix. Using both hands, grasp the loop at two equidistant points and lift it gently out of the water with both sides of the string drawn taut. Now open the strings about ½ inch apart, still keeping the string taut. Lift this string form into the air and *voilà*—a giant bubble!

Store the bubble mix tightly sealed. Be sure to label it. This recipe can be multiplied or divided, as needed.

➡ **Note:** *Glycerin is nontoxic and safe to handle. Buy it at pharmacies and craft supply stores.*

GOOD IDEA!

Distilled water is better than tap water for getting colorful, long-lasting bubbles, although tap water usually works fine. Bubble making is most successful when the air is relatively still.

FLOWER CRAFTS

If you're a beginner at flower crafts, spend an hour in a well-stocked crafts supply store—you'll find straw hats to embellish, wreath forms and baskets to decorate, potpourri jars to fill, plus lots of other doodads that look elegant when decorated with flowers. Or add dried flowers and ribbons to commonplace items like an onion braid, an old tin candle holder, or a lamp shade. You'll find hundreds of ways to use and enjoy the dried treasures from your garden.

Foliage Preservative

Glycerin preservation, a foliage treatment popular even in colonial days, works best with heavy, coarse leaves. Glycerin-treated foliage retains the flexibility and sheen of fresh leaves. Good leaves to try include beech, camellia, euonymus, hemlock, holly, lemon leaf, magnolia, mountain ash, myrtle, oak, peony, rhododendron, and viburnum.

Yield: varies by amount of ingredients chosen

INGREDIENTS

2 parts warm water
1 part glycerin
  plant leaves

SUPPLIES

newspaper
4-quart or larger basin or other container
stirrer
soft cloth
tissues
cardboard box with lid
tissue paper (optional)
floral tape and wire (optional)
bottle or vase (optional)
flower painting spray (optional)

Spread newspaper over the work area. In the basin or other container, mix water and glycerin well. Make enough solution to completely cover the foliage.

Wipe leaves with a damp cloth to clean them. Lay leaves one at a time in the solution. If necessary, place jars or other objects on leaves to keep them completely immersed.

Every few days, shake the container to keep the solution touching all leaf parts. Leaves will turn translucent and dark as they absorb the mixture, some becoming a darker green and others, brown or burgundy.

When two-thirds of a leaf has become translucent and dark, remove it and allow excess solution to drain back into the basin. Leaves left in the solution too long will become limp.

Place the leaves on a layer of newspapers at least seven papers thick. Do not allow the leaves to overlap or touch. Cover the leaves with a layer of seven newspapers. Place a second layer of leaves on top of this, and continue with alternate layers of newspapers and leaves. Leave the stack of foliage and newspapers undisturbed for about a week. Then remove the leaves and wipe them gently with tissues.

Store the leaves in the box, separated by layers of tissue paper, until ready to use. Or use floral tape to attach leaves to wire stems. Stand wired stems upright in a bottle or vase. You may also alter the color of the leaves with flower painting spray.

➥ **Notes:** *Glycerin is nontoxic and completely safe to handle. It is available at pharmacies and craft supply stores. Flower painting spray is available at garden supply stores and craft shops.*

GOOD IDEA!

One way to glycerinize foliage is to place the glycerin solution in a jar and set the leaves upright with their stems in the solution. To help the leaves absorb the glycerin, slit and hammer the bases of woody stems. This is the best method for wood plants, such as cotoneaster.

FLOWER-DRYING GUIDE
Best Drying Methods for Different Flowers

Flower	Air-Dry 1*	Air-Dry 2†	Borax, Cornmeal, Sand	Silica Gel	Silica (microwave)
Ageratum		❀	❀		
Artemisia	❀				
Aster			❀	❀	
Bachelor's-button	❀			❀	
Bells-of-Ireland			❀	❀	
Buttercup			❀	❀	
Carnation				❀	
Chrysanthemum			❀	❀	
Clematis			❀	❀	
Cockscomb	❀				
Dahlia		❀		❀	
Daisy			❀	❀	❀
Delphinium	❀		❀	❀	
Forsythia			❀	❀	
Goldenrod	❀				
Grape hyacinth		❀		❀	❀
Gypsophila	❀				
Hydrangea	❀	❀			
Lavender	❀	❀	❀	❀	
Lilac			❀	❀	
Lily-of-the-valley				❀	❀
Magnolia				❀	❀
Marigold	❀		❀	❀	❀
Peony		❀	❀	❀	
Rose				❀	❀
Strawflower	❀				
Tulip				❀	❀
Zinnia		❀	❀	❀	❀

*Tie stems together in bunches. Hang upside down in a warm, dark, airy place.
†Place stems in a container with 1 inch of water in the bottom. Let sit until dry.

Flower-Drying Tips

The simplest way to air-dry flowers is to hang them in bundles by their stems. A neat trick for tying the bundles for drying uses a rubber band instead of string. Hold the rubber band so that it forms a single strand like a string; do not put the stems *through* the rubber band. Wind it around the lower end of the stems two or three times. Thread one end of the rubber band through the other end to form a loop. Attach a paper clip to the loop. Use the paper clip to hang the stems from a nail or hook. The beauty of using a rubber band instead of string is that as the stems dry and shrink, the rubber band will hold them tight.

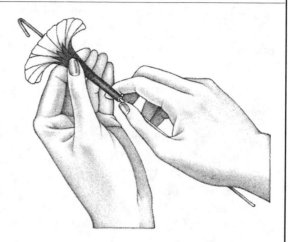

Air-drying works well for many flowers, but other flowers need special drying techniques to preserve their original shape and color. The following tells how to dry blossoms in sand, borax, cornmeal, or silica gel.

To prepare a flower for drying, first cut off the stem leaving a 1-inch stub below the blossom. Remove any leaves remaining on this short stem. Insert a 6-inch wire through the short stem, into the base of the flower, and out through the top. Use needlenose pliers to bend the tip of the wire into a small hook. Gently pull the hook back into the flower center so that it is hidden by petals. After you've dried the flower, you can elongate this short stem with additional wire and floral tape.

Dry flat, open flowers, such as daisies, face down in the drying medium. Dry multi-petaled flowers, such as roses and zinnias, face up in the drying medium. Bend the short wire stem under the flower and then up, so the wire sticks up through the drying mix beside the blossom. Hold each bloom in your hand and begin filling its folds with the drying medium before setting it on the mix. Support the flower petals as you add drying mix around and over them.

When you are ready to use your dried flowers, add longer wire stems. Just twist additional wire around the short wire stem on each flower. Then, beginning at the base of the bloom, wrap floral tape down the entire stem, adding preserved leaves as you wrap. Floral wire and tape are available at floral supply stores and craft shops.

Re-attach any petals that fall off by applying a bit of white household glue or epoxy with a toothpick. Spray dried blooms with an acrylic spray to help keep them intact. If not sprayed with a sealer, flowers dried with silica gel are particularly susceptible to reabsorbing moisture. In a pinch, you can use regular-hold hairspray instead.

Store dried flowers between layers of tissue paper in shoe boxes or gift boxes. Enclose a small amount of silica gel under a paper towel to absorb moisture. Add a few moth flakes or dried lavender or mint to repel insects. Keep the boxes in a cool, dry place.

GOOD IDEA!

To ensure success with flower-drying mixes, follow these tips. A hot, summertime attic works well for drying flowers. Different flower types have different drying rates. To have all flowers in a batch dry at once, dry only one type of flower at a time. Be extra careful to remove borax from dried flowers. Borax residue causes burn spots. Never use cornmeal alone to dry flowers. It attracts weevils, which will feast on the blooms. After sand has been used once, it is no longer sterile. Resterilize it by baking it in a 250°F oven for several hours.

Flower-Drying Mixes

The cornmeal mix is lightweight and useful for delicate flowers. You can use sand alone or combined with other ingredients. To choose a method for your flowers, see the "Flower-Drying Guide" on page 360.

Yield: about 6 cups, enough to dry one layer of daisy-shaped, fairly flat flowers in a 9 × 9-inch container

INGREDIENTS
FOR BORAX/SAND MIX

4 cups borax
2 cups sterilized, fine white sand

INGREDIENTS
FOR BORAX/CORNMEAL MIX

2 cups borax
4 cups cornmeal

INGREDIENTS
FOR BORAX/SALT MIX

4 cups borax
1½ cups table salt

SUPPLIES

clean 1-gallon bucket or disposable container
drying medium
9 × 9-inch baking pan or similar container
teaspoon
tweezers with rounded ends
small camel-hair artist's brush
slotted spoon

☛ **BE SAFE.** Even though borax is a commonly used laundry product, it is poison and can cause death when ingested. Keep it out of the reach of children.

Prepare fresh flowers for drying by cutting and wiring stems as described in "Flower-Drying Tips" on page 361.

Choose a flower-drying mix and combine all ingredients in the bucket or other container. Spread 1 to 2 inches of drying mix in the bottom of the pan or other container. Allowing at least 1 inch of space around each flower head, figure how many flowers will fit on this layer. Place a mound—a teaspoonful—of the mix where each flower will be set.

Place flat, daisylike flowers face down on the mound. Place three-dimensional flowers face up. Then gently pour the drying mix down the sides of the container, so it slides under the petals and around the flower heads, supporting them in a natural way. Carefully straighten any twisted petals with tweezers. Use the paintbrush to sweep the mix over the petals, completely covering each flower.

Leave the pan uncovered in a warm, dry place where humidity is 60 percent or less. Note the date on the container. After a few days, select a flower near the corner or edge of the container and check it for dryness. Test that same flower every few days until the petals feel crisp and papery. Remove each flower by its wire stem or with the slotted spoon. Brush off all traces of drying mix.

➡ **Notes:**   Cardboard boxes with taped seams are ideal for drying flowers. Buy borax (99.5 percent pure sodium borate) in paint supply stores, hardware stores, and the detergent sections of supermarkets. For sterile sand, buy play sand at garden supply stores, toy stores, and home centers.

The When, What, and How of Drying Flowers

To guarantee success when drying flowers, start by picking the right plant at the right time. Dry it using the right drying mix and method.

Flowers placed in sand, borax, or cornmeal mixes usually dry in a week or more. Flowers in silica gel mixes take as little as 48 hours. A microwave can shorten that time to 2 minutes. For the quickest drying by any method, pick plants during dry, sunny weather. Damp flowers need extra time and may mold before they dry. Pick as soon as the dew has lifted from plants.

Drying magnifies blemishes, so choose perfect blossoms and leaves. Gather each flower just before it comes into full bloom. To prevent wilting, put flower stems in a water-filled container as soon as you pick them. If you can't dry flowers immediately, stand them in water in a cool, dark place until you're ready to start.

GOOD IDEA!

Flowers dry faster in gel, but must be removed as soon as they're dry or they become brittle and discolored. The less a gel has been used, the faster it will dry flowers.

GOOD IDEA!

To dry out water-saturated silica gel for reuse, place it in a shallow, oven-proof dish and heat it in a 250°F oven for ½ hour, or until the indicator crystals turn from pink to bright blue. You can "reactivate" silica gel this way innumerable times. Since silica will draw moisture right out of the air, store it tightly sealed.

Silica Drying Mix for Flowers

Flowers to be dried in silica gel must show *not a trace* of surface moisture. Silica will cling to any surface dampness and cause the flower to discolor.

Yield: about 6 cups, enough for one layer of flat flowers in a 9 × 9-inch container

INGREDIENTS

4 cups dry silica gel
2 cups sterilized, fine white sand

SUPPLIES

dust mask
clean 1-gallon bucket or disposable container, such as a milk jug
9 × 9-inch sealable container
teaspoon
tweezers with rounded ends
small camel-hair artist's brush
slotted spoon

☛ **BE SAFE.** It's a good idea to use a dust mask when handling silica gel. Inhaled silica can cause sinus irritation. Keep all equipment for handling silica separate from cooking supplies.

Prepare fresh flowers for drying by cutting and wiring stems as described in "Flower-Drying Tips" on page 361. Wearing a dust mask, combine ingredients in the bucket or other container. Spread 1 to 2 inches of drying mix in the bottom of the sealable container. Allowing at least 1 inch of space around each flower head, figure how many flowers will fit on this layer. Place a mound—a teaspoonful—of the mix where each flower will be set.

Place flat, daisylike flowers face down on the mound. Place three-dimensional flowers face up. Then gently pour the drying mix down the sides of the container, so it slides under the petals and around the flower heads, supporting them in a natural way. Carefully straighten any twisted petals with tweezers. Use the paintbrush to sweep the mix over the petals, completely covering each flower.

Seal the container and place in a warm, dry place where humidity is 60 percent or less. Note the date on the container. After one day, select a flower near the corner or edge of the container and check it for dryness. If it is not ready, reseal the container. Test that same flower daily until the petals feel crisp and papery. Remove each flower by its wire stem or with the slotted spoon. Brush off all traces of drying mix.

➥ **Notes:** *Silica gel is a fine, granular form of colloidal silica that looks like white sand. Although more expensive than some other drying agents, silica gel works quickly and can be used over and over again. Buy it in craft shops and hobby shops. For sterile sand, buy play sand at garden supply stores, toy stores, and home centers.*

GOOD IDEA!

Try the hurry-up method of silica drying. Use a sealable metal container, such as a cookie tin. After covering flowers in silica gel, place the container in a warm (150° to 175°F) oven. After 8 hours, check flowers for dryness. Check again at 3-hour intervals.

Microwaving Flowers

Dry flowers in only minutes with pure silica gel and a microwave. Before you start, remember that metal and microwaves don't mix. Do not add wire stems to flowers until after they have been dried. For best results, microwave only one flower at a time. Microwave drying works best for multi-petaled flowers, such as dahlias or peonies. Small, delicate flowers, such as pansies, don't hold up well to microwaves.

First, select a microwave-safe container with a close-fitting lid, such as a cardboard box or oven-proof glass dish. The container should be at least 2½ inches higher than the flower. Fill the bottom of the container with 1 inch of silica gel. Place the flower face up on the gel and cover carefully with silica, applying gel to its nooks and crannies with a paintbrush. Microwave the flower and gel on high for a total of 1 minute, stopping after 30 seconds to rotate the con-

tainer. If you're using a cardboard box, rest it on a saucer during the microwaving to allow moisture to escape from the bottom of the box.

Remove the container from the microwave. Put the lid on, leaving it open a crack. Cool for 20 to 30 minutes. Lift out the flower and brush off the silica gel.

If the flower is too dry, dry the next one for a total of only 30 seconds, stopping after 15 seconds to rotate the container. If it is not completely dry, put it back in the gel and microwave it for another 15 seconds. If the base of the flower—or some other thick area—is the only part that is not dry, push only that part into the gel for the second microwaving.

Microwave power varies with the model and drying times vary with the type of flower. For future reference, record the drying times for each type of flower you dry successfully.

GOOD IDEA!

Revive the fragrance of old potpourri with essential oils. Add oil of carnation or jasmine to floral potpourri; clove oil to spice mixes; oil of lemon, orange, or tangerine to citrus blends. When dispensing essential oils, use a separate eyedropper to dispense each fragrance.

The airtight container for aging potpourri should be large enough to allow the mix to blend freely when you shake it.

Potpourri Mix

These formulas may inspire you to invent your own blends—look for unique containers and new flowers to try.

Yield: about 2 quarts

INGREDIENTS
FOR ROSE-LILAC MIX

3 cups dried rose petals

2 cups dried lilac petals

2 cups dried marjoram leaves, crushed

¼ cup orrisroot nuggets (1 ounce)

INGREDIENTS
FOR HERBAL BOUQUET MIX

2 cups dried thyme leaves, crushed

1 cup dried rosemary leaves, crushed

½ cup dried lavender petals

1 cup dried mint leaves, crushed

¼ cup dried tansy flowers

¼ cup cloves, crushed

2 tablespoons dried orrisroot nuggets (½ ounce)

INGREDIENTS
FOR SPICY MIX

2 cups dried lemon balm leaves, crushed

1 cup dried thyme leaves, crushed

1 cup ground nutmeg or whole nutmeg seeds

2 tablespoons orrisroot nuggets (½ ounce)

SUPPLIES

2-quart stainless steel or glass bowl

dried flowers and herbs (see "Drying Flowers and Herbs for Potpourri" on the opposite page)

mortar and pestle

2- to 3-quart airtight container

decorative container

Blend all ingredients from one of the mixes above in the bowl. Add decorative dried flowers and herbs as desired. Crush freshly dried leaves with a mortar and pestle before stirring them in. Transfer the mix to the airtight container. Place the container in a cool, dark place.

The fragrance will not be pleasant at first. Gently shake the container every couple of days. Open it after two weeks. You'll know by the aroma whether the mix is ready or not. Continue shaking and checking every few days.

When the potpourri has become fragrant, place it in the decorative container. The aroma will last longest in a sealed container, such as an apothecary jar. Open the jar to release fragrance, when desired.

➺ **Notes:** Orrisroot, a fixative made from florentine iris roots, is available in powder or nuggets, but nuggets work best for potpourri. Powder tends to fall to the bottom of the mix. If you can't find orrisroot nuggets, buy the powder at craft shops, floral supply stores, or pharmacies. As a substitute for orrisroot, try a cellulose fiber fixative made from ground corncobs. You'll find it at floral supply houses.

Drying Flowers and Herbs for Potpourri

Materials for potpourri must be completely dry. Residual moisture encourages mold and spoilage of the potpourri. Also sunlight fades the colors of dried flowers. For best results, set up your drying operations in a warm, dark, dry place, such as an attic or garage loft.

To speed drying, gather flowers and herbs on a warm, dry day. Shorten drying time by separating thick flowers, such as roses or chrysanthemums, into individual petals. Drying reduces plant volume by half. If you need 2 cups rose petals, gather 4 cups to dry.

To air-dry fresh herbs, just tie the stems of the herbs together and hang them upside down in a dry, dark place for two to three weeks. Store them in an airtight container away from sunlight.

Discarded screen doors or windows make handy flower drying racks. Just rest a screen horizontally on cardboard boxes. Scatter petals on the screen to dry. Or place whole flowers face up on the screen by pushing the stems through the screen holes.

DYE CRAFTS

In bygone days, all dyes came from natural materials, usually the roots, leaves, stems, or flowers of wild plants. Even tree bark and heartwood were used. With the development of synthetic dyes in the mid-1800s, the custom of dyeing with natural materials began to wane.

But crafts enthusiasts still enjoy the challenges and surprises of natural dyes. The variations of nature and technique—weather, soil, type of fixative, dyeing time—will produce different colors from the same dyestuffs. And, the same dye applied to different fibers, such as wool versus silk, often yields completely different colors.

Natural dyes work best on natural fibers. Wool is the easiest natural fiber to work with. Other natural fibers require more intense dyes, longer dyeing times, and more careful handling.

The wool-dyeing process described on the following pages relies on three separate steps—conditioning the wool with a chemical called a mordant (see page 370), preparing the dye concentrate (see page 372), and dyeing the wool (see page 374). Until you are completely familiar with dyeing techniques, you may find it easier to schedule a separate work day for each of the three steps.

DYE-GATHERING GUIDE Requirements for 1 Pound of Wool			
Natural Material	**When to Gather**	**Amount Needed**	**Cold-Water Soak Time**
Bark	Spring	2 to 3 lb.	7 days or longer
Berries	When ripe	1½ to 2 lb.	1 to 2 days
Flowers	When in bloom	1½ to 2 lb.	1 to 2 hr.
Leaves and stalks	Spring	1½ to 2 lb.	1 to 3 days
Roots	Autumn	½ to 1½ lb.	3 to 7 days
Spices, coffee, and tea	—	½ to 1 lb.	1 hr.

NOTE: If you plan to dry and store materials for later dyeing, you will get better results if you gather the larger amount shown above.

THE RAINBOW CONNECTION
How Dyes and Mordants Work on Wool

Natural Dyes	Color Produced*
Bedstraw (*Galium verum*) roots	Orange-red (A); red (Ch); purple-red (Ch)
Black walnut (*Juglans nigra*) nuts, leaves, and bark	Brown (A) or (NM); gray-black (I)
Cabbage leaves, purple	Blue-lavender (A)
Carrot tops	Yellow (A); bronze (Ch); green (C)
Chamomile (*Anthemis tinctoria*) flowers	Bright yellow or buff (A); gold (Ch)
Chicory (*Cichorium intybus*) stems, leaves, and flowers	Yellow to beige (A)
Chrysanthemum leaves and stems	Gold-yellow (A)
Coffee beans and grounds	Buff (A); yellow to tan (Ch); gray (I)
Coreopsis (*Coreopsis tinctoria*) flowers	Yellow (A), (NM), or (T); brown, bright green, or gold (NM); burnt orange (Ch)
Crocus (*Crocus vernum*), purple flowers	Green-blue (A); yellow-green (Ch)
Dandelion (*Taraxacum officinale*) flowers	Bright yellow (A); orange (Ch) or (T)
Elderberries (*Sambucus canadensis* or *S. nigra*)	Purple (A); rose (NM)
Goldenrod (*Solidago canadensis*) flowers	Yellow (A); gray-green (I); brown-purple (T)
Logwood (*Haematoxylon campechianum*) heartwood	Blue-purple (A); gray-blue (I); purple (T)
Marigold (*Tagetes* spp.) flowers	Yellow-gold (A) or (Ch)
Marjoram (*Origanum majorana*), whole top	Green (A)
Oak (*Quercus* spp.) bark	Yellow to tan (A); buff-brown (NM); gold (Ch)
Onion, yellow outer skins	Brown-orange (A); yellow (NM)
Pokeweed (*Phytolacca americana*) berries	Red or tan (A)
Rhubarb stalks	Yellow (A)
Sassafras (*Sassafras albidum*) leaves and bark	Red-brown (A) or (Ch); black-gray (I)
Tea leaves, orange pekoe	Taupe (NM)
Yarrow (*Achillea millefolium*) flowers and leaves	Light yellow (A) or (Ch)

*The color produced by a dye depends upon the mordant used to condition the wool. Before dyeing untreated wool yarn, condition it with a mordant indicated by these abbreviations: (A) alum, (C) copper, (Ch) chrome, (I) iron, (NM) no mordant, (T) tannin.

GOOD IDEA!

Wools differ in their reaction to alum. Some wools may absorb too much alum, making them feel sticky when dry. If wool feels sticky, cut back the amount of alum—to as little as 2 ounces per pound of wool, if necessary.

Rainwater and softened tap water work best for mordanting. If you must use hard tap water, add a commercial water softener to it before mixing the mordant bath.

Pre-Dye Wool Conditioner

Before dyeing wool, condition it with a chemical called a mordant. Many different substances are used as mordants (see "The Rainbow Connection" on page 369), but they all work by causing the dye to penetrate or "bite" into the wool. The result is improved colorfastness and enhancement of color quality. Some natural dyes have naturally occurring mordants associated with them. Oak bark, for example, contains the mordant, tannic acid.

The same dye applied with different mordants will give different colors. To be sure that wool skeins dyed in one dye lot will have a uniform color, use skeins that have all been conditioned with the same mordant. After dyeing wool, you may treat it with another mordant to change the color quality. This wool-conditioning formula uses dyeing alum and cream of tartar as the mordants. For instructions on using other mordants, consult a book on fiber-dyeing crafts.

Yield: enough to condition 16 ounces wool yarn

INGREDIENTS

4½ gallons cold softened water
8 scant tablespoons dyeing alum (4 ounces)
2 scant tablespoons cream of tartar (1 ounce)

SUPPLIES

5-gallon or larger enameled, glass, or stainless steel pot
plastic apron
rubber work gloves
wooden, glass, or stainless steel stirrer
portable burner (optional)
16 ounces (dry weight) raw wool yarn
cotton string
mild laundry detergent
water
hot mitts
colander

☞ **BE SAFE.** Mordants and dyes are generally toxic. Store mordants and dyes and equipment away from children. Keep all mordanting and dyeing utensils and chemicals separate from cooking equipment and food. Work in a well-ventilated area, outdoors if possible. Avoid inhaling or ingesting mordant powders. Wear a protective apron and rubber gloves. Always add the mordants to the water. Do not add the water to the mordants. Use hot mitts to handle a hot mordant bath.

Reserving 1 quart, pour water into the pot. Put on apron and gloves. Add alum and cream of tartar to the quart of water and stir to dissolve. Add this to the pot and stir well. Place the pot on a portable burner outdoors or on a stove burner *with the heat off.*

Separate yarn into four equal skeins. Wrap each skein loosely around your hand in continuous loops. Tie string around the loops to keep wool together as you work. Mix detergent in cold water in your sink and wash wool. Rinse well.

Lay wet wool in the cold mordant bath and slowly bring it to a simmer, stirring occasionally. *Do not allow the mordant bath to boil.* Control the heat so the solution just simmers. As the liquid evaporates, add hot water to maintain the original bath level. Simmer for 1 hour. Wearing hot mitts, remove the pot from heat and let stand. When wool is cool enough to handle, use the colander to lift it out, remove it to a sink, and rinse well with warm water. Squeeze it gently to remove water, but do not wring. Lay flat to dry, out of direct sunlight.

➦ **Notes:** Buy raw, unmordanted wool yarn in needlework and knitting supply stores. Do not use alum (ammonium aluminum sulfate) from the supermarket. Alum for dyeing (potassium aluminum sulfate) is available from fiber crafts suppliers. You may also be able to order it through a local pharmacist. See page 444 for other sources of mordanting and dyeing supplies.

GOOD IDEA!

To prevent wet wool from losing its resiliency, use a colander or bowl to lift it from a mordant or dye bath. Never lift wet wool without support. The weight of water will permanently stretch and damage the fibers.

GOOD IDEA!

Use soft water to **prepare natural dye concentrates.** Rainwater and softened tap water are best. If you must use hard tap water, add a commercial water softener to it before preparing the dye concentrate.

Natural Dye Concentrates

To prepare a natural dye concentrate, you'll need anywhere from a few hours to more than a week, depending on which dye you choose. To keep matters simple, you may find it easier to mordant your wool in one work session (see page 370) and prepare the dye concentrate in another work session. Then, do the actual wool dyeing on another day. This formula may be multiplied or divided. If you plan to multiply the formula, be sure you have a large enough pot to accommodate all of the materials.

Yield: enough concentrate to dye 16 ounces dry mordanted wool

INGREDIENTS

natural materials for dye (see "Dye-Gathering Guide" on page 368)

cold softened water

hot water

SUPPLIES

cheesecloth

uncolored string

5-gallon or larger enameled, glass, or stainless steel pot

portable burner (optional)

wooden, glass, or stainless steel stirrer

hot mitts

plastic apron

rubber work gloves

fine sieve

clean basin or bucket

glass or other nonporous, sealable container

☛ **BE SAFE.** Use dyeing equipment only for dyeing. Many natural dyestuffs are poisonous. Always keep them away from food and children. Use separate cleaning equipment for dyeing utensils. The fumes from some vegetable-based dye baths may be harmful. Work in a well-ventilated area, outdoors, if possible.

Avoid inhaling fine-particle dyestuffs or chemicals. Wear a protective apron and rubber gloves. Use hot mitts.

Gather and prepare dye materials, using the "Dye-Gathering Guide" on page 368 for correct amounts and optimum gathering times. If you plan to use leaves or flowers later, air-dry and store them in paper bags. To store berries until dyeing time, freeze them. *Label containers carefully to avoid confusion with food.*

Cut, chop, and crush plant materials into 3-inch pieces to prepare them for soaking. Woody parts, such as roots and bark, may be difficult to cut into small pieces. Soak these in water an hour or two before cutting. Place dry, granular materials, such as coffee, and juicy materials, such as berries, in a cheesecloth "bag" tied with uncolored string.

Place prepared materials in the pot and add enough cold water to barely cover. Let soak for the time indicated in the "Dye-Gathering Guide" on page 368 (it could be more than seven days). After the required soaking time, heat the pot on a portable burner outdoors or on the stove over medium heat until the water simmers. *Do not allow it to boil.* Adjust heat as necessary to keep water just below boiling. Add hot water, as necessary, to keep materials barely covered. Simmer for an hour, stirring occasionally and pressing the cheesecloth bag with the stirrer. Wearing hot mitts, remove from heat and allow to cool.

Don apron and gloves. Strain out dye materials by pouring the dye concentrate through cheesecloth or a fine sieve into the basin or bucket. If a cheesecloth bag held the dyeing agent, squeeze the bag and then discard materials left in the bag. Store dye concentrate in the sealed container until ready to dye. Or pour dye concentrate back into the pot and proceed immediately with dyeing wool as described on page 374.

GOOD IDEA!

If you dye wool fre-quently, keep records for future reference. Note harvest times, materials, mordants, simmering times, and colors pro-duced. Attach a sample of the yarn.

GOOD IDEA!

For gradations of the same color, remove sections of yarn from the dye bath at intervals. For deeper colors, leave wool in the cool dye bath for a longer time before bringing it to a simmer.

Hand-Dyed Wool

You may multiply or divide the formula to accommo-date different amounts of wool. To avoid unwanted color variations, dye all the yarn needed for a project in one batch.

Yield: 16 ounces dyed wool yarn

INGREDIENTS

dye concentrate (see page 372)

cold softened water

16 ounces (dry weight) mordanted wool yarn, tied into skeins (see page 371)

hot water

SUPPLIES

plastic apron

rubber work gloves

5-gallon or larger enameled, glass, or stainless steel pot

portable burner (optional)

wooden, glass, or stainless steel stirrer

colander

hot mitts

☛ **BE SAFE.** Use dyeing equipment only for dyeing. Many nat-ural dyestuffs are poisonous. Always keep them away from food. Use separate cleaning equipment for dyeing utensils. Even the residues of dyes and mordants are generally toxic. Keep dyeing supplies and equipment away from children. The fumes from some vegetable-based dye baths may be harmful. Work in a well-ventilated area, outdoors, if possible. Avoid inhal-ing fine-particle dyestuffs or chemicals. Wear a protective apron and rubber gloves. Use hot mitts.

Don apron and gloves. Use dye concentrate prepared according to directions on page 372. Pour it into the pot and add enough cold water to make a 4-gallon dye bath.

The mordanted wool must be wet before dyeing. If you are beginning with dry wool, let it stand in cold water until thoroughly soaked. Place the wet skeins in the cold dye bath. On a portable burner outdoors or on the stove, slowly bring the dye bath to a simmer, stirring occasionally. *Do not allow the dye bath to boil.* As the liquid evaporates, add hot water to maintain the original level. Lift the yarn up with the colander occasionally to check the color.

Simmer for 1 hour or more, or until wool has reached a shade darker than the desired color. Wearing hot mitts, remove dye bath from heat and let stand until wool is cool enough to handle. Use a colander to lift wool out and drain it. Rinse it well in warm water. Rinse it in slightly cooler water. Rinse several more times in successively cooler water until the rinse water is cold and clear.

Squeeze wool gently, but do not wring. Lay skeins flat to dry in a shady spot, away from direct sun or heat.

➠ **Notes:** Buy untreated wool yarn at needlework and knitting supply stores. Weaving suppliers sell a variety of natural dyes. Gather plants to produce most of the earth tones—yellows, golds, grays, browns, and greens. For brighter shades—blue from indigo, reds and violets from cochineal bugs—order dyestuffs from weaving or crafts suppliers. See page 444 for other sources.

GOOD IDEA!

The dye kettle itself can affect the colors. Iron kettles tend to "sadden" or dull colors, copper kettles give a brighter color, and brass kettles, an even brighter color. Enameled, glass, or stainless steel kettles do not affect the color.

Chapter Nine

Pet Care

by Susan H. Pitcairn, M.S., with Richard Pitcairn, D.V.M.

Preparing your own fresh pet food and health-care products can be invaluable. Diet is particularly important to pet health, so many of the formulas in this chapter cover homemade foods and food supplements.

Maintaining fresh, well-balanced diets for your pets often results in visible improvement in their appearance and health within a few weeks. That's because you can select higher-quality ingredients than those in commercial "least-cost" pet foods. When making dog and cat food, you can include USDA-approved meat and you can eliminate the indigestible fillers, chemical food additives, and rancid grains and fats that are frequently found in commercial foods. A bonus is that you can add quality food supplements, such as nutritional yeast, lecithin, kelp, and bonemeal. Heat processing, which destroys many water-soluble vitamins, is minimal. You can even serve meat raw, the way Mother Nature intended animals to eat it.

In the care of parrots, parakeets, cockatiels, and similar species, proper nutrition and husbandry are the keys to good health. Many people believe that packaged seed mixes provide an adequate diet for birds, but this is not true. Seeds are an important part of an avian diet (particularly for parakeets and cockatiels), but they do not provide adequate amounts of some nutrients, such as vitamins A and C, which help prevent respiratory infections. Home formulation of a healthy diet allows you to provide for all of your bird's nutritional needs and thus assure optimal health.

But formulating a balanced diet for your pet is not easy. A homemade diet often leads to excesses or deficiencies in important vitamins and minerals. The formulas in this chapter spare you the pitfalls and mistakes that can result from developing your own pet nutrition program. The formulas are based on a wealth of observation and practical experience in helping pets maintain optimal health. The bird-feeding program was developed by Yvonne Nelson, an Alabama veterinarian with a special interest in tropical birds. The dog and cat recipes have been carefully formulated by Richard Pitcairn, D.V.M., and Susan Pitcairn, M.S., authors of *Dr. Pitcairn's Complete Guide to Natural Health for Dogs and Cats*.

KEEPING YOUR PET HEALTHY

On the following pages, you'll find a variety of recipes for feeding cats, dogs, birds, and small animals, such as rabbits and gerbils. You'll also find formulas and procedures for solving pet health problems, for grooming, and even for simple problems like odor removal. It is important to use the formulas exactly as they appear. If a formula calls for one ingredient that seems important to you, don't succumb to the temptation to add even more. Likewise don't add ingredients not called for in the recipe, and don't substitute ingredients unless they're specifically mentioned as acceptable substitutes. We've taken a lot of care to give you accurate, thorough, helpful information. Enjoy the information offered here, but better yet, enjoy the enhanced good spirits and well-being your pet will gain from your careful attention to its diet and health.

DOG AND CAT FEEDING GUIDE

It is important to use the formulas and recipes in this chapter accurately. For the dog and cat foods, use a variety of meats, grains, and vegetables. Don't be tempted to just add fresh meat to commercial food, for example. If you do so regularly, your animal will suffer a calcium deficiency.

Another note of caution: Always take up any uneaten food after about 20 minutes. This retards spoilage, of course, and it also is better for your pet. The constant smell of food in the environment overstimulates the parasympathetic nervous system, which governs digestive processes. Animals that smell food throughout the day become sluggish, reduce their grooming activities, and develop an oily coat that separates easily.

Now, here are guidelines for choosing and substituting the basic ingredients.

Meat: We recommend feeding meat raw. (Pork and fish, however, should be cooked to kill parasites.) Use these ground meats interchangeably: chicken, fish, lean chuck, lean hamburger, lean heart, liver, or turkey. But use less than 10 percent of your meat as liver to avoid excesses of vitamin A. Ground meat works best because you can blend it with other ingredients. If you have a food processor, you can grind chunks of meat along with the other ingredients to make a nice texture; otherwise, buy meat already ground.

Dairy: Eggs may be fed raw. You may feed milk, cheese, or yogurt as desired, on the side.

Whole grains and starchy vegetables: You must cook these to help dogs and cats digest them. Use the same amount for any grain within the same group below. All measurements are for cooked amounts, except for Group D. To substitute between groups, first find "1 CUP" beneath your starting ingredient. Equivalent amounts are on the same line. If the dog or cat food recipe calls for 4 cups cooked rice, you may substitute 6⅔ cups cooked oatmeal, 5⅓ cups cooked barley, or 3 cups uncooked rolled oats. To make the calculations yourself, start at the "1 CUP=" below Group C, Rice. Note that 1 cup rice=1⅔ cups cooked oatmeal=1⅓ cups cooked barley=¾ cup uncooked rolled oats. Since the recipe calls for 4 cups, multiply the 1-cup equivalent by 4 to get the total amount needed.

WHOLE-GRAIN AND STARCH EQUIVALENTS FOR DOGS AND CATS			
How to Substitute Different Starches in a Homemade Diet			
Group A*	**Group B***	**Group C***	**Group D**
Whole wheat bread (2 slices=1 cup) Oatmeal Cornmeal Boiled potatoes	Barley Whole wheat pasta Millet Yams Mashed potatoes	Rice Bulgur	Rolled oats, uncooked
1 CUP=	scant ¾ cup=	½+ cup=	½ cup
¾+ cup=	1 CUP=	1⅓ cups=	1¾+ cups
1⅔ cups=	1⅓ cups=	1 CUP=	¾ cup
2¼ cups=	1¾ cups=	1⅓ cups=	1 CUP

*Amounts are for cooked food.

APPROPRIATE VEGETABLES FOR DOGS AND CATS Adding Fiber to Your Pet's Food	
Use These Raw	**Cook These**
Chopped parsley Alfalfa sprouts Finely grated carrots Finely grated zucchini	Broccoli Carrots Corn Green beans Peas

Vegetables: These are valuable for roughage, vitamins, and minerals. Amounts need not be exact; give what your pet will accept. Avoid spinach, Swiss chard, or rhubarb. They are high in oxalic acid, which interferes with calcium absorption.

Flavorings: Most animals will accept the following recipes without additional flavoring. Finicky eaters may appreciate additional flavor from substituting meat drippings or butter for one-third to one-half of the vegetable oil in the recipes. Or, try the guidelines in "How to Bribe Cats to Try New Foods" on page 384. Do not add any salt to these recipes unless called for. You may use iodized potassium chloride, a sodium-free salt substitute.

Pet vitamins: Add these if you wish, or add Healthy Powder from page 382, but avoid feeding cats more than 500 I.U. of vitamin A per day, unless a recipe calls for that much to be added. Also, the calcium-to-phosphorus ratio for dogs and cats should be between 1:1 and 1.3:1.

Supplements

Many of the dog and cat food formulas in this chapter include food supplements, such as vitamin E, vitamin A, or calcium. Supplements provide the additional vitamins and minerals needed to bring the dog and cat food formulas in this chapter to optimum levels. Some supplements are available in several forms—calcium as tablets or powder, for example. When you mix the recipes for dogs or cats, check the table on page 380 to decide what form to buy.

SUPPLEMENTS FOR DOG AND CAT FOOD FORMULAS
Buying the Right Vitamins and Minerals for Your Pet

Supplement	Choose One	Special Instructions	Benefits
Calcium	Tablets or powder	Buy chelated calcium, calcium gluconate, or calcium lactate. Do not buy products that also have phosphorus or magnesium. Grind tablets to powder before mixing into food.	Convenient and easy to use. Prevents calcium deficiency.
	Bonemeal	Buy bonemeal sold as a dietary supplement for humans.	Most natural source of calcium for dogs and cats. Excellent for preventing calcium deficiency.
	Eggshell powder	Make at home using the instructions in "Good Idea!" on page 382. One whole eggshell yields about 1 tsp. eggshell powder or about 1,800 mg calcium.	Cheap, convenient source of calcium. Prevents calcium deficiency.
Healthy powder	Use recipe on page 382.	Add to recipes in the amounts specified. Add to commercial dog or cat food to increase vitamin and mineral content.	Rich in B vitamins, iron, essential fatty acids, iodine, trace minerals, and calcium.
Vegetable oil	Safflower, soy, or corn	Buy cold-pressed oils and keep them refrigerated in a well-sealed container.	Vegetable oils provide essential unsaturated fatty acids, which are necessary for glossy, healthy coats.
Vitamin A*	Cod liver oil	Buy cod liver oil sold for human consumption. Refrigerate after opening. Read label to find out how many teaspoons provide the amount of vitamin A called for in the recipe.	An excellent source of unsaturated fatty acids as well as vitamin A.
	Low-potency A and D capsules	Buy capsules that provide 5,000 I.U. or less of vitamin A. Break open a capsule and use an appropriate portion.	Convenient and easy-to-use source of vitamin A.

Supplement	Choose One	Special Instructions	Benefits
	Liquid A and D drops	Buy drops sold for human consumption that provide 1,600 I.U. of vitamin A per drop.	Most convenient source of vitamin A. Easy to measure.
	Pet vitamins	Use as needed to supply the called for amount of vitamin A.	Adds extra vitamins and minerals as well as vitamin A.
Vitamin E	Capsules or tablets	Buy products that list mixed natural tocopherols on the label.	Both capsules and tablets are a good source for this vitamin, which aids in fighting disease.
Yeast sprinkle	Use recipe below	Tastes good to most dogs and cats. Use as a bribe or condiment to encourage eating.	Rich in B vitamins, calcium, and phosphorus.

*If you choose to omit any of the vegetables in the dog food formulas in this chapter, add about 1,000 I.U. of vitamin A per cup of any omitted vegetable. Cats require an animal source of vitamin A and are also very sensitive to vitamin A deficiency as well as excess. Follow the dietary formulas for cats exactly as given.

Yeast Sprinkle

This "condiment" is full of taste appeal for many cats and dogs. Sprinkle on top of any food to tempt an appetite.

Yield: about 2¼ cups

INGREDIENTS

2 cups nutritional yeast or brewer's yeast

scant 3 tablespoons bonemeal or 1 rounded tablespoon eggshell powder (see "Good Idea!" on page 382) or 5,600 mg calcium

1 to 4 teaspoons unsalted garlic powder (optional)

Mix ingredients right in the measure and sprinkle on top of any food. You may substitute for Healthy Powder in the recipes. Keep in a sealed container.

➡ **Note:** *Buy ingredients at health food stores.*

GOOD IDEA!

To help repel fleas, add a garlic and soy sauce condiment to your cat's food. Mix ⅛ teaspoon tamari soy sauce with ⅛ teaspoon water. Add one crushed whole clove of garlic. Marinate the garlic in the liquid for about 10 minutes and then remove it. Add ¹⁄₁₆ to ⅛ teaspoon soy liquid to each ½ cup cat food. Use the condiment immediately.

GOOD IDEA!

To make eggshell powder to provide calcium carbonate, wash shells out right after cracking the egg. Bake in an oven at 300°F for about 10 minutes to remove a mineral oil coating and make them dry and brittle enough to grind. Then grind to a fine powder with a nut and seed grinder, a blender, or mortar and pestle. Grind well enough so that there are no sharp, gritty pieces. One whole eggshell makes about a teaspoon of powder, which gives you about 1,800 milligrams of calcium.

Healthy Powder

This powder appears in many of the dog and cat food recipes. Yeast provides B vitamins, iron, and other nutrients. Lecithin provides linoleic acid, choline, and inositol, all of which improve coat condition and digestion. Kelp powder provides iodine and trace minerals. Calcium balances the high phosphorus levels in the yeast and lecithin. Adding calcium enables you to add this powder to any diet. Vitamin C is not an official requirement in dog or cat diets, but clinical veterinary experience suggests it's valuable.

Yield: about 3½ cups

INGREDIENTS

- 2 cups nutritional yeast or brewer's yeast
- 1 cup lecithin granules
- ¼ cup kelp powder
- slightly rounded ¼ cup bonemeal or 5 teaspoons eggshell powder (see "Good Idea!") or 9,000 mg calcium
- ¼ teaspoon sodium ascorbate powder or 1,000 mg vitamin C (optional)
- 1 to 4 teaspoons unsalted garlic powder (optional)

SUPPLIES

stirrer

1-quart container with lid

Mix all ingredients in the container, cover, and refrigerate. You may add this to commercial dog or cat food as follows: 1 to 2 teaspoons per day for a cat or small dog; 2 to 3 teaspoons per day for medium dogs; 1 to 2 tablespoons per day for large dogs.

✿ **Variation:** For kelp powder, substitute ¾ teaspoon iodized salt plus ¼ cup alfalfa powder.

➾ **Note:** Buy ingredients at health food stores.

Cat Foods

Once you've made the supplements on pages 381 and 382, you'll be ready to make the food recipes that follow. Cats have a well-deserved reputation for finickiness that sometimes makes it difficult to switch them over to new foods. If you let your cat go without its accustomed food for a few meals, it will get hungry enough to eat something new and will eventually grow to like it. Unless your cat is sick and wasting away, don't be concerned if he misses a few meals. For tips on switching cats to new foods, see "How to Bribe Cats to Try New Foods" on page 384.

Kitten Formula

Use this formula to feed orphaned or lost kittens.

Yield: about 2½ cups

INGREDIENTS

- 2 cups whole cow's milk
- 2 large eggs
- 4 teaspoons protein powder
- 2 teaspoons nutritional yeast
- ⅓ teaspoon bonemeal or ⅛ teaspoon eggshell powder (see "Good Idea!" on page 382) or 220 mg calcium
- 1 to 2 days' worth of balanced cat vitamins (adult dosage)

SUPPLIES

1-quart bowl

hand eggbeater

1-quart saucepan

dairy or candy thermometer

doll bottle or pet nurser

Combine all ingredients in the bowl. Beat lightly until eggs are well-distributed. Pour into the saucepan and heat

(continued)

> ### GOOD IDEA!
>
> **T**o **raise orphaned kittens, think like a mother cat.** To mimic natural feeding at a mother's teat, feed your kittens with a doll bottle, or buy a pet nurser from your veterinarian. After each feeding, moisten a tissue with warm water and gently wipe the genital and anal area. Mother cats lick the same areas to stimulate urination and defecation in their young. Also, massage the kittens' bellies lightly.

to 98°F. It should be warm, *not* hot. Give each kitten just enough to enlarge the belly slightly, without distending it. Feed according to the following schedule.

Begin to introduce solids (high-quality canned food or home recipe for cats) at 3 to 4 weeks. Mix it with the formula to make a thin mush. Weaning can begin at 4 to 6 weeks.

➡ **Notes:** Buy yeast, bonemeal, and protein powder at health food stores. Buy protein powder that is 80 percent animal protein on a dry weight basis.

FEEDING SCHEDULE FOR KITTENS	
Age	**Feeding Frequency**
0 to 2 weeks	every 2 hrs. (total of 2 to 4 Tbs. per day)
3 weeks	every 3 hrs. (total of 4 to 6 Tbs. per day)
4 to 5 weeks	every 4 hrs. (total of 6 to 10 Tbs. per day)
6 weeks	3 times a day (total of 8 to 12 Tbs. per day)

How to Bribe Cats to Try New Foods

One factor that may cause your cat's appetite to lag is simply that we tend to feed cats in a way that is natural to humans but not to cats. Wild cats eat in several-day cycles of alternate feasting and fasting. If a healthy cat goes without eating for a few days, it will probably get hungry enough to try a new food.

Make switching food easy by using bribe foods. Anitra Frazier, author of *The New Natural Cat* suggests the use of special "condiments" that resemble the strong tastes and smells of various cat "junk" foods to which your pet has become accustomed. The bribe food that you use depends upon your cat's former diet.

Add a small amount of the bribe food to the new homemade diet until it may no longer be necessary. Also, make the transition to a new diet gradual by mixing some of your cat's previous food into the new fare. Steadily decrease the proportion of old food over a few days or weeks until your pet has switched totally to the new diet. Be sure to take up uneaten food after each meal. In addition to the bribe foods suggested below, you may also try the Yeast Sprinkle (see page 381) or lightly steamed chicken liver mixed into the new food.

- If the previous diet included highly salted foods or kibble, mix 1/16 teaspoon soy/garlic condiment (see "Good Idea!" on page 381) into the new food.
- If the previous diet included sugary, semi-moist foods, mix 1 tablespoon baby food creamed corn into the new food.
- If the previous diet included tuna or tuna-flavored foods, mix a 1-inch piece of sardine in tomato sauce into the new food.

Turkey Loaf for Cats

This makes a balanced diet for your cat.

Yield: feeds a 7-pound cat for 9 to 10 days

INGREDIENTS

2 pounds raw ground turkey

2 large eggs, lightly beaten

8 slices whole wheat bread, finely crumbled

⅓ cup frozen peas or 1 to 2 tablespoons finely grated carrots or other vegetables (see page 379)

¼ cup Healthy Powder (see page 382)

2 tablespoons vegetable oil

1½ tablespoons bonemeal or 1⅔ teaspoons powdered eggshell (see "Good Idea!" on page 382) or 2,800 mg calcium

2,500 to 3,500 I.U. vitamin A

50 to 100 I.U. vitamin E

1 teaspoon thyme or basil (optional)

water (optional)

SUPPLIES

spoon or paddle

3-quart bowl

freezer containers with lids

3-quart casserole (optional)

Mix all ingredients in the bowl. Add water, if needed, so that the texture resembles canned food. Refrigerate two meals' worth and serve raw. Freeze the rest in meal-size portions. Or bake in the casserole, sprinkled with water, at 350°F for about 20 minutes.

✿ **Variation:** Substitute ground chicken, lean chuck, or beef heart for the turkey.

➤ **Note:** Buy bonemeal and vitamins at health food stores.

GOOD IDEA!

Fill your freezer with feline fare. If you're preparing a week's supply of homemade food for your cat, freeze single portions in small containers, such as recycled sour cream or yogurt containers. Thaw by placing the single-serving container in your refrigerator 24 hours prior to serving. By removing one container every evening, you'll always have a thawed dinner on hand.

Heart-Liver Feast for Cats

Here's a hearty (pun intended!) fare for your feline, especially those that love liver.

Yield: feeds a 7-pound cat for about 8 days

INGREDIENTS

1½ cups rolled oats

water

2 pounds raw lean ground beef heart

1 tablespoon raw ground or chopped beef or chicken liver

2 to 4 tablespoons finely grated carrots or other vegetables (see page 379)

¼ cup Healthy Powder (see page 382)

1½ tablespoons vegetable oil

1½ tablespoons bonemeal or 1½ slightly rounded teaspoons eggshell powder (see "Good Idea!" on page 382) or 2,800 mg calcium

50 to 100 I.U. vitamin E

SUPPLIES

2-quart saucepan

spoon or paddle

freezer containers with lids

Put oats in the saucepan with enough water to cover. Bring to a boil and let sit about 10 minutes, covered. When the oatmeal is done, mix in remaining ingredients and serve one meal warm. Freeze the rest in meal-size portions.

✿ **Variations:** Substitute ground turkey, chicken, or lean chuck for the heart. You may omit the liver and add 2,500 to 3,500 I.U. vitamin A instead. In place of the oats, try six to seven slices whole wheat bread; 2⅔ cups cooked barley, whole wheat noodles, or millet; or 2 cups cooked rice or bulgur.

➦ **Note:** Buy bonemeal and vitamin E at health food stores.

Kitty (and Doggie) Crunchies

Here's a high-quality make-your-own kibble from Joan Harper's *Healthy Dog and Cat Cookbook*.

INGREDIENTS

1 pound raw ground poultry necks and gizzards

16 ounces canned mackerel, including liquid

2 cups full-fat soy flour

1 cup wheat germ

1 cup powdered skim milk

1 cup cornmeal

3 cups whole wheat flour

3 tablespoons bonemeal (5,760 mg calcium)

3 tablespoons kelp or ½ teaspoon iodized salt

¼ cup vegetable oil

1 tablespoon cod-liver oil (less if high potency)

¼ cup alfalfa powder

3 cloves garlic, minced

4 cups water

400 I.U. vitamin E

½ cup chopped onions (optional)

½ cup nutritional yeast

SUPPLIES

4-quart or larger bowl

spoon or paddle

cookie sheet

sealable containers

In the bowl, mix all ingredients except yeast into a firm dough. Press into the cookie sheet about ⅜ inch thick. Bake at 350°F for 30 to 45 minutes. Cool and break into chunks. Sprinkle on yeast. Refrigerate tightly sealed.

➨ **Note:** *Buy ingredients at supermarkets and health food stores.*

GOOD IDEA!

To tempt a finicky **cat to eat a kibble,** try pouring a little bacon fat or gravy over it. If you use kibble as a mainstay diet, supplement it with some raw vegetables (see page 379), cottage cheese, or yogurt.

GOOD IDEA!

To perk up your cat's finicky appetite, turn on your microwave. Cats have been shown to prefer food served at 78° to 103°F. If your cat refuses to try a new food, warming it in the microwave just before serving often aids in curing feline pickiness.

If your cat is overweight, you can also entice him to try a low-calorie diet by adding a pinch of thyme or basil or the garlic/soy sauce condiment found in "Good Idea!" on page 381. This condiment adds taste appeal without calories.

Weight-Loss Diet for Cats

This diet food provides 190 calories per cup.

Yield: about 9 cups

INGREDIENTS

2 cups frozen cooked peas, mashed, or 1 cup finely grated carrots

1½ pounds raw ground turkey

1 large egg

5 slices whole wheat bread, finely crumbled

1 cup oat or wheat bran

2 tablespoons Yeast Sprinkle (see page 381)

1½ tablespoons vegetable oil

5 teaspoons bonemeal or 1¾ teaspoons eggshell powder (see "Good Idea!" on page 382) or 3,200 mg calcium

2,000 to 2,500 I.U. vitamin A

50 to 100 I.U. vitamin E

water (optional)

SUPPLIES

spoon or paddle

3-quart bowl

freezer containers with lids

3-quart casserole (optional)

Mix all ingredients in the bowl. Add water, if needed, to improve texture. Refrigerate two meals' worth and serve raw. Freeze the rest in meal-size portions. Or bake in the casserole for 20 to 30 minutes in a 350°F oven. Ask the vet what your cat's ideal weight is. Feed two meals daily with the total as follows: if the ideal weight is 7 pounds, feed ⅞ cup total; 8 pounds—1 cup; 9 pounds—1⅛ cups; 10 pounds—1¼ cups.

➻ **Note:** Buy ingredients at supermarkets and health food stores.

Force-Feeding Diet for Sick Cats

For cats that are too sick to eat, seek appropriate veterinary care. If your vet recommends force-feeding, try this diet.

Yield: about 1 cup

INGREDIENTS

⅔ cup raw chicken or turkey

about ⅓ cup half milk and half cream or half-and-half

⅔ teaspoon bonemeal or ¼ teaspoon eggshell powder (see "Good Idea!" on page 382) or 400 mg calcium

pet vitamins

SUPPLIES

food processor

towel

dropper or 3cc syringe without needle (optional)

☛ **BE SAFE.** *To avoid getting scratched, wrap your cat firmly in a towel before force-feeding. Refrigerate the food for a maximum of 3 days. If it develops a sour odor during storage, do not use.*

Place all ingredients in the food processor and puree, adjusting the amount of milk and cream, as necessary, to make a thick, smooth paste. Feed ½ to ¾ cup a day. Wrap the cat in the towel. Place a small amount of food at a time on the end of your finger and wipe it on the roof of your cat's mouth, just behind the front teeth. Give the cat plenty of time to swallow before offering the next bit. If necessary, offer a thinner mixture with the dropper or syringe. Administer small amounts every few hours, rather than a large amount less often. Give pets vitamins daily in the dosage recommended on the label.

➻ **Note:** Buy bonemeal at health food stores.

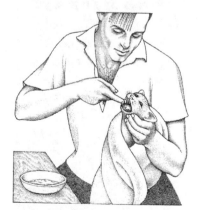

To force-feed a cat without getting scratched, wrap the cat gently but firmly in a towel.

Kidney Diet for Older Cats

This diet is helpful for older cats experiencing beginning kidney failure.

Yield: about 6 cups

INGREDIENTS

⅔ pound raw ground poultry

4 cups cooked white rice (vitamin enriched)

4 large eggs

2 tablespoons vegetable oil

2 tablespoons chopped parsley or finely grated carrots

⅛ teaspoon iodized salt

⅛ teaspoon iodized potassium chloride salt substitute

rounded ¾ teaspoon eggshell powder (see "Good Idea!" on page 382), *not* bonemeal, or 1,500 mg calcium

5 days' worth of cat vitamins

SUPPLIES

spoon or paddle

3-quart bowl

freezer containers with lids

3-quart casserole (optional)

☛ **BE SAFE.** Using bonemeal for the calcium would push the overall phosphorus level too high. The total dosage of cat vitamins for this recipe should not contain more than 7,000 I.U. vitamin A.

Mix all ingredients in the bowl. Refrigerate two meals' worth and serve raw. Freeze the rest in meal-size portions. Or bake in the casserole at 350°F for about 20 minutes. Provide plenty of fresh filtered or bottled water.

✿ **Variations:** Occasionally include 1 to 3 teaspoons liver in the recipe. If more salt flavor is needed, use only iodized potassium chloride, a salt substitute.

Dog Foods

Making fresh food for small and medium-size dogs is practical and fairly easy. Fortunately, dogs need proportionately less protein than cats, so you can feed more grains. Using bread is usually too expensive except for a small dog. That leaves two basic ways to prepare grains for most dogs: cook rolled oats (or other rolled whole grains), which takes only about 10 minutes, or precook large amounts of rice or other whole grains. For larger dogs, consider combining a good-quality commercial kibble with the meat and dairy kibble supplements on pages 392 and 393. No yield lines appear on some of the dog food recipes since the number of meals the recipe produces varies depending on the size of your pet. Use the guidelines that follow to decide how much of the recipe to feed your dog.

APPROPRIATE AMOUNTS FOR DOG FOOD RECIPES	
Dog's Size	Serving Size
Small (15 lb. or less)	Recipe makes 3 to 10 days' supply of food
Medium (20 to 40 lb.)	Recipe makes 1 to 2 days' supply of food
Large (50 lb. and up)	Multiply the recipe 3 to 5 times to make 2 days' supply of food

Supplements for Dog Kibble

If your dog is big, you may come to the conclusion that a cheap bag of dry food may not be optimal, but it's certainly convenient! If you want to provide many of the benefits of fresh foods and extra nutrition without the bother of preparing the entire diet yourself, here's a nice middle ground. Add Meat Supplement for Dog Kibble, on page 392, or Dairy Supplement for Dog Kibble, on page 393, to your dog's dry food. Freeze extra supplement in 1- or 2-day amounts. Thaw in the refrigerator 24 hours before using.

If you're tempted to take a shortcut and throw a slab of meat or a dab of oil on top of your dog's fare, don't do it! Here's why: Extra oil can lower the overall percentage of

(continued)

protein and other nutrients in a marginal-quality kibble to inadequate levels. Meat is dramatically low in calcium, as compared to phosphorus. The added calcium brings the meat into the proper calcium-to-phosphorus balance.

> **GOOD IDEA!**
>
> **If you buy commercial dog food, read the label.** The higher the protein and fat level of the food, the higher the nutritional value. Also, as in human food labeling, pet food ingredients appear on the label in descending order of quantity. Those commercial foods listing meat first are better than those listing grain first. Even though dogs can make do with a minimum protein level of 15 percent, most veterinarians recommend a diet that is 22 to 25 percent protein. A show or working dog, a sick dog, a nursing mother dog, or a growing puppy may need 30 percent protein.

Meat Supplement for Dog Kibble

Use this formula to supplement dry dog kibble.

Yield: enough supplement for 8 to 9 cups of dog kibble

INGREDIENTS

- 4 teaspoons vegetable oil
- 4 teaspoons Healthy Powder (see page 382) or Yeast Sprinkle (see page 381)
- 50 to 100 I.U. vitamin E (can be premixed with oil)
- 1¾ teaspoons bonemeal or slightly rounded ½ teaspoon eggshell powder (see "Good Idea!" on page 382) or 1,080 mg calcium
- 1 pound raw chopped or ground lean chuck

SUPPLIES

spoon or paddle
2-quart bowl
freezer containers with lids

Mix oil, powder, vitamin E, and bonemeal or eggshell powder in the bowl. Stir in meat, coating it. To use, add ¼ cup per 1 cup kibble when you feed your dog (you'll feed proportionately less kibble). Refrigerate two meals' worth. Freeze the rest in meal-size portions. Alternate this recipe with the Dairy Supplement for Kibble, on the opposite page, which is higher in vitamin A. If you prefer to feed this meat version exclusively, add 1,000 to 2,000 I.U. vitamin A supplement to it.

✿ **Variation:** Instead of chuck, use lean hamburger or ground dark meat turkey or chicken.

➾ **Note:** Buy vitamins and bonemeal at health food stores.

Dairy Supplement for Dog Kibble

Eggs, one of the most balanced and high-quality protein sources available, are also helpful for skin conditions.

Yield: enough supplement for 1 to 2 cups dog kibble

INGREDIENTS

1 teaspoon vegetable oil

1 teaspoon Healthy Powder (see page 382)

⅓ teaspoon bonemeal or ⅛ teaspoon eggshell powder (see "Good Idea!" on page 382) or 225 mg calcium

2 medium eggs

SUPPLIES

spoon or paddle

1-pint bowl

Mix oil and powders in the bowl and stir into the kibble. Serve the eggs raw or cooked, either separately or mixed into the dry food.

➤ **Note:** Buy bonemeal at health food stores.

GOOD IDEA!

Try adding milk to your pet's kibble. You can moisten dry food with 1 part milk (or ½ part milk) to 4 parts dry kibble. Like egg, milk adds protein, fat, and taste. Milk won't cause diarrhea if it's reintroduced later in life over a period of five to six days.

Supplements for Dog Skin Conditions

If your dog is plagued by a dry, itchy, scaly coat or hair loss, a marginal diet may be a big part of the problem. Just switching to homemade dog food recipes may bring about a marked improvement. In addition to using either the recipes or kibble supplements, follow these guidelines for at least one month before deciding on further veterinary care.

- Double the amount of Healthy Powder (see page 382). Always use this in preference to the Yeast Sprinkle. It provides lecithin, kelp, and vitamin C, all important to healthy skin.
- Add ½ teaspoon regular-potency cod-liver oil to the standard recipes or ¼ teaspoon per cup of kibble. Use half this amount of cod-liver oil if the oil contains significantly more than 5,000 I.U. vitamin A per teaspoon.
- Add 10 to 20 milligrams chelated zinc to the basic dog food recipes. Or, feed or pill a small dog 5 to 10 milligrams of zinc a day. Give medium dogs 10 to 20 milligrams and large dogs 20 to 40 milligrams daily.
- Avoid wheat and corn, possible allergens. Use brown rice, oats, or millet. Emphasize raw foods, except for the grain.
- Avoid exposure to toxic products, including flea sprays and shampoos. If the coat is greasy, use a natural shampoo.

Dog Food Recipes

These recipes include the supplements Yeast Sprinkle and Healthy Powder. You'll find the recipes for these supplements in the previous section.

Kidney Diet for Older Dogs

Feed a dog with failing kidneys minimal levels of protein, phosphorus, and sodium in a maximally usable form.

Yield: about 4 cups

INGREDIENTS

½ cup regular (fatty) hamburger, raw or cooked

2¾ cups cooked white rice (vitamin enriched)

1 large egg

2 tablespoons vegetable oil

2 tablespoons chopped parsley, finely grated carrots, or other vegetables (see page 379)

⅛ teaspoon iodized salt

⅛ to ¼ teaspoon iodized potassium chloride salt substitute

⅓ teaspoon eggshell powder (see "Good Idea!" on page 382), *not* bonemeal, or 600 mg calcium

garlic or onion (optional)

dog vitamins, providing 1 day's worth for a 40-pound dog

SUPPLIES

spoon or paddle

2-quart bowl

freezer containers with lids

2-quart casserole (optional)

☛ **BE SAFE.** *Using bonemeal for the calcium would push the overall phosphorus level too high.*

Mix all ingredients in the bowl. Serve raw and freeze leftovers in meal-size portions. Or bake in the casserole at

---

GOOD IDEA!

If you buy commercial kibble for an older dog, select a food that meets your dog's needs. Food for older dogs should not contain excess protein, phosphorus, or sodium; excesses may worsen existing kidney or heart disease. If the kibble says "high pro" or "high protein," don't buy it for an older dog.

Older dogs also need fewer calories because they're usually less active than younger animals. But, don't attempt to reduce your dog's calorie intake by giving him less food. You may cause a nutrient deficiency. Instead, choose a lower-calorie food sold for senior dogs or ask your vet how to meet the dog's dietary needs.

350°F for 20 to 30 minutes. Use the table below to determine how much special diet to feed your dog daily.

➜ **Note:** Buy bonemeal at health food stores.

FEEDING DOGS WITH KIDNEY PROBLEMS		
Dog's Weight	**For 1 Day, Multiply Recipe By**	**Comments**
10 lb.	⅓	This recipe = about 3 days' worth
25 lb.	⅔	2 × this recipe = about 3 days' worth
40 lb.	1	This recipe = 1 days' worth
60 lb.	1¼	5 × this recipe = 4 days' worth
85 lb.	1½	3 × this recipe = about 2 days' worth

Weight-Loss Diet for Dogs

This recipe provides about 60 percent of the calories needed to maintain ideal weight.

Yield: about 12 cups

INGREDIENTS

4 cups carrots, broccoli, peas, green beans, or corn

3 to 4 cups water

2 cups rolled oats

1 cup oat or wheat bran

1 cup raw or cooked ground or chunky lean beef heart, hamburger, or poultry

1 cup uncreamed cottage cheese

2 rounded tablespoons bonemeal or 2¼ teaspoons eggshell powder (see "Good Idea!" on page 382) or 4,000 mg calcium

1 to 2 teaspoons vegetable oil

2 tablespoons nutritional yeast

garlic or onion (optional)

GOOD IDEA!

If you buy a commercial weight-loss food for your pet, be sure it provides good-quality protein and nutrients, including a minimal but adequate amount of unsaturated fatty acids (oil). Feeding poor-quality dog food can cause a dog to gain weight—in an effort to get nutrients, the dog may overeat.

(continued)

GOOD IDEA!

If your chubby dog begs for food, offer low-calorie snacks, such as carrot sticks or leftover vegetables. A good weight-loss program provides bran, vegetables, and other high-fiber foods to assuage hunger, while providing about 60 percent of the calories needed to maintain ideal weight.

SUPPLIES

4-quart saucepan
spoon or paddle
freezer containers with lids
complete dog vitamins

Place vegetables in the saucepan, add water, and cook. When done, add oats and bran. Cover and let sit for 10 minutes until oats are soft. Add remaining ingredients and stir well. Refrigerate two meals' worth and serve raw. Freeze the rest in meal-size portions. Feed dog vitamins daily, as directed on the label, using the amount that fits your dog's ideal weight, or slightly more. Check with your veterinarian on what your dog's ideal weight should be. Feed your dog two meals a day, using the total amount of food from the table below.

➡ **Note:** Buy bonemeal at health food stores.

FEEDING OVERWEIGHT DOGS	
Dog's Ideal Weight	**Daily Total Intake**
10 lb.	about 2 cups
25 lb.	about 4 cups
40 lb.	about 5½ cups
60 lb.	about 7½ cups
85 lb.	about 9¼ cups

Hearty Food
for Puppies and Mother Dogs

When a dog is growing, pregnant, nursing pups, or under stress, it needs a high-protein, high-energy diet chock-full of good nutrition. Use this recipe as a regular food in any situation where more protein is desirable. Mothers and pups require 1½ to 2 times more food per body weight than the quantities listed on the table on page 391. Let puppies and mother dogs feed freely.

Yield: 6 to 7 cups

INGREDIENTS

4	cups cooked brown rice, room temperature
½	cup cooked vegetables (see page 379), room temperature
2	cups lean hamburger or ground lean beef heart or turkey, raw or cooked
2,500	I.U. vitamin A (with D)
1	tablespoon Healthy Powder (see page 382)
1	tablespoon Yeast Sprinkle (see page 381)
1	teaspoon eggshell powder (see "Good Idea!" on page 382) or 2¾ teaspoons bonemeal or 1,800 mg calcium
50	to 200 I.U. vitamin E

SUPPLIES

spoon or paddle
3-quart bowl

Thoroughly mix all ingredients in the bowl. Serve immediately. Discard any uneaten food at the end of the day.

✿ **Variation:** Occasionally omit the vitamin A and add 1 tablespoon liver.

➥ **Note:** Buy bonemeal and vitamins at health food stores.

GOOD IDEA!

If you have a new puppy, consider neutering your pet. The best time to neuter a puppy is usually between 6 and 8 months of age. Check with your veterinarian for the most appropriate timing for your pet. Neutering your puppy has several benefits. If you don't breed your pet, you increase the chances for adoption for the thousands of homeless pets in shelters right now. Neutering also eliminates unwanted behaviors. In male dogs, neutering eliminates the sex hormone testosterone, which is largely responsible for roaming, mounting, urine marking, and fighting with other dogs. Spaying a female eliminates the reproductive heat cycle. You won't have to contend with carpet stains from the discharge that occurs at that time.

GOOD IDEA!

Don't make your dog a finicky eater. Dogs are attracted to sweets, which are not good for them. Dogs that frequently receive sweets or table scraps often hold out for something better than dog food. To cure a finicky eater, don't leave uneaten food out and don't overindulge your dog by feeding excess table scraps or by hand feeding. Dogs get used to being hand-fed and are reluctant to give this habit up. If you give your dog table scraps, make the "human food" no more than 10 percent of its diet.

To unspoil a fussy eater, gradually introduce a well-balanced, palatable dog food over a period of a few weeks. And don't give into your dog's whims. If you do, you only train your pet to be more finicky. Keep in mind that, barring real illness, your dog will not starve himself.

Meatloaf for Dogs

Bake this recipe like a meatloaf or serve it raw, which will better preserve the nutrition. It ranges between 26 to 29 percent protein, depending on which meat and grain you use. Poultry, lean beef, oats, and bread are higher in protein than fatty meats and rice.

INGREDIENTS

¼ pound raw ground turkey, chicken, hamburger, chuck, or beef heart

6 slices whole wheat bread, crumbled, or 1½ cups rolled oats or 1⅔ cups cooked rice

½ to 1 cup whole milk (1 cup if you use bread or raw rolled oats)

2 large eggs

½ cup chopped vegetables (see page 379)

1 tablespoon vegetable oil

1 tablespoon Healthy Powder (see page 382)

1⅓ teaspoons bonemeal or scant ½ teaspoon eggshell powder (see "Good Idea!" on page 382) or 850 mg calcium

50 to 100 I.U. vitamin E

garlic or onion (optional)

SUPPLIES

2-quart bowl

spoon or paddle

freezer containers with lids

2-quart casserole (optional)

Combine all ingredients in the bowl and mix well. Refrigerate two meals' worth and serve raw. Freeze the rest in meal-size portions. Or press into the casserole 1 to 2 inches thick and bake at 350°F until lightly browned, 20 to 30 minutes. See page 391 for feeding guidelines.

↠ **Note:** Buy bonemeal and vitamins at health food stores.

Deluxe Dog Biscuits

Here's a real treat—fresh, homemade dog biscuits!—from Joan Harper's *Healthy Dog and Cat Cookbook*.

INGREDIENTS

2 cups whole wheat flour
¼ cup corn meal
½ cup soy flour
½ cup sunflower or pumpkin seeds
1 teaspoon iodized salt
1 teaspoon bonemeal
2 tablespoons corn oil or soy oil
¼ cup unsulfured molasses
   garlic or onion (optional)
2 large eggs mixed with ¼ cup milk

SUPPLIES

spoon or paddle
2-quart bowl
rolling pin
pastry brush
pastry wheel or knife
cookie sheets

Mix all dry ingredients in the bowl. Add oil and molasses, garlic or onion, if desired, plus all but 1 tablespoon of the egg/milk mixture. Knead together a few minutes to make a firm dough, adding more milk if needed. Let dough rest ½ hour or more. Roll out to ½ inch. Brush with remaining egg/milk mixture and cut into biscuit-size pieces with a pastry wheel or knife. Bake on cookie sheets at 350°F for 30 minutes or until lightly toasted. To make the biscuits harder, turn off the heat after baking and leave in the oven for an hour or more. See page 391 for feeding guidelines.

➼ **Note:** Buy bonemeal at health food stores.

GOOD IDEA!

Don't rely on dog biscuits to keep your pet's teeth clean. Many pet owners think that dogs clean their own teeth with hard dog biscuits. In reality, both dogs and cats fare best if they are examined annually by a veterinarian for evidence of periodontal disease. Your veterinarian may recommend a program of home dental care that includes daily brushing of your dog's teeth. He may even recommend that you have your dog's teeth cleaned professionally on a regular basis.

As for the old notion that dog biscuits make good toothbrushes, it's a half-truth. Dog biscuits help clean teeth somewhat, if the dog chews the biscuit slowly and thoroughly. Most larger dogs will simply break the biscuit into manageable pieces and then gulp it down.

GOOD IDEA!

If your dog won't eat vegetarian fare, try weaning him from the old food gradually. At first, mix only a small portion of vegetarian fare into the old preferred food. Each day, gradually increase the proportion of vegetarian food until your dog has grown accustomed to the new diet.

Dogs are social animals and prefer to eat when people or other animals are around. To encourage your dog to finish a new food, try praising and petting him while he eats.

Vegetarian Diet for Dogs

Dogs are somewhat omnivorous and can get along on a vegetarian diet if it includes ample dairy products. Do not feed a meatless diet to cats, however, or they will develop deficiencies in several nutrients.

INGREDIENTS

2   cups rolled oats
     water or broth
2   large eggs
1   cup creamed cottage cheese
¼   cup chopped vegetables (see page 379)
2   tablespoons Healthy Powder (see page 382)
1   tablespoon vegetable oil
2   teaspoons bonemeal or ¾ teaspoon eggshell powder (see "Good Idea!" on page 382) or 1,400 mg calcium
50 to 100 I.U. vitamin E
     garlic or onion (optional)

SUPPLIES

2-quart saucepan
spoon or paddle
sealable container (optional)

Put oats in the saucepan and cover twice as deep with water or broth. Bring to a boil, turn off the heat, and let sit about 10 minutes. When the oats are soft, but still hot, mix in the eggs. After it coagulates, add remaining ingredients and serve warm. Immediately refrigerate leftovers tightly sealed. See page 391 for feeding guidelines.

✿ **Variations:** For cottage cheese and one egg, substitute 8 ounces tofu and three eggs. For flavor, add a little cheese or Yeast Sprinkle (see page 381). If you omit the vegetables occasionally, add 1,500 to 2,000 I.U. vitamin A supplement, like cod-liver oil.

➡ **Note:** Buy bonemeal and vitamins at health food stores.

Dog Oats 'n' Meat

This basic recipe, which can be varied with different meats, grains and vegetables, is easy to fix and is well-accepted. The protein level averages 29 percent of dry weight, which is higher than the minimal recommendations (22 percent) found in many dog foods.

INGREDIENTS

2 cups rolled oats

water or broth

1 cup raw ground chicken, turkey, hamburger, chuck, or beef heart

¼ cup chopped vegetables (see page 379)

2 tablespoons Healthy Powder (see page 382)

1 tablespoon vegetable oil

2 slightly rounded teaspoons bonemeal or ¾ teaspoon eggshell powder (see "Good Idea!" on page 382) or 1,400 mg calcium

50 to 100 I.U. vitamin E

garlic or onion (optional)

SUPPLIES

2-quart saucepan

spoon or paddle

sealable container (optional)

Put oats in the saucepan and cover twice as deep with water or broth. Bring to a boil, turn off the heat, and let sit about 10 minutes. When the oats are soft, but still hot, mix in remaining ingredients and serve warm. Immediately refrigerate leftovers tightly sealed. See page 391 for feeding guidelines.

✿ **Variation:** If you omit the vegetables occasionally, add 1,500 to 2,000 I.U. vitamin A supplement, like cod-liver oil.

➺ **Note:** Buy bonemeal and vitamins at health food stores.

GOOD IDEA!

For optimum results in a homemade pet diet, use only organically raised and minimally processed foods. If you find it too difficult to find organic sources for everything, use the best whole, fresh foods you can afford. They will be a vast improvement over commercial products, which can be laced with anything from preservatives to moldy grains or sugar.

Also aim for variety. Don't always use the same cut or type of meat, the same grain, or the same vegetable. By changing the contents of the basic diet, you'll ensure the best balance of nutrients for your dog's health.

PET HEALTH AND GROOMING

Combine commercial grooming products with home-made formulas to give your pet's skin and coat extra good care. You can also soothe motion sickness and "hot spots".

Dry Shampoo

Here's a way to clean a pet that resists water bathing.

Yield: 1 shampoo

SUPPLIES

bran, oatmeal, and/or cornmeal

cookie sheet

bath towel

pet brush

Place the grain(s) on a cookie sheet and warm in the oven on low heat. Remove a small amount at a time, so that it stays comfortably warm, *not* hot. Rub into the fur with the towel concentrating on greasy, dirty areas. Then thoroughly brush out.

After-Bath Rinse for Dogs and Cats

This formula removes soap residue and helps prevent dandruff.

Yield: 1 rinse

INGREDIENTS

1 tablespoon white vinegar

1 pint warm water

Add vinegar into the measure of water. When you have thoroughly rinsed the shampoo off your pet, pour on the solution and rub throughout the fur. Rinse again with plain water.

GOOD IDEA!

To remove grease spots, such as those cats get on their heads and backs from lurking under cars, rub a small amount of Murphy's Oil Soap and warm water onto the spot. Rinse thoroughly with warm water.

GOOD IDEA!

For a glossy coat, try a rosemary coat conditioner. Add 1 teaspoon dried rosemary to 1 cup boiling water. Let steep for 10 minutes. Strain out rosemary and let cool to body temperature. Pour over your dog or cat after the final shampoo rinse.

Abscess Irrigation Formula

An abscess, most commonly found in cats, is a pus-filled swelling that resembles a boil. Unlike a boil, it results from the premature closing and subsequent infection in a puncture wound. After your pet's abscess has been opened by your veterinarian, use this formula twice a day to gently flush out debris and infectious material from the wound.

Yield: 1 cup

INGREDIENTS

¼ teaspoon sea salt (or table salt)
1 teaspoon Betadine solution
1 cup distilled or spring water

SUPPLIES

stirrer
bowl of hot water
infant ear syringe or bulb-type poultry baster

Mix salt and Betadine into the cup of water. Warm to body temperature by setting the cup in the bowl of hot water. Fill the syringe or baster with the formula. Gently place your cat in a bathtub and stroke it reassuringly. If your veterinarian has inserted a drain tube, gently insert just the tip of the syringe or baster into the tube opening, taking care not to wiggle the tube. Slowly inject the solution into the abscess pocket. If you inject it too forcefully, it will tickle and cause your cat to struggle. Gently press the abscess pocket flat, expressing the fluid and abscess contents out. Repeat this procedure two or three times.

✿ **Variation:** *Instead of Betadine, use 10 drops goldenseal extract or tincture of echinacea to help cleanse and reduce swelling.*

↔ **Notes:** *Buy Betadine solution at your pharmacy. Buy goldenseal extract or tincture of echinacea at health food stores and herb shops.*

GOOD IDEA!

If your pet is recovering from an abscess, provide nutritional and herbal support to help heal the wound. For three days following the opening of an abscess, give your pet 250 milligrams of vitamin C three times a day plus 5,000 I.U. of vitamin A once a day. Also give your pet 1 drop of tincture of echinacea every 4 hours throughout the three-day treatment period.

Echinacea stimulates the immune system to fight infection. Buy it at health food stores and herb shops. When buying vitamin C, buy it as sodium ascorbate powder and sprinkle it on your pet's food. Vitamin C sold as ascorbic acid has a highly acidic taste that many pets reject.

Healing Mouthwash

Periodontal disease in pets is caused by a buildup of plaque on the teeth, a condition that is more likely to occur when the teeth are overcrowded or the jaw is oddly shaped. As plaque accumulates, it causes inflammation, swelling, and receding. If your pet has bleeding gums, foul breath, excess salivation, painful chewing, or loss of appetite and weight, have a veterinarian examine its mouth. After teeth cleaning, your pet's gums will be sore and inflamed. To speed healing, use this mouthwash.

Yield: 1 cup

INGREDIENTS

1 teaspoon fresh echinacea root or ½ teaspoon dried
1 cup water

SUPPLIES

stainless steel, enamel, or glass saucepan
strainer
bulb-type poultry baster, syringe without needle, or eyedropper

In the saucepan, boil echinacea in water for 10 minutes. Cover, remove from heat, and let steep for an hour. Strain and apply it to the gums with the baster, syringe, or eyedropper.

✿ **Variation:** Boil 2 cups water and add 1 teaspoon powdered goldenseal root. Remove from heat and steep until the water is cool. Strain and apply the clear liquid.

➥ **Note:** Buy echinacea and goldenseal at health food stores and herb shops.

Cut and Abrasion Treatment

You can easily treat slight cuts or abrasions at home.

Yield: 1 cup

INGREDIENTS

1 cup warm distilled or spring water

¼ teaspoon sea salt (or table salt)

1 teaspoon calendula solution or tincture

SUPPLIES

1-pint bowl

stirrer

washcloth

vitamins A and E

Place water in the bowl. Mix in salt and calendula. Soak the washcloth in the solution and hold it against the wound for 2 minutes. Treat two or three times a day. Once a scab forms, stop treatment. Give 2,500 to 10,000 I.U. vitamin A (depending on your pet's size) once a day for three days and give 100 to 500 I.U. vitamin E (depending on size) once a day for five days.

➡ **Note:** Buy sea salt and calendula tincture at health food stores, herb shops, and homeopathic pharmacies.

GOOD IDEA!

To speed healing, don't bandage minor wounds. Also, don't worry if your pet licks a wound. Animal saliva promotes healing and repair.

GOOD IDEA!

Use a bar of soap to stop bleeding from a claw. If you accidentally trim your pet's nail too short, simply press the bleeding nail into a bar of soap. It stops the bleeding almost immediately.

"Hot-Spot" Relief

"Hot spots" are moist, highly inflammed skin erruptions that bother many dogs and even some cats. To offer your pet hot-spot relief, all you need is a teabag of black or green tea. The tannic acid in these two types of tea helps heal hot spots.

Simply dunk a teabag briefly in scalding water, just as if you were making a cup of tea. Remove the tea from the water and let it cool to a comfortable temperature. Press it gently against the hot spot for a few minutes while holding and petting your animal. Or, if your pet will tolerate the minor annoyance, tie the teabag in place with a strip of cloth and leave it on the hot spot for up to an hour. If hot spots fail to improve, see your veterinarian.

GOOD IDEA!

Apply skin treatments to pets right before meals or walks. If you do, your pet will often be temporarily distracted by the activity so that the relief may be in effect by the time it would usually get preoccupied with its skin again.

GOOD IDEA!

Treat your pet's itch with colloidal oatmeal. The colloidal oatmeal commonly sold in health food stores and pharmacies not only relieves itching for people but also for dogs and cats. Mix 2 tablespoons colloidal oatmeal with 2 gallons cold water and use to rinse and wet down the affected areas over the entire body. Applied as a cold rinse, colloidal oatmeal will often give itch relief for 24 to 36 hours.

Itch and Eczema Relief

Many animals have trouble in the summer with itching and scratching from fleas or allergies. Completely curing the problem requires help from your veterinarian. However, it helps to have some safe and simple things to do at home to relieve the worst aspects of the skin irritation.

Yield: 1 pint

INGREDIENTS

1 rounded tablespoon dried chickweed (*Stellaria media*)

1 rounded tablespoon dried plantain (*Plantago lanceolata*)

1 rounded tablespoon dried yellow dock (*Rumex crispus*)

1 pint boiling water

SUPPLIES

teapot or covered 1-quart casserole
cotton balls

Place herbs in the teapot or casserole. Add boiling water and let steep, covered, for 20 minutes. When cool, store in the refrigerator until quite cold. Apply the cold herbal infusion to the irritated skin areas with a saturated cotton ball several times a day, as needed.

✿ **Variation:** If this treatment doesn't provide relief, try aloe vera. Break off a small piece of aloe vera leaf and apply it several times a day directly to the affected skin or buy a ready-made aloe vera gel. It will not harm your animal to lick it off.

➡ **Notes:** Buy ingredients at health food stores and herb shops. Unprocessed aloe vera gel is more effective than the "stabilized" variety.

Herbal Flea Powder

Fleas have become very resistant to chemicals. At this point, it is not clear who is going to win the Great Flea Wars. However, it can be helpful to use herbal repellents even if you can't completely get rid of the fleas. Like most creatures, fleas don't like to be where it doesn't smell good to them.

Yield: varies by amount of ingredients chosen

INGREDIENTS

1 part eucalyptus powder
1 part fennel powder
1 part pennyroyal powder
1 part yellow dock powder (*Rumex crispus*)

SUPPLIES

shaker-topped jar with big holes, such as a jar for dried parsley flakes
pet comb (optional)

☛ **BE SAFE.** *Use sparingly in cats since they lick themselves so much. Avoid getting powder in your pet's eyes or nose. Do not use in large amounts. Do not use this formula on pregnant animals.*

Combine all ingredients in the jar and shake to mix. Apply to your pet's coat by brushing backward with your hand or the comb and sprinkling the powder into the roots of the hairs. Concentrate on the neck, back, and belly. Use just enough to add a little odor to the hairs. In severe flea infestations, treat daily; otherwise, two or three times a week is sufficient.

➠ **Note:** *Buy ingredients at health food stores and herb shops.*

GOOD IDEA!

To repel fleas, give your pet fresh garlic and brewer's yeast mixed with food. About 25 percent of animals will be more repellent to fleas if you use garlic and brewer's yeast in the diet regularly. On a daily basis, give 1/2 clove of garlic to cats and 1/2 to 2 cloves to dogs, depending on their size. Give 1 teaspoon yeast to a cat and 1 teaspoon to 3 tablespoons to a dog. Some animals like these flavors and some don't, so experiment.

Ear Mites in Cats

Ear mites, small parasitic creatures that infest cats' ears, cause itching and a dark, dry crusty material inside the ears.

Treat ear mites with almond oil and dried yellow dock (*Rumex crispus*), both of which are available at health food stores and herb shops. First, heat the almond oil to body temperature. While someone holds the cat, clean out its ears with warm oil. Hold the ear tip to prevent shaking and put ½ eyedropperful into the ear. Carefully massage around the base of the ear. Then press in at the base of the ear to push the oil up to the opening, using a tissue to remove the excess oil. Repeat every other day for a total of three treatments.

Six days after the first treatment, begin yellow dock infusions. Steep 1 rounded teaspoon in 1 cup boiling water for 15 minutes. Cool to body temperature. Clean the ear with this infusion, just as you did with the almond oil. Repeat the yellow dock treatment every other day for three treatments.

GOOD IDEA!

Take extra care with floppy-eared dogs. Dogs with this type of ear have the most frequent swimmer's ear infections. The drooping ear flap holds moisture in the ear and leads to infection. To dry the ears of a floppy-eared dog, gently clothespin or tie the ears up behind the head. Don't pin or tie the skin, just any extra hair that may extend from the end of the ears.

Canine "Swimmer's Ear" Formula

If your dog swims often, clean the ears with this solution after swimming.

Yield: 1 cup

INGREDIENTS

juice from ½ lemon
1 cup lukewarm water

SUPPLIES

eyedropper, infant ear syringe, or small cup
cotton balls

Add lemon juice into the water. Using the eyedropper, syringe, or cup, introduce it into the ear. Gently massage the ear canal (feels like a small plastic tube in the area underneath the ear) from the outside. Allow your dog to shake its head, then *gently* blot up extra moisture with cotton balls. Do *not* use cotton swabs because they could push wax against the eardrum or damage it.

Mange Parasite Treatment

Mange, a skin irritation caused by a skin parasite, should be identified and treated by your veterinarian. This simple treatment provides additional relief.

Yield: 1 pint

INGREDIENTS

1 lemon, thinly sliced
1 clove garlic, peeled and grated
2 cups boiling distilled or spring water

Add lemon and garlic to the boiling water. Let sit until room temperature. Pour over the affected skin twice a day until the problem is resolved.

Ringworm Treatment

Ringworm, a fungus that grows on the skin, can be easily treated if it is not too extensive. Ringworm that covers a large area requires veterinary care.

SUPPLIES

small scissors
cotton swabs
tincture of goldenseal

Clip the hair around the ringworm patch. Once a day, dip a cotton swab into the goldenseal tincture and paint the entire affected area. Limit the treated area to a dime-size spot in cats and small animals and up to a quarter-size spot in larger dogs. If there is more than one spot, alternate daily treatments from one spot to the other.

➤ **Note:** Buy goldenseal tincture at health food stores and herb shops.

GOOD IDEA!

To prevent infecting people, take a dog with mange symptoms to a vet. Mange is caused by two different skin mites. Demodex canis usually results in mild hair loss; Sarcoptes scabei mange causes intense itching, scaling, and hair loss and is extremely contagious to people and animals.

GOOD IDEA!

If your pet has ringworm, keep children away. Ringworm is contagious and can be passed from your pet to people or other animals. If you are treating your pet for ringworm, check your own skin frequently for signs of the infection. If you develop ringworm lesions yourself, see your doctor for treatment.

Cleansing Drops for Eyes and Nose

In response to dust or disease, dogs and cats often develop an uncomfortable discharge from the nose or eyes. For persistent nose or eye discharge, see your veterinarian for a diagnosis and appropriate medical treatment. In addition to prescribed medical treatment, you can provide important nursing care for your pet by gently cleansing the eyes and nose with a warm saltwater solution. To prepare the solution, dissolve ¼ teaspoon salt in 1 cup boiling distilled water. Let the solution cool to body temperature before using.

For safety, apply nose and eye drops using a saturated cotton ball and your index finger rather than an eyedropper or syringe. If your pet should move suddenly, it won't be poked in the eye with a pointed object. Be sure your fingernails are short.

To practice applying drops to the eyes, saturate a cotton ball with the solution and squeeze it out just a little. Place the saturated cotton ball between your thumb and index finger and let the solution dribble out of the cotton, down your index finger, and off your fingertip. Practice this drip technique until you can accurately drip solution one drop at a time onto a target about an inch below your hand.

When you're sure of your technique, pick up your pet and face it away from you, gently but firmly holding it between your legs so that it can't back up. Stroke your pet soothingly. With your left hand, tilt its head back, placing your fingers and thumb under the cheekbone. With your right hand, dip a cotton ball into the solution and gently dribble three or four drops onto the inner corner of the eye, in the manner you just practiced.

If your pet closes its eye when the drops hit, put the cotton swab down and coax the eye open by gently massaging upward on the skin above the eye. After the fluid runs into the eye, immediately blot off any excess with a tissue.

Release the head, petting and praising your animal. If its tongue flicks out briefly, the solution has passed through the tear duct into the back of the throat. This means you have opened the tear duct. If your pet doesn't flick its tongue, repeat the procedure up to three times. Treat both eyes.

To cleanse the nose, use a very similar position and procedure. With your pet's head tilted back and nostrils facing the ceiling, dribble three or four drops of the salt solution into one nostril only. Hold the head back five or six seconds so that the drops will go down into the sinuses. Wipe with a tissue. After your pet swallows and relaxes a bit, do the other nostril.

For convenience, you can refrigerate the salt solution in a sealed jar for a week or two. Before you use it, put a tablespoon or two in a small cup and warm it to body temperature by placing the cup in a larger bowl of hot water.

If you like, you can add herbal extracts to the basic saline solution just before you use it. Add 1 drop goldenseal extract per 2 tablespoons salt solution to help disinfect and shrink swollen tissues. To help soothe inflamed tissue, add 1 drop eyebright extract (*Euphrasia officinalis*) per 2 tablespoons salt solution.

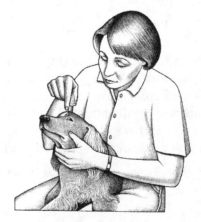

Eye Ointment

Use one of these oils as a soothing eye ointment.

SUPPLIES

olive oil (for mild irritations), castor oil (for more
    irritated, inflamed eyes), or cod-liver oil (for dry or
    ulcerated eyes)
tissues

First, cleanse irritated eyes with saltwater as described
on the opposite page. Choose the appropriate oil and apply
one drop to the inner corner of each eye. Use the same finger drop technique that you used to apply the saltwater.
Blot off excess oil with tissues.

Nose Care Ointment

Use this remedy for a sore, plugged-up nose.

SUPPLIES

petroleum jelly or petroleum jelly mixed with pow-
    dered goldenseal root; almond oil; or 2 tablespoons
    olive oil mixed with 2 drops tincture of calendula
tissues

If your pet has a plugged-up nose, apply saltwater
drops as described on the opposite page. Then, holding
your pet from behind as you did for the nosedrops, dip
your finger in one of the above ointments and apply to the
nose two or three times a day. Blot off excess with tissues.

➥ **Note:** Buy calendula tincture at health food stores, herb
shops, and homeopathic pharmacies.

GOOD IDEA!

To remove dried,
**hard secretions from
your pet's eyes,** use saltwater. Mix ½ teaspoon
sea salt (or table salt) with
1 pint warm, distilled
water. To soften secre-
tions, saturate soft gauze
or cotton in the salt solution and gently wipe the
eyes.

GOOD IDEA!

To remove hardened
**secretions from your
pet's nose,** wipe the
nose with cloth or a
gauze pad dipped in
warm water. If the mate-
rial is so hardened that it
is difficult to remove,
apply warm, damp cloths
in several short sessions,
softening and removing
small amounts each time.

First-Aid for Poisoning

Pets are usually poisoned two ways—by licking a toxic substance off the coat or by swallowing a toxin directly. To be prepared for accidental poisoning, keep a bottle of activated charcoal on hand. This nonprescription item is available at most pharmacies. When an animal gets poisoned, time is of the essence; having activated charcoal may save its life.

If your pet is poisoned, call your veterinarian for instructions. He may recommend that you immediately administer activated charcoal. Make a very thick mixture of charcoal and water—like thick soup. Give 2 tablespoons to a cat or small dog. For medium and large dogs, give 3 tablespoons to 2 cups, depending on size—a little too much won't harm your animal.

If your pet won't drink this antidote, administer it with a spoon, a bulb syringe, or a bulb-type poultry baster. Do not force your pet to swallow large amounts at one time. Proceed slowly to prevent choking. Do not give any poison antidote to an unconscious animal.

If you don't have activated charcoal, give your pet whole milk. Give 2 tablespoons to a cat or small dog; 3 tablespoons to 2 cups to a medium or large dog. If you have no milk, use water as a last resort; milk is much more effective.

If a poison is on your pet's skin or coat, immediately bathe the animal, repeatedly shampooing and rinsing with water until you can no longer see or smell the toxin.

Weaning Formula

The mother may still produce milk when weaning. This formula should help with the "drying off" process.

Yield: 1 cup

INGREDIENTS

2 teaspoons dried stinging nettle
1 cup boiling distilled or spring water

Add nettle to the boiling water. Let steep for 20 minutes. When cool, give a cat ½ teaspoon three times a day for three to five days (or until milk production stops). Give a dog ½ teaspoon to 2 tablespoons, depending on size.

➻ **Note:** Buy stinging nettle at health food stores and herb shops.

Tick Prevention and Removal

This herbal powder may repel ticks enough that they don't sign up for a ride on your pet.

Yield: varies by amount of ingredients chosen

INGREDIENTS

1 part powdered rosemary
1 part powdered rue
1 part powdered wormwood

SUPPLIES

shaker-topped jar with big holes, such as a jar for dried parsley flakes
flea comb (optional)

☛ **BE SAFE.** Do not use this powder as continuous prevention. Also, avoid getting it in your pet's eyes or nose. Dog ticks can transmit Rocky Mountain spotted fever to humans. Thoroughly wash your hands after handling ticks.

Mix herbs in the jar and shake to combine. Store in a dark, cool place. Before you take your animal out in a tick-infested area, groom its coat, removing loose hair and mats. Then dust the coat with this powder. Work it in thoroughly with your fingers, concentrating on the neck, back, and legs, and underneath the tail and ear flaps. After you return from the outing, examine your pet and remove any ticks that have attached themselves. Also, use the comb to capture ticks that haven't yet attached. If you accidentally break off a tick's body and can't get the head out of your pet's skin, don't worry. It may fester a little, but it's not a serious problem. Treat a buried tick head with calendula tincture.

➥ **Note:** Buy ingredients at health food stores and herb shops.

GOOD IDEA!

To remove stubborn ticks from your dog or cat, use the old-fashioned hot match trick. Light a match and blow it out. Place the hot match head on the tick's back. The heat will cause the tick to release its grip. Take care not to singe your pet and don't try this on an animal that is jumpy or hard to keep still.

To remove newly attached small ticks, grasp the head of the tick with a pair of tweezers. Use a very slow, steady pull with a slight twist to remove the tick. This technique usually gets the whole tick out, head included.

Remedy for Gastrointestinal Upsets

If a dog or cat is experiencing temporary gastrointestinal upset, such as diarrhea, vomiting, or gas, this herbal treatment is very soothing.

Yield: 1 cup

INGREDIENTS

1 cup distilled or spring water

1 teaspoon slippery elm powder

1 tablespoon honey (for dogs)

SUPPLIES

1-pint saucepan

spoon or paddle

teaspoon, baby ear syringe, or bulb-type poultry baster

Place water in the saucepan and mix in powder, stirring well to remove all lumps. Bring to a boil, stirring constantly. After mixture reaches a boil, turn down to simmer and stir a few more minutes until it thickens slightly. Remove from heat. Allow to cool. Add honey for dogs. Mix it in food at mealtime; otherwise, you can give it with the teaspoon, syringe, or baster. Give ½ teaspoon three or four times a day to a cat. Give 1 teaspoon to 3 tablespoons (depending on size) three or four times a day to a dog.

➻ **Note:** *Buy slippery elm powder at health food stores and herb shops.*

Help for Your Constipated Pet

Constipation can be caused by inadequate dietary fiber, lack of exercise, stress, or poor-quality food. A dirty litter box or not being let out enough may discourage pets from engaging in normal bowel habits. If your pet suffers from frequent constipation, see your veterinarian for a diagnosis. For occasional constipation, add psyllium seed powder to each meal. Psyllium seed adds fiber to your pet's diet. Give a cat ¼ to ½ teaspoon; a dog, depending on size, should get ½ teaspoon to 1 tablespoon. Always feed moist food with psyllium, either fresh home-prepared food, canned food, or kibble moistened with water or broth.

Worming Aid

Many different kinds of worms afflict dogs and cats. Most worms bother younger animals—especially those under 6 months of age. However, others, such as hookworms and whipworms, can plague animals of any age. Complete elimination requires an individualized veterinary program for each type of parasite. However, there are several things you can do that will aid the process by discouraging the worms and making your pet more resistant. Try adding some or all of these to the daily food (whatever your pet will accept), along with regular treatment, until your veterinarian finds no more worm eggs in the stool.

Yield: 1 treatment

INGREDIENTS
FOR CATS

½ clove garlic

½ teaspoon raw, unprocessed diatomaceous earth

1 tablespoon fresh ground meat

INGREDIENTS
FOR DOGS

½ to 2 cloves garlic

½ teaspoon to 1 tablespoon raw, unprocessed diatomaceous earth

1 tablespoon to ¼ cup fresh ground meat or Meat Supplement for Dog Kibble (see page 392)

Combine all ingredients and mix with your pet's regular food. Serve with each meal. Choose the amount of ingredients for dogs based on size.

➻ **Note:** Diatomaceous earth must be in the raw, unprocessed form. Do not use diatomacous earth sold for use with swimming pool filters. See page 444 for a source.

GOOD IDEA!

Have your dog checked for heartworms. Heartworms are spread by mosquitoes and are an extremely common cause of heart disease in dogs.

To prevent the spread of heartworm infestation, ask your veterinarian to perform a simple blood test to determine if your pet is already infested. If the test is positive, your vet will begin treatment for the worms right away. If the test is negative, your veterinarian will begin treatment with a drug that prevents heartworms. The newest preventive drug, Ivermicten, is so effective your dog needs only a single tablet once a month. Treatment usually begins in the spring, continues throughout the summer months, and ends 60 days after mosquito season is over.

GOOD IDEA!

Before a trip, consider fasting (plenty of water but no solid food) for a susceptible pet. Begin fasting 24 hours before departure, particularly if going by public transit. Fasting also helps to prevent a pet traveling in a container from getting soiled with its own excrement.

Motion Sickness and Travel Stress Treatment

Traveling can cause motion sickness in some animals. This regimen can help to prevent these problems.

SUPPLIES

B-complex, low-potency vitamins (5 to 20 mg)

$\frac{1}{16}$ teaspoon sodium ascorbate powder (250 mg vitamin C)

10,000 I.U. vitamin A capsules (with 400 I.U. vitamin D)

peppermint tea or capsules

Starting two weeks ahead of the trip, give your pet the B-complex and vitamin C every day. Give about 5 milligrams of B complex to a cat; 5 to 20 milligrams to a dog, depending on size. Give a single vitamin A and D capsule once a week. Double or triple these dosages for larger dogs. If motion sickness begins to occur during the trip, give your pet some peppermint tea (available at many restaurants!) or peppermint capsules, which will help to settle its stomach. Use one capsule for a cat; one to three capsules for a dog.

Help for Gas and Diarrhea

If your dog or cat has temporary gas or foul diarrhea, try this treatment described in Anitra Frazier's book, *The New Natural Cat.*

Give your pet one capsule of activated charcoal (two or three for large dogs). Charcoal helps to absorb impurities and toxic wastes from the intestines. Repeat the next day, if needed, but do not continue beyond that because charcoal absorbs digestive enzymes.

After the charcoal treatment, mix 1 part liquid chlorophyll and 2 parts liquid acidophilus. Feed $\frac{1}{4}$ teaspoon of this mixture twice a day in the food (up to 1 teaspoon for larger dogs). If your pet won't eat it, mix with a little chicken broth and give as a liquid medication. The chlorophyll helps to purify the intestines, and the acidophilus introduces "friendly" bacteria into the gastrointestinal tract. If the problem continues for more than a few days, consult your veterinarian. You can buy all the ingredients for this treatment at health food stores.

Herbal Cough Treatment

See a veterinarian for diagnosis of persistent cough. This formula may soothe the symptoms.

Yield: 1 cup

INGREDIENTS

1 cup distilled or spring water
1 teaspoon slippery elm powder

SUPPLIES

1-pint saucepan

spoon or paddle

teaspoon, infant ear syringe, or bulb-type poultry baster

sealable container

vitamin C (250 to 1,000 mg)

Place water in the saucepan, mix in powder, and stir well to remove all lumps. Bring to a boil, stirring constantly. Then reduce heat, simmer, and stir a few minutes until mixture thickens slightly. Remove from heat. Allow to cool. To soothe the throat, give ½ teaspoon three or four times a day to a cat. For a dog, give 1 teaspoon to 3 tablespoons (depending on size) three or four times a day. Mix it in food or give it with the teaspoon, syringe, or baster. Refrigerate leftovers, tightly sealed, for a few days. Give vitamin C, 250 milligrams three times a day to a cat. Give a dog 250 to 1,000 milligrams (depending on size) three times a day. Continue treatment until pet is well.

GOOD IDEA!

Use steam to relieve your pet's cough. Run a very hot shower for a few minutes until the bathroom is steamy. Then place your pet in the bathroom until the coughing ceases. You can repeat this several times a day.

GOOD IDEA!

Use a long-handled scrub brush to clean a litter box. Be sure it's reserved for this purpose only. Put used cat litter (without chemical additives) in your compost heap, unless your soil already contains too much clay (which is what litter is).

Litter Box Cleaner and Disinfectant

This keeps your cat's litter box germ-free.

Yield: 1½ cups

INGREDIENTS

1 tablespoon liquid hand soap or scented liquid castile soap

1 tablespoon chlorine bleach

1½ cups water

SUPPLIES

1-pint plastic spray bottle

Add soap and bleach to the spray bottle. Add water and shake. Spray the empty, rinsed box thoroughly and let it sit for 2 minutes. Rinse, dry, and refill.

➥ **Note:** Castile soap is made from olive oil and is available at health food stores and specialty gift shops.

GOOD IDEA!

To the odor from a pet-urine stain on carpets, mix 2 cups corn-meal with 1 cup borax and sprinkle on the spot after using carpet sham-poo. Let sit for 1 hour; vacuum. (Borax is toxic. Keep it away from chil-dren.) To keep a cat from respraying the area, thor-oughly wash out the orig-inal stain. Spray the spot with white vinegar.

Rosemary Spot Remover

This homemade soap removes pet stains and odors.

Yield: one 8-ounce tub

INGREDIENTS

1 bar castile soap, grated

1 ounce rosemary oil

1 ounce rubbing alcohol

SUPPLIES

double boiler

spoon or paddle

8-ounce margarine tub with lid

Melt soap in the top part of a double boiler. Stir in oil and alcohol. Pour in the tub and let set.

➥ **Note:** Castile soap is made from olive oil and is available at health food stores and specialty gift shops.

FEEDING SMALL ANIMALS

These recipes promote good health for birds, rabbits, and gerbils. The best diet for small animals begins with fresh ingredients without additives or preservatives.

Parakeet and Cockatiel Mix

Parakeets and cockatiels thrive best on a diet that is primarily seeds. Here's a good combination.

Yield: varies by amount of ingredients chosen

INGREDIENTS

2 parts millet
2 parts whole oats
1 part safflower seeds
1 part buckwheat, wheatberries, or sunflower seeds

SUPPLIES

sealable container

Mix ingredients in the container and store, tightly sealed, in a dark, cool place. Use as the main food source, supplementing it with fresh fruits and vegetables daily.

> **GOOD IDEA!**
>
> **Y**our parakeet may enjoy dog food. An all-natural dry kibble for older dogs makes a good supplement to the everyday fare for your parakeet or cockatiel. In addition, you may treat your bird with small chunks of apple, orange, banana, grapes, corn on the cob, green beans, or okra.

Rabbit Fare

Supplement pelleted rabbit food with these fresh foods: apples; cabbage; carrots; fresh clover, grass, alfalfa, or any leafy hay; stale (but not moldy) bread; sweet potatoes; and turnips.

Feed your rabbit all the hay or alfalfa he wants. If you use fresh grass or clover from your yard, be sure it has not been treated with herbicides or pesticides. Introduce new foods slowly, one at a time. Feeding excessive greens can cause diarrhea. Do not feed young rabbits (under six months) fresh greens.

GOOD IDEA!

Offer your parrot a relaxing shower from your plant mister. Wild parrots bathe in the rain. To duplicate a refreshing afternoon rain, fill your plant mister with lukewarm water and lightly mist your pet until its feathers are damp. Then sit back and watch your parrot preen and groom. To complete your parrot spa treatment, stand an ordinary incandescent lamp next to a corner of the cage. Your pet may enjoy basking in the mild heat of the lamp while its feathers dry.

Parrot Custard

This simple custard is an excellent treat for parrots. It is especially valuable for sick birds. Besides being yummy, it is high in protein and is easily digested.

Yield: 2½ cups

INGREDIENTS

2 cups pasteurized milk

2 to 3 tablespoons honey or sugar

2 large eggs, beaten well

hot water

SUPPLIES

1-quart bowl

four 6-ounce custard cups

folded towel or wire cooling rack

roasting pan

Place milk and honey or sugar in the bowl and blend well. Add beaten eggs and whip ingredients together. Pour into custard cups. Place the towel or wire rack in the pan. Cover with an inch of hot, not boiling, water. Set the cups on the towel or rack and bake at 325°F for 30 to 45 minutes. Insert a knife near the edge of the cup. If it comes out clean, the custard is set. Let cool. Store leftovers in the refrigerator.

Happy Hamsters and Gerbils

Gerbils and hamsters have similar dietary needs. Feed a packaged mix from the pet store or mix your own food using these ingredients: 3 parts each millet, rolled barley, rolled oats, and sunflower seeds, *plus* 4 parts each rabbit pellets and rolled corn.

To supplement the basic diet, offer your pet hard foods for gnawing, such as rabbit pellets or dog biscuits, as well as fresh raw foods and trimmings, such as carrots, potatoes, apples, watermelon rinds, banana peels, dandelion greens, and clover.

Pampering Your Parrot

Good nutrition and husbandry are the keys to good health for any pet bird. Many people believe that packaged seed mixes provide an adequate diet for birds, but according to avian veterinarian Yvonne Nelson of Daphne, Alabama, this is not true. While seeds are an important part of an avian diet (particularly for parakeets and cockatiels) she says, they do not provide adequate amounts of some nutrients, such as vitamins A and C. Dr. Nelson notes that the lack of such nutrients is the underlying cause of avian respiratory infections.

In addition, parrots need less fat and more protein than seeds provide. There are special pelleted bird foods for these needs, but Dr. Nelson thinks they may contain high levels of ethoxyquin, a food preservative, and other objectionable ingredients. Dr. Nelson has created a feeding regimen for her own 24 parrots. Follow these steps.

For 4 or 5 days, feed a mainstay diet of a high-quality natural kibble for older dogs. Then for 2 or 3 days feed a seed mix consisting of equal parts of buckwheat, millet, safflower seeds, sunflower seeds, wheat berries, and whole oats.

Some birds will not eat millet; you may omit it. When it is cold and birds have higher energy needs, increase the proportion of seed mix in the diet. If a bird is reluctant to try new foods, change the diet gradually. On alternate days, feed the pellets your bird is accustomed to and then the seed mix. Gradually add dog kibble to the pellets, steadily increasing the proportion.

In addition to the diet of seed mix and kibble, offer fresh, bite-size chunks of raw fruits or vegetables daily. These should make up 20 to 35 percent of the daily diet. To get a bird to try a fruit, insert sunflower seeds into chunks of fruit. The bird will taste the fruit when it eats the seed. Choose a variety, including apples, bananas, carrots, cherries, corn on the cob, grapes, green beans, greens, okra, oranges, and raisins.

Parrots are very companionable and enjoy the attention and affection shown through occasional treats such as nuts, peanut butter on crackers, or cooked sweet potatoes. They are intelligent birds that thrive in a stimulating environment, which you can provide by offering a variety of appropriate toys and activities.

One simple toy enjoyed by most parrots is a length of rawhide tied at intervals around small tree branches or bones. To make a rawhide toy, buy strips of natural rawhide with no preservatives or softeners added. At intervals along the strip, tie small, nontoxic tree branches (apple branches are a good choice) or bones. Bones should be disks 1 to 2 inches in diameter and sturdy enough for a dog to chew on. Tree branches should only come from pesticide-free trees. Branches, bones, and rawhide are available at well-stocked pet supply stores. Tie the rawhide toy near the top of your parrot's cage. Your pet will enjoy manipulating and untying the rawhide knots.

Chapter Ten

Outdoor Life

by Cindy Ross, with Todd Gladfelter, and Kate Delhagen

On the following pages, you'll find a collection of formulas for outdoor life, including a formula for making your own high-energy "candy" bars, ideas for caring for sports equipment, and even a recipe for making your own fluid-replacement drink. Most of the formulas in this chapter will increase your enjoyment of hiking, camping, and backpacking.

At first glance, hiking and backpacking seem like simple activities requiring only boots, a tent, and a sleeping bag. But novice hikers soon discover that this sport requires more than fancy footgear and a taste for adventure. The formulas in this section provide the extra advice and wisdom that make the difference between a smooth, enjoyable trip and a miserable one. You'll find a wide selection of camp kitchen recipes—all developed to keep pack weight down and appetites satisfied. And you'll find quick, practical advice on necessary chores, like boot care and equipment repair.

These backpacking formulas are the fruits of more than 6,000 miles of hiking experience, including end-to-end hikes on both the Appalachian Trail and the Pacific Crest Trail. Everything here has been trail-tested and selected to increase your hiking enjoyment. According to the legendary nineteenth-century backwoodsman, Nessmunk, "You don't go out there to rough it, you go out there to smooth it. You get it rough enough at home." We think the formulas here will smooth the way for many great hikes to come.

CAMP COOKING

There's no rule that says roughing it has to include boring food. The recipes here are fast and easy, but also delicious enough to serve to company at home.

Gorp

Gorp, an acronym for "good old raisins and peanuts," provides instant energy for strenuous hiking. Backpacking lore describes dozens of different versions of this all-time favorite trail food.

Yield: varies by amount of ingredients chosen

INGREDIENTS

1 part raisins
1 part peanuts
1 part M & M's candy

Choose any:
assorted nuts, broken or chopped
banana chips
carob chips
chocolate chips
chopped dried fruit
pumpkin seeds
shredded coconut
sunflower seeds

SUPPLIES
sealable plastic bags

Combine the first three ingredients in equal volumes in a large bowl. Add any combination of remaining ingredients, to taste. Toss with your hands or with a large mixing spoon. Package in plastic bags.

GOOD IDEA!

When preparing **food and snacks for hot-weather hiking,** keep in mind that milk-chocolate chips melt faster than semi-sweet chocolate chips. If you're using banana chips, avoid those fried in coconut oil; they become rancid more quickly than dried chips.

GOOD IDEA!

Try hot carob drink instead of hot chocolate. You'll sleep better without the caffeine that comes with chocolate. Combine 1 tablespoon carob powder (available at health food stores), 1/2 cup water, and 2 teaspoons honey in a saucepan and bring to a boil. Reduce heat and simmer 1 to 2 minutes. Pour in 1 cup nonfat dry milk reconstituted in 1 1/2 cups water and heat, but do not boil. Remove from heat. Stir in 1/2 teaspoon vanilla extract and a dash of cinnamon. This recipe makes two 1-cup servings.

High-Energy Carob/Chocolate Chunks

Chocolate's high fat content makes it especially useful for winter camping when just staying warm requires plenty of extra calories. Carob, however, is a wonderful, nutritious alternative to chocolate.

Yield: varies by amount of ingredients chosen

INGREDIENTS

chunks of carob or chocolate (milk or semi-sweet)

Choose any:

assorted nuts, broken or chopped

raisins

Rice Krispies cereal

sesame seeds

sunflower seeds

SUPPLIES

double boiler

flexible, disposable aluminum pie plates or recycled aluminum frozen food trays

sealable plastic bags

Melt carob or chocolate in the top part of a double boiler. When it is completely melted, add any combination of remaining ingredients and mix thoroughly. Pour into aluminum pans to desired thickness—3/4 to 1 inch is best. Place pans in the freezer for several minutes, or until the bar cools enough to be sliced with a table knife. The chocolate/carob should be soft enough to score with a knife but stiff enough that the score lines remain. Score the bar into a grid of chunk-size pieces.

Return the pan to the freezer and cool until hard. Bending back the pan to ease removal, break the bar along the score lines. Store in plastic bags.

↦ Note: Purchase sweetened carob or chocolate chunks at candy-making supply stores. If not available, the largest-size plain Hershey bar will do.

Pow! Bars

Pow! Bars can take the edge off your hunger on those last miles into camp, or they can power you up a mountain just when you think you've run out of steam. These energy bars are easy to make and require no baking.

Yield: 6 bars

INGREDIENTS

½ cup honey or molasses
½ cup natural peanut butter, crunchy or smooth
    about 1 cup dry milk (noninstant preferred)
    chocolate chips
    raisins
    chopped dried fruit
    shredded coconut
    confectioners' sugar (optional)

SUPPLIES

electric mixer
sealable plastic bags

Beat honey or molasses and peanut butter together in a 1-quart bowl until well-combined. Beat in enough dry milk to make a stiff but not crumbly dough. Mix in remaining ingredients, to taste. Mixture will be stiff. Knead together with your hands and shape into logs 2 to 3 inches long and about 1 inch in diameter. Roll logs in dry milk, confectioners' sugar, or coconut. Store in plastic bags.

✿ **Variation:** *Use cashew or almond butter in place of the peanut butter.*

➡ **Note:** *Buy cashew and almond butter as well as noninstant dry milk at health food stores.*

GOOD IDEA!

Warm up after a long day on the trail with Russian spiced tea. Combine 2 cups orange-juice flavored instant drink mix, ¾ cup unsweetened lemonade-flavored instant drink mix, ¾ cup unsweetened instant tea (plain or with lemon), 1 cup sugar, 2 teaspoons ground cinnamon, 1 teaspoon ground allspice, and 1 teaspoon ground cloves. Pack the mix in plastic bags. To serve, stir 2 teaspoons of mix into 1 cup hot water. This recipe makes about 4½ cups, enough for 100 servings of tea.

Beef Jerky

One of the most valuable American Indian foods was slices of sun-dried game—jerky. In fact, Alaskan Indians still preserve meat this way. Many convenience stores sell jerky, but it's usually laced with chemical additives. This recipe makes a more wholesome alternative. It's a great high-protein trail snack.

Yield: 12 ounces

INGREDIENTS

3 pounds lean beef, such as flank steak
1 tablespoon onion powder
1 teaspoon garlic powder
½ teaspoon black pepper
   small bottle of Worcestershire sauce
   small bottle of soy sauce or tamari

SUPPLIES

9 × 13-inch glass or enameled baking dish
colander or strainer
wire cooling racks
brown paper lunch bags
sealable plastic bags

Partially freeze meat. To prevent spoilage, remove all visible fat. To ensure tenderness, remove all visible membrane. Slice the steak horizontally with the grain—in broad ½- to ¼-inch-thick slabs. Cut thin strips of meat from these slabs, being sure to cut across the grain. To ensure even drying, make the strips as thin and uniform as possible.

Mix remaining ingredients to make a marinade. Lay meat strips in the bottom of a glass baking dish, cover with marinade, and refrigerate overnight.

The next day drain meat strips in a colander or strainer and lay them on wire racks set directly on the oven rack. Pieces may be close together but should not be touching. Set the oven door partially open at the first stop. If your oven is electric, set it at the lowest possible setting; if gas, simply use the pilot light for heat. The jerky will dry in 12 to 24 hours in an electric oven, up to 48 hours for a gas oven. It's ready when it snaps as you bend it.

Wrap finished jerky in paper bags to protect it from light. Store brown-bagged jerky in sealed plastic bags. Keeps for up to a year without refrigeration.

✿ **Variations:** You can make jerky from pork, but you must first boil the meat slices until they are cooked through. This destroys trichina larvae, the source of trichinosis, a serious muscular disease. If you like hot, spicy jerky, add red-pepper sauce or cayenne pepper to the marinade. Or eliminate the garlic powder and rub the meat with fresh garlic before placing in marinade.

Pemmican

Pemmican, the original American Indian "traveling" food, is as valuable and easy to make today as it was years ago. Indian pemmican contained buffalo, elk, or venison jerky, plus berries, nuts, and, honey. Choose ingredients from this list.

- beef jerky
- raisins
- dried blueberries
- dried cranberries
- dried apricots
- dried peaches
- unroasted peanuts or pecans
- honey
- peanut butter
- cayenne pepper

Pound beef jerky into powder or grind using a blender. Mix jerky with raisins, dried fruits, and nuts in any combination, ending up with a ratio of 1 part meat to 2 parts nuts and fruit.

Combine honey and peanut butter in a saucepan and heat on low to soften. Mix in cayenne pepper to taste. Blend this into the jerky/nut mixture, adding just enough to make a mixture with the consistency of bread dough. Store the mixture in plastic bags in a cool, dry place. Pemmican keeps for a long time and is an excellent lunch or trail snack.

GOOD IDEA!

Take fruit leather on your next hiking trip. Start with peaches, pears, apples, or berries. Peel and slice fresh fruit until you have 3 to 3½ cups. Using a cookbook to check correct times, blanch to prevent discoloration. In a saucepan, mix each cup of blanched fruit with 1½ tablespoons sugar or honey. Bring just to boiling; cook until tender. Remove from heat and when it's cool, put it through a sieve or food mill. Line cookie sheets with foil or plastic freezer wrap—enough to extend past the ends and sides—and oil. Spread on the pulp and dry at 130°F for an hour, then increase to 145°F and cook until the surface is no longer tacky (about 45 minutes). Keep the oven door open at the first stop for the drying process. When the leather is dry, remove from oven, cool, and roll it up in the liner.

Hiker's Basic Tomato Leather

For a backpacking trip, try sauce made from tomato leather; this one adds only 6 ounces to your pack weight.

Yield: 6 ounces leather; enough sauce for 6 servings

INGREDIENTS

⅓ onion, minced

2 cloves garlic, finely minced

1 tablespoon olive oil and 1 tablespoon margarine, or 2 tablespoons of either

2 cans tomato paste (6 ounces each)

1 teaspoon salt

pinch of sugar

2 teaspoons chopped parsley

ground black pepper

pinch of basil

pinch of oregano

SUPPLIES

skillet

cookie sheet(s) with sides

nonstick cooking spray

sealable plastic bag(s)

Sauté onions and garlic in oil and/or margarine until soft and golden. Do not allow them to brown. Add remaining ingredients and cook slowly for about 10 minutes.

Spray a cookie sheet with nonstick spray and spread the mixture over the sheet in as thin a layer as possible, using two cookie sheets if necessary. Dry in a 140°F oven for about 6 hours with the door open at the first stop. Roll up leather and store in a plastic bag.

To reconstitute, add a volume of water that is three times the volume of the leather. For example, for a piece of leather that fills ½ cup, add 1½ cups water. Cook and stir over low heat until sauce is warm and smooth.

Hiker's Granola

Granola with instant milk is a fast yet nutritious trail breakfast.

Yield: about 5½ cups

INGREDIENTS

2½ cups rolled cereal grains (use oatmeal alone or combine with rolled wheat and rolled rye)

¼ cup sesame seeds

¼ cup sunflower seeds

½ cup shredded coconut

¼ cup raw wheat germ

½ cup sliced almonds

⅛ cup date sugar or ¼ cup brown sugar

½ cup water

⅓ cup honey

⅓ cup soy or safflower oil

chopped dried fruit, such as apricots, peaches, or prunes, to taste

raisins, to taste

SUPPLIES

cookie sheet with sides

sealable plastic bags

Combine cereal grains, seeds, coconut, wheat germ, almonds, and sugar in a mixing bowl and set aside. Combine water, honey, and oil and beat lightly just to combine. Stir into dry ingredients and mix until uniformly moistened. Spread on a cookie sheet. Bake 2 hours at 225°F. Cool. Add dried fruit and raisins. Store in plastic bags.

✿ **Variations:** For a moister granola, use more honey and oil. Just before serving, add brewer's yeast, lecithin granules, and whey powder to boost the granola's nutritive value.

➦ **Note:** Buy all ingredients at supermarkets or health food stores.

GOOD IDEA!

Make your own instant breakfast drink without the flavorings and chemicals of the commercial kind. Simply mix 1 cup water with ⅔ cup instant milk powder in a wide-mouthed water bottle. Shake vigorously, add flavoring, then shake again. Choose one of these flavoring mixes: 1 teaspoon carob powder, ¼ teaspoon vanilla, a dash of cinnamon, ½ teaspoon honey; 1 teaspoon cereal beverage, such as Postum or Caffix, 1 tablespoon honey; ¼ teaspoon almond extract, ¼ to ½ teaspoon nutmeg, plus honey, to taste; 1 teaspoon instant coffee, 1 tablespoon honey; 1 tablespoon molasses; ½ teaspoon vanilla and 1 teaspoon honey; 1 tablespoon jam or preserves. To use sugar in place of honey, double the honey measurement.

GOOD IDEA!

To make Logan bread even more nutritious, substitute 1 cup wheat germ for 1 cup white flour. To boost the iron content, add chopped apricots and about ¼ cup brewer's yeast.

Logan Trail Bread

Logan bread is a dense, chewy bread, very high in calories and almost impervious to spoilage. It originated in 1950 with a University of Alaska expedition to climb 19,000-foot Mount Logan. Expedition leader Gordon Herreid persuaded a baker to make an indestructible, high-energy bread for the party. The result of the baker's inspiration became known as Logan bread. This recipe, a variation of the original, has an unusually high fat content and is extremely rich and nutritious. A single serving (4 inch square) provides 718 calories and 10.4 grams usable protein. It's an excellent choice for cold-weather trips.

Yield: four 9 × 9-inch loaves

INGREDIENTS

3 cups whole wheat flour
3 cups white flour
½ cup dry milk
2½ cups rolled oats
1½ cups brown sugar
3 teaspoons baking powder
2 teaspoons salt
1 cup soy grits
1¼ cups broken or chopped nuts
2 cups raisins
1 cup honey
½ cup molasses
2 cups margarine
1 cup oil
6 eggs

SUPPLIES

8-quart or larger mixing bowl
medium mixing bowl
four 9 × 9 baking pans

Combine dry ingredients in the large mixing bowl and stir well. Combine remaining ingredients in the medium bowl and beat until well-combined. Fold into dry mixture and stir until well-combined. Divide equally among four pans and bake at 350°F for 45 minutes or until done. The bread does *not* rise to the top of the pan. The final product is dense and chewy.

➥ **Note:** *Buy soy grits at most health food stores.*

Hiker's Potato-Cheese Soup

Hot soup is a wonderful way to end your hiking day, especially if it's cold and damp. It's also a good choice when your main dish is a little on the skimpy side.

Yield: two 2½-cup servings

INGREDIENTS

½ pound cheese, such as Parmesan or cheddar
4 cups water
1 tablespoon oil or butter
½ cup instant potatoes
½ cup dry milk
¼ cup flour
1 tablespoon wheat germ
1 tablespoon dried minced onion
1 teaspoon parsley flakes
½ teaspoon salt (or to taste)

SUPPLIES

2-quart soup pot

Cut cheese into small bite-size chunks and set aside. Place water in the pot and stir in all ingredients except cheese. Bring to a boil while stirring continuously. Simmer for 5 to 10 minutes more, stirring occasionally. Remove from heat, add cheese, and stir until melted.

GOOD IDEA!

Before your trip, pre-measure all the dry ingredients for your meal recipes and pack them in labeled and sealed plastic bags or containers.

Hiker's Ground Beef Mix

If you're not fond of the soy granules that pass for ground beef in backpacking circles, take along this tasty real ground beef mix.

Yield: 4 servings

INGREDIENTS

1	pound lean ground beef
2	cloves garlic, finely minced
½	cup finely chopped onion
	fresly ground black pepper, to taste
¼	teaspoon rosemary leaves (optional)
1½	packages instant beef bouillon, 1½ beef bouillon cubes, or 1½ teaspoons beef-flavored Bovril
¼	teaspoon Worcestershire sauce
2	tablespoons flour
1	teaspoon salt

SUPPLIES

large frying pan
cookie sheet with sides
nonstick cooking spray
sealable plastic bag

In the pan, brown beef with garlic and onions. Tilt the pan and spoon out all the fat. Add remaining ingredients and cook over medium heat, scraping the flour off the bottom of the pan to brown it evenly. Spread mixture in a thin layer on the cookie sheet coated with nonstick spray. Dry for about 6 hours in a 140°F oven with the door open at the first stop. Mixture is crumbly when dry.

Store in a plastic bag in the freezer until your trip. To reconstitute, add 1¾ cups water, bring to a boil, and simmer 5 minutes.

➡ **Note:** Buy Bovril, a concentrated beef- or chicken-flavored bouillon, at specialty food stores.

Trail Gravy

Make camp stews or soups more hearty with gravy. Or stretch a ground beef dish to feed more people. This hearty gravy is ready to serve in only 3 minutes, and the ingredients are light enough to pack for a long backpacking rip.

Yield: 1 cup

INGREDIENTS

2 beef bouillon cubes, 1 oversize Knorr beef bouillon cube, or 1 package Herb-Ox beef bouillon powder
1 cup boiling broth or water
1½ tablespoons flour
2 to 3 tablespoons cold water

SUPPLIES

small pan (1 pint)
small cup or measure (¼ cup)

In the pan, dissolve bouillon in broth or water. In the cup or measure, make a thin paste of flour and cold water. Stir into the hot liquid. Cook and stir over low heat for 2 to 3 minutes, or until the gravy is thick.

✿ **Variation:** Bovril makes a nice trail gravy. Carry Bovril in a small, watertight container, such as a film canister. To make gravy using Bovril, make a paste of 2 tablespoons cold water, 1½ tablespoons flour, and 1 teaspoon Bovril. Stir this into a cup of boiling broth or water, and cook slowly, stirring for 2 to 3 minutes until the gravy is thick.

➥ **Note:** Buy Bovril, a concentrated beef- or chicken-flavored bouillon, at specialty food stores.

GOOD IDEA!

When you pack for a hike, measure the amount of gravy flour you need for the whole trip and store it in film canisters or sealed plastic bags. Keep in mind that 1½ tablespoons flour thickens 1 cup liquid.

GOOD IDEA!

Make a sauce mix to keep on hand so you can have back-home tummy fillers. Use it for macaroni and cheese, chicken à la king, or creamed chipped beef, for example. For 1 cup sauce, mix 1 table-spoon Butter Buds (a butter substitute found in grocery stores), 1½ tablespoons flour, 2 table-spoons dry milk, and a pinch of salt in a moisture-proof container. To make the sauce, place the mix in a small sauce-pan and slowly add 1 cup water, stirring con-stantly to prevent lumps. Heat the sauce over low heat, stirring constantly until smooth and warm. If you plan to use the sauce over salty foods, like clams or ham, omit the salt from the mix and season to taste at serving time.

Hiker's Seafood Supper

This simple dish is equally at home served on china in your dining room or dished out on a tin plate around a campfire.

Yield: 2 servings

INGREDIENTS

water
about ⅓ pound thin pasta, such as linguine
1 can minced clams (6½ ounces)
2 cloves garlic, minced
2 tablespoons butter
1 tablespoon parsley flakes
½ tablespoon flour

SUPPLIES

small saucepan
medium-size saucepan with lid
can opener or pocketknife with can-opening blade

In the medium pot, bring water to a boil and add pasta. In the smaller pot, sauté garlic in butter for a few minutes over low heat. Add parsley and flour and cook for 3 to 4 minutes, but do not brown. Add clams, including the juice, to the garlic/butter mixture. Increase the heat to bring the mixture to a boil. As soon as a boil begins, reduce heat to simmer, and continue stirring until sauce thickens. Drain the cooked pasta using the pot lid and serve with thickened clam sauce.

OUTDOOR SKILLS

Don't get lost and above all, don't get blisters. The Boy Scouts have a rank for boys inexperienced in backwoods ways—Tenderfoot. You can bypass the Tenderfoot rank by following the advice on these pages.

Blister Remedy

Boy Scouts, mail carriers, backpackers, and infantry all suffer from the same miserable ailment—blisters! When you pack for your next hiking trip, include the blister remedy kit here.

SUPPLIES

small manicure scissors or pocketknife with scissors
moleskin
soap and water

Carry blister treatment supplies together in a plastic bag or small container in an outer pocket of your pack for quick access. If you feel a "hot spot" forming as you walk, stop immediately and treat it before it becomes a blister. Inspect the place where your foot feels hot. If the skin is merely reddened with no blister formed, cut a patch of moleskin larger than the irritated area. Apply the moleskin directly to the hot spot for protection against further friction.

If a blister has formed, wash the affected area with soap and water. Cut a piece of moleskin in the shape of a doughnut and fit the hole around the blister. Shape several more doughnuts and stack them on top of the first. They will keep pressure off the blister and prevent it from breaking.

➥ **Note:** *Moleskin comes in sheets that you cut to fit. Buy it in the foot-care section of your pharmacy.*

GOOD IDEA!

Use the preventive approach to blister care. Before starting out on the trail, break in your boots at home. Blisters are most often caused by shoes that are ill-fitting or not broken in. To reduce friction that promotes blisters, coat blister-prone areas of your feet with petroleum jelly before hiking. Or sprinkle cornstarch or baby powder on your feet before putting on your socks.

A pair of thin socks worn under woolen hiking socks will also reduce the friction on your feet. If your feet sweat heavily, you may want to change socks several times a day. Letting your feet air out during rest stops also helps.

Boot Care

A good pair of leather hiking boots costs a bundle. Mud left to dry on boots dries out the leather. From time to time, treat boots to retain water repellency and preserve the leather. To get the most mileage out of leather boots, follow this simple, effective boot-care routine.

SUPPLIES

scrub brush

cool water

old toothbrush

newspapers or paper towels

clean rag

boot oil or wax

☛ **BE SAFE.** Overly frequent applications of boot oil or wax will soften leather too much. Never dry wet boots by a campfire or other heat source. Excess heat can permanently damage leather.

After a hiking trip, clean dirt from your boots by washing them with the scrub brush and water. Use the toothbrush to scrub dirt from the seam where the upper is sewn to the sole. Stuff the boots with crumpled newspaper or paper towels and let them dry, either outside in the sun or inside at room temperature.

With a clean rag, briskly rub oil or wax into the boot. Make sure to completely cover the entire outside of the boot, especially the seam where the upper is stitched to the sole. Then put the treated boots in the sun to melt the oil or wax into the boot.

➥ **Notes:** When you buy leather boots, make sure you find if they are oil-tanned leather, chrome-tanned leather, or vegetable-tanned leather. Treat oil-tanned leather with oil-based products only. Treat chrome-tanned and vegetable-tanned leather with wax- or silicone-based products only. If you have an old pair of boots you want to condition, ask an experienced salesperson about your brand of boots. Most experienced salespeople know what type of leather is used by various boot manufacturers.

You'll find the greatest selection of boot treatment products at backpacking supply stores and in specialty mail-order catalogs, such as L. L. Bean or REI. Wax- or silicone-based products include Sno Seal, Bee Seal, and Biwell. Oil-based products include any brand of neat's-foot oil, L. L. Bean's SuperDry, and REI's Ultra-Seal.

SUPER SUBSTITUTES How to Make Do with Available Equipment	
Item	**Substitution**
Boot deodorizer	Baking soda
Candle lantern	Soda can with side cut out
Clothesline and clothespins	Shower hooks hung from branches
Cook kit	Cake pans with pie plate as a lid
Dish cleaner	Campfire ashes or sand, plus water
Drinking cup	Plastic yogurt container
Emergency sunglasses for glaciers or snow	Paper with a slit cut out
Fire extinguisher	Baking soda
Foil for baking potatoes	Several layers of wet newspaper wrapped around potato
Gloves	Plastic bags or bread bags
Ground cloth	Plastic shower curtain
Map case	Ziploc storage bag
Pack rain cover	Plastic garbage bag
Shoelace	Nylon cord
Tent stakes	Rocks and tree limbs or half of a wire coat hanger
Toothpaste	Baking soda carried in a plastic bag
Water bottle	1-liter plastic seltzer bottle

GOOD IDEA!

To give yourself the best possible chance of not getting lost, spend the money to buy a good compass and topographic map. Some of the best maps are those put out by the Department of the Interior's Geological Survey. Know at all times where you are. Before you leave home, plan your route and mark it on your map. Study the map to familiarize yourself with the countryside, and while you're hiking, look over your shoulder often—you will see your route as it will look on your return. In addition to the compass and map, carry these supplies: pencil, flashlight with spare batteries and bulb, extra food (candy bars, raisins, jerky), water, matches in a waterproof container, pocketknife, bright-colored waterproof cover (poncho), extra shirt or sweater, and a metal whistle on a string around your neck.

Band-Aid-Box Repair Kit

These items will help to see you through nearly every equipment breakdown you can imagine. What's more, everything fits into a Band-Aid box!

SUPPLIES

extra flashlight bulb and batteries

2 to 4 feet of thin flexible wire

needle and thread assortment

small square of sandpaper

Super Glue or Crazy Glue

clevis pins and split rings

nylon cord

extra stove parts

safety pins

large metal Band-Aid box or similar sealable container

electrical tape

Flashlight bulbs *do* burn out. To avoid breakage, carry a spare bulb in its original plastic packaging. Carry only brand-new spare batteries. Include wire to repair broken pack joints or to hold the sole of a boot to its leather upper. To secure the sole, simply run a single strand of wire through the lug grooves around to the boot top and twist off. Include needle and thread for fabric repairs—heavyweight thread for repairing equipment and lightweight thread for clothes. Pack sandpaper to clean dirt off of equipment before applying glue. Extra clevis pins and split rings will replace lost or broken ones on your pack. Use nylon cord as a shoelace, a tent line, or a clothesline. Examine your stove for parts that are easily lost or broken. Buy duplicates and pack them in your kit. Include safety pins to replace broken tent zippers and lost buttons. Pack all repair kit items in the Band-Aid box or other container. Wrap several yards of electrical tape around the container. Use electrical tape for fabric tears that are too difficult to sew. In a pinch, electrical tape can even hold a pair of broken eyeglasses together.

Mosquito Repellent

Here's a sweet-smelling substitute for commercial insect repellents.

Yield: about 4 ounces

INGREDIENTS

1 cup safflower or peanut oil
½ cup sweet orange oil
½ cup dried chamomile flowers
½ cup dried nettle leaves
½ cup dried pennyroyal
¼ cup fresh sweet basil
1 teaspoon boric acid

SUPPLIES

large double broiler
funnel lined with cheesecloth
clean bottle with lid

☛ **BE SAFE.** Oils are flammable. Heat oils only in a double boiler; never over direct heat. Boric acid is poisonous if ingested. Keep away from children.

Place all ingredients in the top part of a double boiler, pressing and mashing the herbs down into the oil. Heat for ½ hour to an hour, or until oils are very hot. Cover with lid, turn off heat, and remove to a heat-proof surface. Set aside until cool. Dump the oil-soaked herbs and oil into the lined funnel. Press and mash the herbs so that oil is strained through the cheesecloth, down the funnel, and into the bottle. Seal tightly. Use sparingly. To prevent oils from turning rancid, store in the refrigerator between outings.

➥ **Notes:** Buy orange oil and herbs at health food stores. See page 444 for other sources. You can also grow all of the herbs in your garden. Buy boric acid at pharmacies.

GOOD IDEA!

To keep mosquitoes and gnats away from your face when you hike, tie a branch of fresh witch hazel high on your pack above your head. Mosquitoes are repelled by witch hazel and will usually stay away. Witch hazel also attracts gnats, so the pesky insects should hover near the branch and away from your face.

SPORTS

A wise athlete once said: "It's not whether you win or lose, it's how *comfortably* you play the game." The formulas here help banish the little problems that bring discomfort and distraction instead of fun. In this section, you'll find help for windburned skin or sore muscles. And you'll find a few hints on caring for equipment, like shoes or skis. After all, staying ahead of the little problems helps keep you in the game.

Athlete's Foot Remedy

If the skin on your feet—especially between and around the toes—becomes dry, red, cracked, itchy, or blistered, you probably have the common fungal infection, athlete's foot. Fortunately, it's easy to treat.

Yield: 1 soak

INGREDIENTS

about 2 quarts warm water
8 teaspoons table salt
1 tablespoon baking soda

SUPPLIES

pan or bucket large enough to accommodate foot
hair dryer (optional)

Place 2 quarts water in the pan or bucket. Dissolve salt in water and soak your foot in the warm solution for 5 to 10 minutes. Dry your foot. Make a baking soda paste in the palm of your hand by mixing a few drops of warm water with 1 tablespoon baking soda. Apply the paste to the affected area. Leave it on for a minute or so; then rinse and dry gently. Use a hair dryer, if necessary, to dry between your toes. Treat your foot twice a day.

GOOD IDEA!

To avoid recurring athlete's foot, don't walk barefoot in moist areas, especially around swimming pools and locker rooms. These places usually harbor athlete's foot fungus. Keep your feet dry. Dust the insides of your shoes daily with cornstarch or with a medicated anti-fungal powder. If possible, place your shoes outside to dry in sunshine. Avoid shoes that make your feet sweat. Wear open, breathable shoes or sandals. And finally, if you've been wearing old, worn-out sneakers, throw them out. They could be the source of repeated infections.

Chapped Skin Relief

If you participate in any outdoor sport in cold weather—skiing, bicycling, running, ice skating—you may find yourself with reddened, irritated skin blotches on your cheeks, hands, or legs. Treatment is simple.

SUPPLIES

warm water

warm, moist towels

Choose one:

cocoa butter

liquid lanolin

mineral oil

vegetable oil

vegetable shortening

Soak the affected area in warm water for a few minutes. If your face is chapped, apply warm, moist towels. Pat the area dry, and gently rub a small amount of any of the ingredients above into the chapped skin.

➥ **Note:** Buy liquid lanolin and cocoa butter at pharmacies and health food stores.

GOOD IDEA!

If you're prone to dry skin, avoid frequent hand-washing, bathing, and swimming. Repeated bathing removes the natural skin oils that protect against chapping. To treat severely chapped hands, apply a treatment at bedtime and wear light cotton gloves to bed. Also, if you must wash dishes, wear light cotton gloves under rubber gloves. Wearing rubber gloves alone makes the problem worse. And if the cotton gloves get wet, replace them immediately.

Shampoo for Swimmers

Chlorine and other pool chemicals dry and damage your hair. To prevent chlorine damage, apply about ½ teaspoon mineral oil to your hair before swimming. The oil prevents chlorine from attacking the hair shafts.

Wear a rubber swim cap and shampoo after every swim with this natural shampoo: Mix 1 cup liquid castile soap and ¼ cup almond, avocado, or olive oil in a 1-pint container. Add ½ cup distilled water and shake until mixed. Castile soap is made from olive oil. Buy it, as well as almond and avocado oils, at health food stores and specialty gift shops. If you can't find liquid castile soap, make your own. Grate a bar of castile soap into a blender and blend with just enough distilled water to make a creamy liquid soap.

GOOD IDEA!

Do not dry athletic shoes near a heat source; they may shrink. To speed drying, stuff the shoes with newspaper. Every ½ hour or so, remove damp paper and replace with more dry newspaper.

Athletic Shoe Cleaner

This cleans and deodorizes shoes that are fabric mesh with leather trim, such as tennis and jogging shoes.

Yield: enough solution to clean 1 pair shoes

INGREDIENTS

1⅓ cups baking soda

4 cups warm water

SUPPLIES

2-quart bowl

scrub brush

old toothbrush

Mix baking soda and water in the bowl. Scrub onto shoes thoroughly. Use the toothbrush for crevices. Remove and scrub the insoles, if possible. Let stand for a few minutes, then rinse well. Repeat, if necessary, and air-dry.

High-Energy Snack Mix

This high-energy snack mix travels well.

Yield: about 7 cups

INGREDIENTS

6 cups rolled oats

½ cup raw wheat germ

¼ cup honey

¼ cup vegetable oil

1 cup raisins

Choose any:

    assorted nuts, broken or chopped

    sesame seeds

    shredded coconut

    sunflower seeds

SUPPLIES

cookie sheets with sides

small saucepan

sealable plastic bags

Preheat the oven to 300°F. Grease cookie sheets. In a large bowl, mix oats and wheat germ. In the saucepan, heat and stir honey and oil until well-combined. Add to oat mixture and combine well. Spread evenly on cookie sheets and bake for 15 minutes, or until lightly browned. Cool. Spoon into a large bowl, mix in raisins and any combination of the remaining ingredients. Store in plastic bags.

Fluid-Replacement Drink

Prolonged exercise calls for replacement of body fluids lost through sweating. If you exercise for longer than 30 minutes, you might benefit from a fluid-replacement drink. This formula provides about 7 grams of carbohydrate (for quick energy) and 50 percent of the adult Recommended Dietary Allowance for vitamin C per 8-ounce serving.

Yield: about 1 gallon

INGREDIENTS

4 cups freshly squeezed orange juice or one can frozen concentrate (6 ounces)

2 tablespoons freshly squeezed lemon juice

1 tablespoon freshly squeezed lime juice

¾ teaspoon salt (optional)

water

Mix all ingredients, using enough water to make a gallon, and serve cold.

✿ **Variations:** For extra flavor, replace half the water with diet lemon-lime soft drink or flavored seltzer. Replace half the orange juice with other juices.

GOOD IDEA!

Fluid-replacement **drinks may taste too sweet if you drink them while exercising.** Try diluting them with additional water, or add some ice to the container before you begin exercising. As the ice melts, the drink will become diluted.

Supply Sources

Supplies are grouped in combinations as needed for the formulas. The following lists combinations of ingredients available from the same supplier(s).

Chapter 3

Gardening

For colloidal phosphate, cotton-seed meal, and granite dust:

Growing Naturally
P.O. Box 54
Pineville, PA 18946
(215) 598-7025

I.F.M.
333 Ohme Gardens Rd.
Wenatchee, WA 98801
1-800-332-3179

The Necessary Trading Co.
8320 Salem Ave.
New Castle, VA 24127
(703) 864-5103

For fish emulsion and seaweed extract (liquefied kelp):

Gardens Alive!
P.O. Box 149
Sunman, IN 47041
(812) 623-3800

Peaceful Valley Farm Supply
P.O. Box 2209
Grass Valley, CA 95945
(916) 272-GROW

For bonemeal, diatomaceous earth, and rock phosphate:

Harmony Farm Supply
P.O. Box 460
Graton, CA 95444
(707) 823-9125

The Necessary Trading Co.
8320 Salem Ave.
New Castle, VA 24127
(703) 864-5103

Ohio Earth Food, Inc.
5488 Swamp St.
Hartville, OH 44632
(216) 877-9356

For fish oil:

Peaceful Valley Farm Supply
P.O. Box 2209
Grass Valley, CA 95945
(916) 272-GROW

For neem seeds:

The Banana Tree
715 Northampton St.
Easton, PA 18042
(215) 253-9589

For chinaberry seeds:

J. L. Hudson, Seedsman
P.O. Box 1058
Redwood City, CA 94064

Richters
P.O. Box 26
Goodwood, Ontario
CANADA L0C 1A0
(416) 640-6677

For apple maggot lures and commercial trap glue:

Gardens Alive!
P.O. Box 149
Sunman, IN 47041
(812) 623-3800

Great Lakes IPM
10220 Church Rd. NE
Vestaburg, MI 48891
(517) 268-5693

The Necessary Trading Co.
8320 Salem Ave.
New Castle, VA 24127
(703) 864-5103

For Bacillus thuringiensis, commercial pyrethrin, pyrethrum, and rotenone:

Harmony Farm Supply
P.O. Box 460
Graton, CA 95444
(707) 823-9125

Peaceful Valley Farm Supply
P.O. Box 2209
Grass Valley, CA 95945
(916) 272-GROW

For bordeaux powder:

Growing Naturally
P.O. Box 54
Pineville, PA 18946
(215) 598-7025

The Necessary Trading Co.
8320 Salem Ave.
New Castle, VA 24127
(703) 864-5103

Ohio Earth Food, Inc.
5488 Swamp St.
Hartville, OH 44632
(216) 877-9356

Peaceful Valley Farm Supply
P.O. Box 2209
Grass Valley, CA 95945
(916) 272-GROW

For dried blood and powdered wettable sulfur:

Growing Naturally
P.O. Box 54
Pineville, PA 18946
(215) 598-7025

Peaceful Valley Farm Supply
P.O. Box 2209
Grass Valley, CA 95945
(916) 272-GROW

For bloodmeal, bonemeal, greensand, kelp meal, and rock phosphate:

Growing Naturally
P.O. Box 54
Pineville, PA 18946
(215) 598-7025

The Necessary Trading Co.
8320 Salem Ave.
New Castle, VA 24127
(703) 864-5103

Ohio Earth Food, Inc.
5488 Swamp St.
Hartville, OH 44632
(216) 877-9356

For bonemeal and dolomitic lime:

Ohio Earth Food, Inc.
5488 Swamp St.
Hartville, OH 44632
(216) 877-9356

Peaceful Valley Farm Supply
P.O. Box 2209
Grass Valley, CA 95945
(916) 272-GROW

For bloodmeal, calcitic lime-stone, cottonseed meal, and rock phosphate:

Growing Naturally
P.O. Box 54
Pineville, PA 18946
(215) 598-7025

Harmony Farm Supply
P.O. Box 460
Graton, CA 95444
(707) 823-9125

Orol Ledden & Sons
P.O. Box 7
Center & Atlantic Aves.
Sewell, NJ 08080
(609) 468-1000

The Necessary Trading Co.
8320 Salem Ave.
New Castle, VA 24127
(703) 864-5103

Ohio Earth Food, Inc.
5488 Swamp St.
Hartville, OH 44632
(216) 877-9356

For soy meal:

Bountiful Gardens
19550 Walker Rd.
Willits, CA 95490

For bonemeal and cottonseed meal:

Harmony Farm Supply
P.O. Box 460
Graton, CA 95444
(707) 823-9125

Orol Ledden & Sons
P.O. Box 7
Center & Atlantic Aves.
Sewell, NJ 08080
(609) 468-1000

The Necessary Trading Co.
8320 Salem Ave.
New Castle, VA 24127
(703) 864-5103

Ohio Earth Food, Inc.
5488 Swamp St.
Hartville, OH 44632
(216) 877-9356

For yellow beeswax suppliers, see chapter 7 entry.

Chapter 5

Health

For herbs:

The Herb and Spice
Collection
Rte. 1, Box 118
Norway, IA 52318
1-800-365-4372

Nature's Herbs Co.
1010 46th St.
Emeryville, CA 94608
(415) 601-0700

Chapter 6

Home Repair and Remodeling

For Penetrol:

Flood Co.
P.O. Box 399
Hudson, OH 44236
1-800-321-3444
Manufacturers of Penetrol.
Call toll-free number to find
where to buy Penetrol in
your area.

For dry artist's pigments, Japan colors, and powdered aniline dyes:

Wood Finishing Supply Co.,
Inc.
100 Throop St.
Palmyra, NY 14522
(313) 597-3743

For turkey feathers:

Janovic/Plaza
30–35 Thomson Ave.
Long Island City, NY 11101
(718) 786-4444

For yellow beeswax suppliers, see chapter 7 entry.

Chapter 7
Housekeeping

For carnauba wax and paraffin oil:

Wood Finishing Supply Co., Inc.
100 Throop St.
Palmyra, NY 14522
(315) 597-3743

For stearic acid:

Early American Candle Shoppe
5573 Hamilton Blvd.
Wescosville, PA 18106
(215) 395-3995

Earth Guild
33 Haywood St.
Asheville, NC 28801
1-800-327-8448

Pourette
6910 Roosevelt Way NE
P.O. Box 15220
Seattle, WA 98115-0220
(206) 525-4488

For beeswax and yellow beeswax:

Point Phillip Honey Farm
2764 W. Scenic Dr.
Danielsville, PA 18038
(215) 837-6038

Surma Company
11 E. 7th St.
New York, NY 10003
(212) 477-0729

For herb suppliers, see chapter 5 entry.

Chapter 8
Crafts

For dyes for batik and pysanky:

Surma Company
11 E. 7th St.
New York, NY 10003
(212) 477-0729

Taws Art Supply
1527 Walnut St.
Philadelphia, PA 19102
(215) 563-8742

Yost's Art & Drafting Supply, Inc.
1202 Walnut St.
Allentown, PA 18102
(215) 432-5668

For beeswax, candle molds, candlewick, and stearic acid:

Early American Candle Shoppe
5573 Hamilton Blvd.
Wescosville, PA 18106
(215) 395-3995

Earth Guild
33 Haywood St.
Asheville, NC 28801
1-800-327-8448

Pourette
6910 Roosevelt Way NE
P.O. Box 15220
Seattle, WA 98115-0220
(206) 525-4488

For plaster molds and mold release sprays:

Deep Flex Plastic Molds, Inc.
1200 Park Ave.
Murfreesboro, TN 37129
(615) 896-1111

For dyes and mordants:

Creek Water Wool Works
P.O. Box 716
Salem, OR 97308
(503) 585-3302

Earth Guild
33 Haywood St.
Asheville, NC 28801
1-800-327-8448

Mannings Creative Crafts
P.O. Box 687
East Berlin, PA 17316
(717) 624-2223
Supplies only alum mordants.

Serendipity Shop
2 Prairie St.
Park Ridge, IL 60068
(708) 692-7177

The Yarn Barn
Box 334
918 Massachusetts St.
Lawrence, KS 66044
(913) 842-4333

For beeswax suppliers, see chapter 7 entry.

Chapter 9
Pet Care

For diatomaceous earth:

Herbal Animal
Eco-Safe Products Inc.
P.O. Box 1177
St. Augustine, FL 32085
(904) 824-5884

Chapter 10
Outdoor Life

For orange oil and other herbs:

The Herb and Spice Collection
Rte. 1, Box 118
Norway, IA 52318
1-800-365-4372

Meadowbrook Herb Garden
93 Kingstown Rd.
Wyoming, RI, 02898
(401) 539-7603

Index

Page references in *italic* indicate illustrations. **Boldface** references indicate tables.